Science and H   e Medicine

09

Derek S. Wheeler, Hector R. Wong, and Thomas P. Shanley (Eds.)

Science and Practice of Pediatric Critical Care Medicine

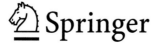 Springer

Editors

Derek S. Wheeler, MD
Assistant Professor of Clinical Pediatrics
University of Cincinnati College of Medicine
Division of Critical Care Medicine
Cincinnati Children's Hospital Medical Center
Cincinnati, OH, USA

Hector R. Wong, MD
Professor of Pediatrics
University of Cincinnati College of Medicine
Director, Division of Critical Care Medicine
Cincinnati Children's Hospital Medical Center
Cincinnati, OH, USA

Thomas P. Shanley, MD
Ferrantino Professor of Pediatrics and
  Communicable Diseases
University of Michigan Medical Center
Director, Division of Critical Care Medicine
C.S. Mott Children's Hospital
Ann Arbor, MI, USA

100858949

ISBN 978-1-84800-920-2   e-ISBN 978-1-84800-921-9
DOI 10.1007/978-1-84800-921-9

British Library Cataloguing in Publication Data
A catalogue record for this book is available from the British Library

Library of Congress Control Number: 2008940129

Springer Science+Business Media
springer.com

Preface

The field of critical care medicine is in the midst of a dramatic change. Technological and scientific advances during the last decade have resulted in a fundamental change in the way we view disease processes, such as sepsis, shock, acute lung injury, and traumatic brain injury. Pediatric intensivists have been both witness to and active participants in bringing about these changes. As the understanding of the pathogenesis of these diseases reaches the cellular and molecular levels, the gap between critical care medicine and molecular biology will disappear. It is imperative that all physicians caring for critically ill children in this new era have a thorough understanding of the applicability of molecular biology to the care of these patients at the bedside in order to keep up with the rapidly evolving field of critical care medicine. To the same extent, the practice of critical care medicine is in the midst of fundamental change. In keeping with the Institute of Medicine's report "Crossing the Quality Chasm," the care of critically ill and injured children needs to be safe, evidence-based, equitable, efficient, timely, and family-centered [1,2]. In the following pages, these changes in our specialty are discussed in greater scope and detail, offering the reader fresh insight into not only *where we came from*, but also *where we are going* as a specialty. Once again, we would like to dedicate this textbook to our families and to the physicians and nurses who provide steadfast care every day in pediatric intensive care units across the globe.

Derek S. Wheeler
Hector R. Wong
Thomas P. Shanley

References

1. Institute of Medicine Committee on Quality of Health Care in America. Crossing the Quality Chasm: A New Health System for the 21st Century. Washington, DC: National Academy Press, 2001.
2. Slonim AD, Pollack MM. Integrating the Institute of Medicine's six quality aims into pediatric critical care: Relevance and applications. Pediatr Crit Care Med 2005;6:264–269.

Preface to *Pediatric Critical Care Medicine: Basic Science and Clinical Evidence*

The field of critical care medicine is growing at a tremendous pace, and tremendous advances in the understanding of critical illness have been realized in the last decade. My family has directly benefited from some of the technological and scientific advances made in the care of critically ill children. My son Ryan was born during my third year of medical school. By some peculiar happenstance, I was nearing completion of a 4-week rotation in the newborn intensive care unit (NICU). The head of the pediatrics clerkship was kind enough to let me have a few days off around the time of the delivery—my wife, Cathy, was 2 weeks past her due date and had been scheduled for elective induction. Ryan was delivered through thick meconium-stained amniotic fluid and developed breathing difficulty shortly after delivery. His breathing worsened over the next few hours, so he was placed on the ventilator. I will never forget the feelings of utter helplessness my wife and I felt as the NICU transport team wheeled Ryan away in the transport isolette. The transport physician, one of my supervising third-year pediatrics residents during my rotation the past month, told me that Ryan was more than likely going to require extracorporeal membrane oxygenation (ECMO). I knew enough about ECMO at that time to know that I should be scared! The next 4 days were some of the most difficult moments I have ever experienced as a parent, watching the blood being pumped out of my tiny son's body through the membrane oxygenator and roller pump, slowly back into his body (Figures 1 and 2). I remember the fear of each day when we would be told of the results of his daily head ultrasound, looking for evidence of intracranial hemorrhage, and then the relief when we were told that there was no bleeding. I remember the hope and excitement on the day Ryan came off

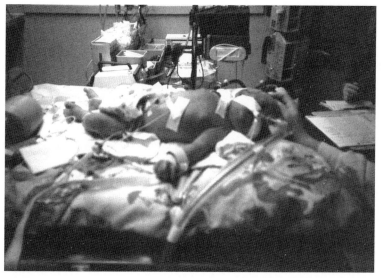

FIGURE 1

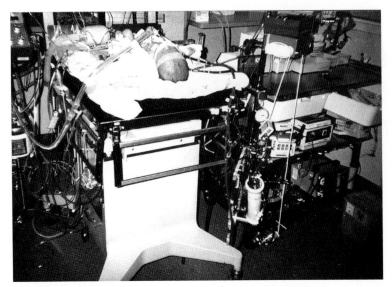

FIGURE 2

ECMO, as well as the concern when he had to be sent home on supplemental oxygen. Today, Ryan is happy, healthy, and strong. We are thankful to all the doctors, nurses, respiratory therapists, and ECMO specialists who cared for Ryan and made him well. We still keep in touch with many of them. Without the technological advances and medical breakthroughs made in the fields of neonatal intensive care and pediatric critical care medicine, things very well could have been much different. I made a promise to myself long ago that I would dedicate the rest of my professional career to advancing the field of pediatric critical care medicine as payment for the gifts with which we, my wife and I, have been truly blessed. It is my sincere hope that this textbook, which has truly been a labor of joy, will educate a whole new generation of critical care professionals and in so doing help make that first step toward keeping my promise.

Derek S. Wheeler

Contents

Contributors

Susan L. Bratton, MD
Associate Professor of Pediatrics
Division of Critical Care Medicine
Primary Children's Hospital
Salt Lake City, UT, USA

Franco A. Carnevale, RN, PhD
Associate Professor, School of Nursing
McGill University
Coordinator, Critical Care Services
Montreal Children's Hospital
Montreal, Quebec, Canada

Thomas J. Cholis III, MD
Division of Critical Care Medicine
Children's National Medical Center
Washington, DC, USA

Timothy T. Cornell, MD
University of Michigan Medical Center
Division of Critical Care Medicine
C.S. Mott Children's Hospital
Ann Arbor, MI, USA

Mary K. Dahmer, PhD
Department of Molecular Sciences and
    University of Tennessee Health Science Center
Memphis, TN, USA

Girish G. Deshpande, MD
University of Illinois College of Medicine at
    Peoria
Division of Pediatric Critical Care Medicine
Children's Hospital of Illinois
Peoria, IL, USA

Lesley A. Doughty, MD
Associate Professor of Clinical Pediatrics
University of Cincinnati College of Medicine
Division of Critical Care Medicine
Cincinnati, OH, USA

John J. Downes, MD
Professor of Anesthesia and Critical Care
University of Pennsylvania School of Medicine
Children's Hospital of Philadelphia
Philadelphia, PA, USA

Lorry R. Frankel, MD, MBA
Associate Professor of Pediatrics
Stanford University School of Medicine
Division of Pediatric Critical Care Medicine
Lucile Packard Children's Hospital
Palo Alto, CA, USA

Sol J. Goldstein, MD
Child Psychiatrist, Private Practice

Mary E. Hartman, MD
Division of Critical Care Medicine
Children's Hospital of Pittsburgh
Pittsburgh, PA, USA

K. Sarah Hoehn, MD, MS
Assistant Professor of Anesthesia and
    Pediatrics
Department of Anesthesiology and
    Critical Care Medicine
University of Pennsylvania School of Medicine
The Children's Hospital of Philadelphia
Philadelphia, PA, USA

Gwen Lombard, PhD
University of Illinois College of Medicine at
    Peoria
Division of Pediatric Critical Care Medicine
Children's Hospital of Illinois
Peoria, IL, USA

James P. Marcin, MD, MPH
Associate Professor of Pediatrics
University of California, Davis
Sacramento, CA, USA

Robert M. Nelson, MD, PhD
Associate Professor of Anesthesia and Pediatrics
Department of Anesthesiology and
    Critical Care Medicine
University of Pennsylvania School of Medicine
The Children's Hospital of Philadelphia
Philadelphia, PA, USA

William M. Novick, MD
Nemir Endowed Professor
University of Tennessee Center for
    Health Sciences
International Children's Heart Foundation
Memphis, TN, USA

Murray M. Pollack, MD, MBA
Professor of Pediatrics
Executive Director, Center for Hospital-Based
    Specialties
George Washington University School of
    Medicine
Chief, Critical Care Medicine
Children's National Medical Center
Washington, DC, USA

Michael W. Quasney, MD, PhD
Associate Professor of Pediatrics
Director, Fellowship Training Program
Division of Critical Care Medicine
LeBonheur Children's Medical Center
St. Jude Children's Research Hospital
University of Tennessee Health Sciences Center
Memphis, TN, USA

Adrienne G. Randolph, MA, MD, MSc
Associate Professor of Anesthesia
    (Pediatrics)
Harvard Medical School
Senior Associate in Critical Care Medicine
Children's Hospital Boston
Boston, MA, USA

Daniel G. Remick, MD
Professor of Pathology
Assistant Dean of Admissions
University of Michigan Medical School
Ann Arbor, MI, USA

Thomas P. Shanley, MD
Associate Professor of Pediatrics and
    Communicable Diseases
University of Michigan Medical Center
Director, Division of Critical Care Medicine
C.S. Mott Children's Hospital
Ann Arbor, MI, USA

Anthony D. Slonim, MD
Assistant Professor of Internal Medicine and
    Pediatrics
Vice Chairman, Clinical Effectiveness
George Washington University School of
    Medicine
Executive Director, Center for
    Clinical Effectiveness
Division of Critical Care Medicine
Children's National Medical Center
Washington, DC, USA

Gregory L. Stidham, MD
Professor of Pediatrics
University of Tennessee Health Sciences Center
Director, Critical Care Medicine
St. Jude Children's Research Hospital
LeBonheur Children's Medical Center
Memphis, TN, USA

David C. Stockwell, MD
Division of Critical Care Medicine
Children's National Medical Center
Washington, DC, USA

Kenneth Tegtmeyer, MD
Assistant Professor of Pediatrics
Division of Critical Care Medicine
Doernbecher Children's Hospital
Oregon Health and Science University
Portland, OR, USA

I. David Todres, MD
Professor of Paediatrics
Harvard Medical School
Chief, Ethics Unit
MassGeneral Hospital for Children
Boston, MA, USA

Adalberto Torres, Jr., MD
Assistant Professor of Pediatrics
University of Illinois College of Medicine at
    Peoria
Division of Pediatric Critical Care Medicine
Children's Hospital of Illinois
Peoria, IL, USA

R. Scott Watson, MD, MPH
Assistant Professor of Critical Care Medicine
University of Pittsburgh School of Medicine
Department of Critical Care Medicine
Children's Hospital of Pittsburgh
Pittsburgh, PA, USA

Hector R. Wong, MD
Professor of Pediatrics
University of Cincinnati College of Medicine
Director, Division of Critical Care Medicine
Cincinnati Children's Hospital Medical Center
Cincinnati, OH, USA

Basilia Zingarelli, MD, PhD
Associate Professor of Pediatrics
Division of Critical Care Medicine
Children's Hospital Research Foundation
Cincinnati Children's Hospital Medical
    Center
Cincinnati, OH, USA

1

Development of Pediatric Critical Care Medicine—How Did We Get Here and Why?

John J. Downes

Medicine arose out of the primal sympathy of man with man; out of the desire to help those in sorrow, need and sickness.
From *The Evolution of Modern Medicine*, the 1913 Silliman Lectures at Yale University by Sir William Osler (1842–1919)

If the science of medicine is not to be lowered to the rank of a mere mechanical profession, it must pre-occupy itself with its history.
Emile Littre (1801–1881)

Introduction

Pediatric critical care represents a small, albeit vital, component of health care in this nation, but it has been part of the long stream of medical history for only 50 years. Yet when one thinks about the current state of critical care for children, do we not wonder why and how we got here, how we are doing, and where we are going? This chapter aims to provide at least some answers to these questions. First, however, let us define our subject. *Pediatric critical care medicine*, a subspecialty of pediatrics and of critical care medicine, focuses on clinical care, education, and research regarding vital system surveillance and support for infants, children, and adolescents with potential or existing life-threatening illnesses or injuries. The goals of pediatric critical care are to restore the child who is suffering from a life-threatening condition to health with a minimum of pain, anxiety, and complications and to provide comfort and guidance to the child's family. The usual locus for this activity is the pediatric intensive care unit (PICU), a specialized hospital location first devised for children in 1955 in Europe and in 1967 in North America. In most PICUs the medical and nursing staff provide full-time attendance in the unit. These medical practitioners generally are called *pediatric intensivists,* and their subspecialty is *pediatric critical care medicine.*

The philosophical, scientific, and clinical concepts leading to the imperative for physicians, nurses, and other health professionals to rescue and care for critically ill and injured children has evolved in western culture over at least 2,000 years. In the biblical story of Elijah [1], the prophet resuscitated a young boy believed by his mother to be dead. Elijah lay upon the boy and breathed into him, and the boy began to breathe, awakened, and recovered. In 117 CE, the Greek physician Antyllus related in great detail the technique for tracheotomy with insertion of a hollow reed as the tube in a child with upper airway obstruction and the child's recovery [2]. The French obstetrician Desault in 1801 [3] described in his obstetrics textbook how to successfully resuscitate the apneic or limp newborn by digital orotracheal intubation with a lacquered fabric tube and blowing into the tube. He also mentions using this technique of intubation for an older infant with life-threatening *croup* to relieve airway obstruction; the tube was left in place for several days to allow the obstruction to subside, then was removed and the infant recovered. Thus, prolonged tracheal intubation for croup, thought to be an innovation of the early 1960s, began much earlier. Unfortunately, this information about effective infant resuscitation and prolonged intubation remained buried in a textbook read by a limited group for over 150 years. This is only one of many examples of such failure of wide dissemination of vital information throughout medical history, even into the 20th century. These and other reports [4], however, reflect the commitment of some physicians to the rescue of desperately ill children despite limited knowledge and resources.

In order to understand *why and how we got here* in the current era, we need to consider certain monumental contributions to medicine occurring from 1540 to 1900 and then to examine in more detail the four areas of 20th century medicine that provided the basis for the development of pediatric critical care in the past 50 years. What follows reflects my own reading and study, my personal observations and biases, and those persons and events I view as important to the development of modern medicine that forms the basis for the critical care of children. I also include some recollections of cherished colleagues who attended the birth of pediatric critical care medicine in the mid-20th century. Insofar as possible, these individuals are cited, as are the papers and chapters of which I am aware that deal with this part of medical history. My focus herein is on the subspecialty's evolution in North America, although I cite its European roots. For a more complete story of this field in Europe and elsewhere in the world, I refer the interested reader to

D.S. Wheeler et al. (eds.), *Science and Practice of Pediatric Critical Care Medicine,*
DOI 10.1007/978-1-84800-921-9_1, © Springer-Verlag London Limited 2009

a recently published, authoritative global historical account [5]. History tends to be messy, with conflicting information and opinions and inadvertent errors. I welcome from readers any criticisms, corrections, or additions that would enhance the historical record of our subspecialty.

Origins of Modern Medicine Before 1900

The scientific and philosophical bases of the astounding achievements of late 19th and 20th century medicine evolved out of the intellectual revolutions of the 17th and 18th centuries in England, France, the Netherlands, and Germany, a period termed *the Enlightenment*. The preservation of classical Greek and Roman writings by Irish monks and Arab scholars after the fall of Rome (410 CE), and their return to Western Europe through the monasteries of the early Middle Ages led to the rediscovery of the great classical Greek philosophers in the 13th century by Thomas Aquinas (1226–1274) and others. The emphasis on rational thinking, coupled with the artistic, religious, and scientific achievements of the Italian Renaissance and the Protestant Reformation in the 15th and 16th centuries, resulted in this prolific epoch. The great intellectuals of the Enlightenment liberated man's thinking from the theological and feudal constraints of the previous 1,500 years and placed the highest priority on advancement through human reason. Francis Bacon defined the scientific method, and Isaac Newton established the fundamental laws of motion and gravity, as well as the calculus. Rene Descartes, Thomas Hobbes, and David Hume challenged existing authority with new ideas about the mind and man's relation to society. John Locke, Joseph Priestly, and Jeremy Bentham in England, François Marie Arouet (Voltaire) in France, and Thomas Paine and Thomas Jefferson in the American colonies provided a rational basis for a revolutionary new concept—the right of each individual to be free to think and worship according to conscience and the duty of the state to ensure that right. The inclusion of persons of all races, religions, and classes in these rights remains an ongoing project for the developed as well as the developing world.

It can be difficult for us in the 21st century to conceive of life before 1700 CE with the constraints placed by religious authority, the aristocracy, and tradition on people's freedom to think for themselves; to question, to investigate, and to observe; and to reach their own conclusions about fundamental causes, proper laws, and their human rights. These new ideas of the Enlightenment regarding individual rights also formed the basis for a cardinal duty of the modern health professional, the *imperative to rescue* any person with life-threatening illness or injury, the underlying philosophy for emergency and critical care medicine. All the great medical scientists of the Enlightenment and the 18th century whose discoveries relate to pediatric critical care medicine and cardiopulmonary resuscitation are too numerous to discuss in a single chapter. However, several stand out as pivotal to the evolution of modern medicine. These are cited below with a brief discussion about their unique contributions in a chronology from 1543 to 1900. The facts and interpretations expressed in this sweep through three centuries of medical and scientific history have been derived from several historical texts, review articles, and classical works, [6–10], and from occasional landmark publications as referenced in the text.

Sixteenth Century

1543

Andreas Vesalius (1514–1564), a brilliant Flemish surgeon and anatomist, became Professor of Anatomy at the University of Padua while in his twenties. He inaugurated the revolution of medical science by introducing his results of precise experimental observation and human anatomic dissection with the publication of *De Humani Corporis Fabrica, Libri Septum* (Figure 1.1) [11]. He refuted the erroneous anatomic and physiologic doctrines of Claudius Galen (129–216? CE), whose teachings had been held virtually infallible by western physicians and the church for nearly 1,400 years. Thereafter, the great innovators in medicine would trust their eyes and minds rather than authority and would be looking inside human bodies for the truths of structure, function, and disease. He also wrote in the *Fabrica* about collapse of the lungs when the thorax of a mammal is opened and how positive pressure ventilation through a tracheostomy tube (a hollow reed) could restore the heart beat and living color to an asphyxiated fetal lamb. This is the first record in western literature of these phenomena. Unfortunately, under pressure from medical and church authorities, and the need for income, Vesalius left Padua in 1544, moving to Madrid to become physician to Emperor Charles V. He carried out no further published research. While returning from a pilgrimage

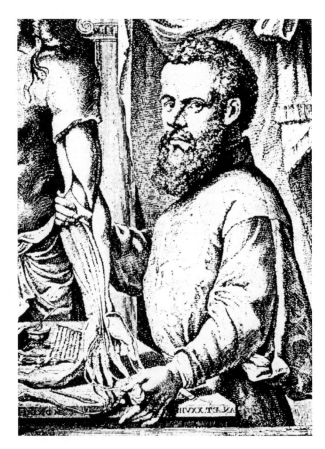

FIGURE 1.1. Andreas Vesalius. Frontpiece illustration from *De Humani Corporis Fabrica Liber Septum*, Basel, 1543. (Photograph from a first edition printed in 1543, courtesy of the Library of the College of Physicians, Philadelphia, PA.)

to Jerusalem, he died on a remote Greek island at the age of 50 years.

1553

Michael Servetus (1511–1553), Spanish theologian and physician living in Paris, mixed his theological beliefs and anatomic discoveries in the 700-page tome *Christianismi Restitutio*. Therein he denounced belief in the Holy Trinity as well as Galen's teachings on circulatory system anatomy and function. In correctly describing the pumping action of the heart's ventricles and the circulation of blood from the right heart through the lungs to the left heart, he laid the foundation for the later discoveries of William Harvey and others. For his theological and anti-Galenic views he was condemned by both Catholic and Protestant authorities. Upon traveling to Geneva, he unfortunately was captured by John Calvin's forces, was condemned as a heretic, and was burned at the stake along with most copies of his book. This certainly was the most damaging editorial review in the history of medical literature.

1559

Matteo Realdo Colombo (1515?–1559), student of and successor to Vesalius as Professor of Anatomy at Padua, also described the pulmonary circulation and function of the heart in his posthumously published *De re Anatomica* (1559). Whether he possessed a copy of Servetus's work and plagiarized his findings or made independent discoveries remains unsettled. He did add the concept that the lungs added a *spirituous* element to the blood by the admixture of air. Nonetheless, it was Colombo's book that almost surely was read by William Harvey during his years in Padua, as well as by anatomists and physicians throughout Europe.

1559

Hans and *Zacharius Jansen*, father and son, both Dutch optical lens grinders, invented the single-lens microscope. Some 74 years later, their countryman, Antoni van Leeuwenhoek, using a multi-lens compound microscope, discovered, defined, and classified microscopic life.

Seventeenth Century

1628

William Harvey (1578–1657), the next great pioneer in modern medical science after Vesalius, studied at Cambridge and Padua (1600–1602). He returned to London, becoming a Fellow of the College of Physicians and a physician at St. Bartholomew's Hospital and in 1618 a physician to the Royal Court. Despite all these responsibilities, yet with the income they produced, he was able to continue his laboratory animal research and human clinical investigations into the circulation of the blood in man and other mammals. His experience at Padua had taught him the principles of investigation. His genius and perseverance provided the other elements essential for a monumental achievement in correctly delineating the systemic and pulmonary circulation of blood in man and thereby founding modern physiology. His publication *De Motu Cordis (On the Motion of the Heart)* [12] in 1628 thrust medicine into the modern era of disciplined scientific investigation as the means to achieving understanding of the body's functions and disease. The explanations missing from his work, gaps that he acknowledged, included the mechanism for transfer of blood from the arterial to the venous systemic or pulmonary circulation (he lacked a microscope to observe capillaries) and the gas exchange function of the lungs. These were soon forthcoming. Although criticized and declared in error by some, Harvey successfully defended his theory and findings in subsequent writings. He also served as elder member of the renowned Oxford Philosophical Club of philosophers, scientists, and scholars who helped found the Enlightenment in Great Britain during this period.

1661

Marcello Malpighi (1628–1694), Professor of Medicine at Pisa, using a compound lens microscope to study dried frog lungs, correctly described, in his most important paper, *De Pulmonibus (On the Lungs)* (1661), the alveolar–capillary membrane and the tiny vessels connecting the pulmonary arteries and veins. This provided one of the two missing links in Harvey's work, and it refuted the prior theory that air and blood freely mixed in the lungs. Malpighi also made numerous other microanatomic and physiologic discoveries, including the bile-secreting function of the liver.

1664

Thomas Willis (1611–1675), a devout Anglican physician and royalist during the English civil war, was a founding member of the Oxford Philosophical Club, along with Robert Boyle, the father of modern chemistry and his co-worker Robert Hooke, anatomic artist and architect Christopher Wren, physiologist Richard Lower, and philosopher of the English Enlightenment John Locke. In this fertile atmosphere Willis lectured, cared for patients, conducted studies on nervous system functions in animals, and dissected with precision the brains and nervous systems of sheep and humans. Despite his religious convictions, he placed consciousness and mental functions, emotions, personality, and the soul of man in the brain. While specializing in the care of patients with mental and neurologic disorders, he made detailed observations that could be correlated at times with postmortem pathologic abnormalities in the brain. His two major publications were *Cerebri Anatomi* (Anatomy of the Brain) (1664) and *Pathologiae Cerebri et Nervosi Generis Specimen (Pathology of the Brain and Nature of the Nerves)* (1667). Willis can thus be regarded as the father of neurophysiology, neuropathology, and the clinical specialty of neurology [13].

1669

Richard Lower (1631–1691) studied medicine at Oxford with Boyle, Hooke, and Willis. He became fascinated with the circulation and functions of blood while conducting animal studies with Robert Hooke. He subsequently proved that it was passage of blood through the lungs, ventilation of the lungs, and gas exchange with blood that *vivified* the blood and turned its color red. Thus Lower defined clearly the true function of the lungs, providing the second missing link in Harvey's work. He published these landmark findings in *Tractatus de Corde (Treatise on the Heart)* (1669). Lower also was among the first to study blood transfusions. He transfused blood from a healthy dog directly through a cannula into one that had been severely exsanguinated with resuscitation of the latter and survival of both. He later transfused blood from the carotid artery of a lamb directly into an arm vein of a mentally ill man in hopes of improving the man's condition. His patient survived the procedure twice but his mental state deteriorated. A French group tried a similar experiment, killing their patient. The Royal Society then proscribed transfusions in humans, and 250 years would pass until safe and effective blood transfusions became established in clinical practice.

Eighteenth Century

1711

Stephen Hales (1677–1761), Anglican clergyman and physiologic investigator, cannulated the femoral artery of a horse with a brass tube that he attached to a 9 foot tall glass tube; upon releasing a ligature around the artery, blood rose over 8 feet in the tube above the level of the heart, the first documented observation of arterial blood pressure. Hales also measured the lower venous pressure and related these pressures, heart rate, vascular resistance, and ventricular volume (postmortem) to the sizes of various animals and man. After Harvey, he was the greatest of cardiovascular physiologists of the Enlightenment. It would be 185 years before a clinically practical noninvasive method of measuring arterial blood pressure would be developed by Riva-Rocci in 1896, and improved by Korotkoff in 1905, resulting in the same method used worldwide today.

1754

Joseph Black (1728–1799), the great Glasgow physicist and chemist, isolated and identified carbon dioxide as a separate gas arising from soda lime and as expired gas from human beings, labeling it *fixed air*. He published his findings in *Dissertatio de Humore Acido a Cibo Orto (Dissertation on Acid Fluid Arising from Food)* (1754). To a physicist, gas and liquids are *fluids*. Black also defined specific heat and latent heat, concepts used by engineer James Watt in improving the early Savery-Newcomen steam engine to develop the modern powerful steam engine that fueled the industrial revolution.

1757

Albrecht von Haller (1708–1777), Swiss physician and polymath, conducted numerous anatomic and physiologic studies on blood vessels, muscles, and nerves, but his greatest contribution was an eight-volume compendium synthesizing what then was known about functional anatomy, *Elementa Physiologiae Corporis Humani (Elements of the Physiology of the Human Body)* (1757–1766). This served as an encyclopedic reference for decades and placed physiology among the major medical sciences.

1759

Caspar Friedrich Wolff (1733–1794), German physician and father of modern embryology, demonstrated that embryologic tissues and organs differentiate and develop from undifferentiated primitive tissues, thus refuting the long espoused theory that the embryo held the fully developed human baby in miniature. His classic work was published as *Theoria Generationis (Theory of Generation)* in 1759.

1768

Humane Societies in Amsterdam and Copenhagen were organized to promote resuscitation of victims of near-drowning using mouth-to-mouth breathing and digital blind orotracheal intubation with positive pressure breathing with a bellows [4]. In 1774, the Royal Humane Society formed in London for the same purpose. Unfortunately, these efforts were mixed with useless practices of the time, including rectal insufflation of smoke. This combined with inadequate appreciation of upper airway obstruction in the unconscious person resulted in discouraging outcomes, although there were certified rescues reported. Eventually the alternative techniques of prone positioning and arm lift or back pressure gained favor and remained the recommended methods of resuscitation for near-drowning or other causes of apnea until proven virtually useless in the mid-1950s by Peter Safar, who also proved the efficacy of mouth-to-mouth ventilation, which became the standard of care nationally in 1958 [14].

1772

Karl Wilhelm Scheele (1742–1786), Swedish apothecary and chemist, obtained and isolated oxygen by heating mercuric oxide and labeled the gas, which clearly supported combustion, *fire air*.

1774

Joseph Priestly (1733–1804), English chemist, Unitarian minister, scholar learned in eight languages including Arabic, liberal thinker of the Enlightenment, supporter of the French Revolution, political activist, and scientific genius, independently isolated oxygen, labeling it *de-phlogisticated air*. He determined its vital role in supporting combustion by observing a lit candle in an airtight bell jar become extinguished over time in contrast to the candle that would burn more brightly when exposed to the gas derived from heating mercuric oxide. *Phlogiston* was a hypothetical vaporous substance allegedly liberated by burning metals or other materials; the phlogiston theory confounded scientists great and small from 1660 onward until demolished by Lavoisier. Priestly was persecuted in England for his religious and political beliefs and fled to the new United States in 1794, settling in Northumberland in central Pennsylvania. He continued with investigations and discussions with American chemists, dying in 1804. His gravesite remains a local attraction.

1777

Antoine Laurent Lavoisier (1743–1794), the brilliant Parisian chemist, through careful animal experiments and remarkable insight, demonstrated that the component gas in air discovered by Priestly and Scheele indeed was the vital element taken up by the lungs that maintains life. Lavoisier named this gas *oxygen* (*oxy* for *acid* and *gen* for *generator*, believing that acids were the vital chemicals of life). He further proved that oxygen is converted by the body into carbon dioxide that is exhaled from the lungs. He published these findings in 1777 as *Experiences sur la Respiration des Animaux (Experience with Animal Respiration)*. Unfortunately, this aristocratic genius fell victim to the Terror and was executed in 1794 at the age of 51 years.

Nineteenth Century

Modern medicine with its effective therapeutics and surgery, and the ability of physicians to successfully rescue critically ill and injured persons, begins in 1842 and 1846 with the discovery of surgical anesthesia and in the 1850s to 1870s with the establishment of hygienic and compassionate nursing care, aseptic surgery, and the discovery of microorganisms as the cause of infections. These advances led quickly to the establishment of hospitals, including children's hospitals, serum treatment and chemotherapeutics for infections, and modern public health and surgery. Also, the mysteries of oxygen transport and gases in the blood were explored and partially explained.

1819

Rene T. H. Laennec (1781–1826) invented the first stethoscope and described in his classic 900-page *Treatise on Mediate Auscultation* the use of this single wooden tube to diagnose the known range of maladies affecting the chest. His work laid the foundation for clinical pulmonology, and he described accurately the auscultatory findings in phthisis, or white plague (tuberculosis), a disease to which he would succumb at 45 years of age. In 1852, George P. Cammann, an American physician, developed the two-ear stethoscope similar to that in use today.

1842

Crawford Long (1815–1878) observed the insensibility to pain exhibited by injured participants in the recreational inhalation of diethyl ether *(ether frolics)* while a medical student at the University of Pennsylvania. Subsequently, as a rural general practitioner

in Jefferson, Georgia, Long made the gigantic leap in reasoning that inhalation of *sulfuric ether* (diethyl ether) might prevent the perception of pain during surgery. He successfully anesthetized a young man with an ether-soaked towel for removal of a small neck tumor on March 30, 1842, and repeated this use of ether on an 11-year-old slave boy for a toe amputation in July of that year, the first pediatric anesthetic. Unfortunately, Long did not publish his accomplishments with ether anesthesia in eight patients until 1849 [15]. *William Thomas Green Morton* (1819–1868), a dentist and controversial figure in history, used both nitrous oxide and ether for anesthesia in dental procedures. He then obtained an opportunity to demonstrate its efficacy in an operation to remove a mandibular tumor in a young man performed by the nation's leading surgeon, J. Collins Warren, at the Massachusetts General Hospital. Fortunately for all concerned, including succeeding generations of mankind, the anesthetic worked perfectly, leading to Warren's comment, "This is no humbug!" Morton soon delivered a second successful surgical anesthetic at the Massachusetts General Hospital. Henry Jacob Bigelow, a senior associate of Dr. Warren's, presented these two cases to a November 9, 1846, meeting in Boston and published his lecture in the *Boston Medical and Surgical Journal* (later the *New England Journal of Medicine*) (Figure 1.2) [16]. Within a few weeks the story was known worldwide, and the use of ether for surgical anesthesia was undertaken with great relief on every continent.

1854

Florence Nightingale (1820–1920), an extraordinary woman of aristocratic birth in England, decided early in life to be of service to humanity. She observed the nursing care in hospitals on the

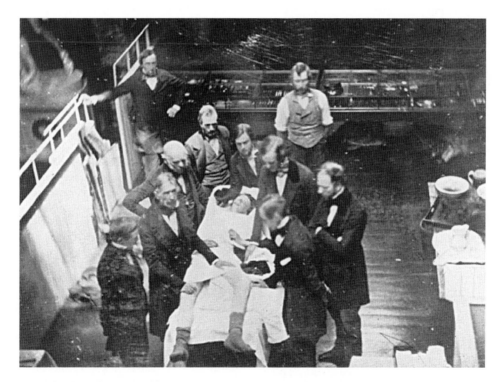

FIGURE 1.2. Dr. Henry Bigelow (second from left), senior author of the first paper on ether's efficacy in November 1846, operating in the "Ether Dome" of the Massachusetts General Hospital (MGH) on a patient under ether anesthesia being administered by a surgical house officer at the head of the table (face mask off at the moment). Date presumed to be early 1847. Note the lack of aseptic conditions. (Photograph from MGH archives, courtesy of Dr. Warren Zapol, Professor and Chair of the Department of Anesthesiology.)

continent, which emphasized cleanliness and hygienic care of patients, and then became Supervisor of Nursing at King's College Hospital (London) (Figure 1.3). Shortly thereafter the Crimean War erupted, and in 1854 she agreed to become the nurse in charge at a British military hospital in Skutari, Turkey, where 4 out of 10 wounded soldiers died. With her 38 English nursing colleagues, Nightingale reduced that mortality rate to 2% within 6 months of their arrival through intense environmental cleanliness and elimination of vermin, daily clean bed linens and wound dressings, and proper sewage and waste disposal. She became a national hero upon return to England in 1856, and funds were raised across the nation in support of a school of nursing under her direction. The school opened at St. Thomas Hospital in 1860 with the goal of training *matrons*, those who would train and supervise others in the profession of nursing. Nightingale insisted on careful tabulation of data, especially outcomes, and thus can be regarded as one of the founders of modern epidemiology. Graduates of this school established the leading nursing education programs in Sweden, Australia, Canada, and the United States within 10 to 15 years and set the standards for nursing care worldwide. This movement changed hospitals into safe and effective places for the care of the

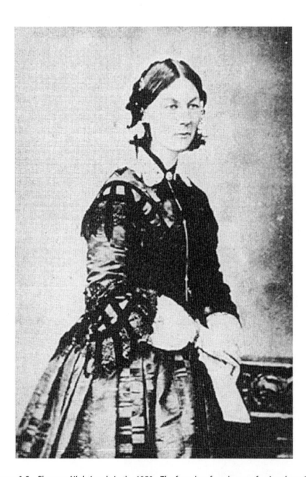

FIGURE 1.3. Florence Nightingale in the 1850s. The founder of modern professional nursing is seen here as a young woman in her thirties. Her phenomenal success in reducing mortality rate through hygiene and compassionate nursing care to wounded British soldiers in Turkey during the Crimean War proved the value of cleanliness and skilled nurses in medical care. (From the Library of Congress Collection of Portraits; www.loc.gov/rr/print/list/235.)

sickest patients of all social classes. Although Nightingale withdrew from public life at a relatively young age, through her writings and personal interviews with numerous leaders of the day, she remained a potent force in the advancement of health care until her death in 1920 [17].

1867

Joseph Lister (1817–1911), whose father produced one of the best microscopes of the day and was one of the founders of modern histology, trained as a surgeon in London and Edinburgh and was soon appointed to the Chair Surgery in Glasgow. He became unpopular with his surgical colleagues because of his dissatisfaction with the frequency of postoperative wound infection (so-called *laudable pus*), gangrene, and sepsis. Current wisdom held that pus was a normal part of the wound-healing process and that serious infections were caused by *miasmas* in the air. Lister regarded these complications akin to the *putrefaction* or rotting of organic material caused by bacteria described by Louis Pasteur (1822–1896). Carbolic acid, when added to raw sewage, was known to *purify* the water so that it did not stink and foul the rivers. Lister reasoned that bacteria were the source of the both bad odor of sewage and of the pus in surgical wounds and that carbolic acid sprayed over the surgical field during operations might eliminate bacteria from the wounds. This indeed proved to be correct, although the dilute carbolic acid was an irritant to the eyes and respiratory passages of the surgeons and others in attendance. In addition to spearheading operative antisepsis, Lister removed blood clots from open wounds, packed the wounds with lint soaked in carbolic acid, and covered the area with tin foil, periodically lifting the foil to inspect and cleanse the wound. Lister's patients subsequently experienced only rare postoperative wound infections or sepsis, resulting in much higher survival rates than experienced by his colleagues. He published his procedures and remarkable results in *The Lancet* in 1867 [18]. Despite severe criticism and disbelief from many sources, gradually Lister and others convinced the surgical leaders in Europe and North America to change their practices to relatively aseptic techniques. However, modern surgical asepsis did not become the norm worldwide until well into the 20th century.

1862

Felix Hoppe-Seyler (1825–1895), considered the father of modern medical biochemistry, and his colleagues in the 1870s at the University of Strasburg focused their research on the transport of oxygen in blood. Building on the first measurements of blood gases by the German physical chemist Heinrich Gustav Magnus (1802–1870) and his successors, they applied the new analytic techniques of colorimetry and spectrometry in 1862 to isolate the pigment hemoglobin as a crystalline structure. They then defined its role in the reversible transport of oxygen in mammalian blood. Hoppe-Seyler also devised a colorimetric method of estimating hemoglobin concentration in blood. Thus, by extending the discoveries of Priestly and Lavoisier, Hoppe-Selyer vastly improved our fundamental understanding of vital gas exchange in the body. However, thorough understanding of gas transport and acid–base balance in blood and tissues would have to wait more than three decades for the concepts of ionization (Arrhenius), blood pH (Sorenson), the dissociation of CO_2 and the bicarbonate ion (Henderson and Hasselbach), and measurement of blood oxygen and CO_2 content in the clinical laboratory (VanSlyke) in the early 20th century [19].

1865

Claude Bernard (1813–1878), the most influential of all French bioscientists, established the foundation of modern medical laboratory research with publication of his *Introduction to the Study of Experimental Medicine* in 1865. This brilliant polymath not only described functions of the autonomic nervous system in regulating blood flow, hepatic synthesis of glucose, the mechanism by which carbon monoxide kills through displacement of oxygen from hemoglobin, the effects of the new South American alkaloid curare on muscular activity, and the role of the pancreas in digestion, but he also defined the principle of the *milieu interieur.* Bernard proposed that higher organisms, through complex and interacting physiologic processes, regulate their vital systems in internal harmony to achieve a high degree of autonomy. These ideas proved extraordinarily prescient. Harvard physiologist Walter Cannon (1871–1945) in 1932 described the body's autoregulation as *homeostasis.* In the 1930s and 1940s, McGill endocrinologist Hans Selye (1907–1982) further amplified these concepts by defining the body's response to stress and the disorders altering that response. Bernard finally advocated that physiology constituted the central science of clinical medicine, with pathology and disease being the results of altered physiology and with pharmacology being the use of drugs to restore physiologic processes toward normal function. This overarching view of medicine prevails today, with physiology extending to the cellular and molecular levels. In addition to these monumental achievements, Bernard served as Professor at the Sorbonne, President of the French Academy, and an elected member of the Assembly, the French parliament [20].

1882

Robert Koch (1843–1910), although less well known than Pasteur, made lasting contributions to the evolution of modern medicine and thus to critical care medicine. Paramount among these is the concept that diseases have a specific and discoverable etiology, especially infectious disorders. His formulas for identifying the cause of a specific infection are referred to as *Koch's Postulates,* formalized in 1882, setting the stage for the development of medical microbiology. He and his colleagues in Berlin isolated and identified *Mycobacterium tuberculi* as the organism causing tuberculosis, one of the leading causes of premature death and disability throughout the world in the 19th century. Working in Egypt with cholera victims, he and his team isolated and identified *Vibrio cholerae,* the comma bacillus, as the cause of this common and often fatal disorder. Koch's co-workers and students went on to discover the organisms causing numerous widespread infectious diseases, including diphtheria, typhoid, pneumococcal pneumonia, gonorrhea, syphilis, leprosy, plague, and pertussis. Unfortunately, Koch became the victim of his own fame, stopped doing research, and adopted an imperious style. Then, on very shaky grounds, he promoted tuberculin as the vaccine for tuberculosis for which he was prematurely honored and then defamed and ridiculed for many years. Despite this personal tragedy, Koch's Institute for Infectious Diseases in Berlin continued to produce astounding discoveries through laboratory animal research and clinical trials. Koch quite appropriately

received the Nobel Prize in 1905 for his discovery of the tubercle bacillus.

1891

Emil Behring and *S. Kitasato* achieved a landmark on December 25, 1891, with the first effective treatment of an infectious disorder, giving diphtheria serum antitoxin to a child to combat the toxic effects of that disease on the upper airway and the heart. This soon extended to serum therapy for a variety of disorders, including tetanus (used through the 1950s), pneumococcal pneumonia, and snake bites (still used). Not until the introduction of widely available antibiotics in the late 1940s would serum therapy become a rarity.

1895

Wilhelm Konrad von Roentgen (1843–1923), a Professor of Physics at the University of Wurzburg, while studying cathode rays, noticed that under certain focused conditions the rays penetrated soft tissues and illustrated the bones in his hand. He termed the phenomenon x-*rays* because he could not explain them on then-known theories of energy radiation. He recognized their potential value in clinical medicine, and his report the following year changed medicine for centuries to come. He received the Nobel Prize in Physics for this achievement.

1896

Scipione Riva-Rocci (1863–1937) reported in 1896 his use of a sphygmomanometer for indirect measurement of systolic pressure by palpation. Nikolai Korotkoff, in 1905, introduced the auscultatory method currently used to determine systolic and diastolic pressures.

With these discoveries and advances, as well as numerous others, the stage was set for the unprecedented improvement in public health and care of the sick and injured over the last two decades of the 19th century and in the years leading up to World War I in the 20th century. The development of the experimental method and its application to anatomy, physiology, physiologic chemistry, and microbiology combined with the discovery of general anesthesia, surgical asepsis, and professional nursing resulted in (1) new and modern hospitals including children's hospitals, (2) rapid expansion of medical knowledge through laboratory research, (3) consequent medical specialization, (4) the development of public health departments in major cities, and (5) the expectation that many if not most individuals could survive to *old age* (then regarded as beyond 50 years).

Origins of American Pediatrics—1860 to 1900

Founders of Pediatrics in the United States

Establishing a group of physicians dedicated to the care of infants and children proved essential for the application of these advances to acutely ill or injured pediatric patients. This occurred in New York City in the last half of the 19th century under the leadership of one of America's most remarkable physicians. *Abraham Jacobi* (1830–1919), a German physician, fled his native country after the failed revolution of 1848 and two years in prison for promoting socialist causes and human rights [21]. He arrived in the United

States in 1853 and established a family practice in a German section of Manhattan. In 1860, Jacobi founded a free children's clinic at New York Medical College, the first in the nation, and was given the academic title *Professor of Infantile Pathology and Therapeutics*, also the first such appointment in America. There he instituted bedside teaching of students and physicians, again the first recorded in this country. Thus began the specialty of clinical and academic pediatrics in the United States.

Jacobi, a physically small man with phenomenal energy and exceptional organizing abilities, devoted his career to advocacy for the well being of infants and children. In that he was the consummate advocate, extending his influence first over the city and eventually over the nation. He worked tirelessly establishing free children's clinics and children's hospitals in New York City, training physicians, and writing chapters in textbooks as well as numerous papers. In addition, he advocated for public health laws and practices to ensure clean milk and sanitary conditions in housing and schools in order to reduce the appalling mortality rate of more than 33% for children under the age of 5 years because of infections. From 1870 to 1899, he served as Professor of Pediatrics at the College of Physicians and Surgeons of Columbia University. He was the prime mover to establish the Section on Pediatrics of the American Medical Association (1871), as well as a founder and first president of the American Pediatric Society (1888), this nation's first independent pediatric organization. In 1912, at the age of 82, he served as president of the American Medical Association, the first immigrant physician to achieve this position. In all these efforts, Jacobi had a powerful compatriot in Mary Putnam Jacobi, his wife and an extraordinary academic pediatrician in her own right. Two recent biographical reviews of Jacobi's life and achievements provide inspiring reading about him and the other remarkable individuals of that seminal period [22,23].

Joseph O'Dwyer (1841–1898), also of New York City, devoted most of his career to the care of children and was a founding member of the American Pediatric Society. At this time, diphtheria killed thousands of children in our major cities each year by obstructing the upper airway. O'Dwyer, Jacobi, and other pediatric physicians would perform a tracheostomy, but this was accompanied by significant morbidity and mortality. O'Dwyer is best remembered for a laryngeal tube he developed in the 1880s for the nonsurgical management of infants and children with severe airway obstruction. This brass hollow tube with a proximal flange was attached to a metal rod and inserted blindly or with digital guidance through the glottis and was placed in the subglottic lumen, with the flange above the vocal cords preventing the tube from slipping down the trachea [24,25]. A tethered string attached to the flange was taped on the child's cheek so that the tube could be pulled out if it became occluded or for a trial extubation. The nose and pharynx served as a natural filter and humidifier of the inspired air. The physician or other caretaker had to be taught the procedure for insertion, and the tubes could be accidentally displaced by vigorous coughing or pulling on the tether. Nonetheless many children appear to have been saved from fatal asphyxia by the O'Dwyer tube. This clever device was used throughout the country until the 1930s, when surgeons competent to perform a tracheostomy on a child and provide airway care became more widely available.

Job Lewis Smith (1827–1897) was primarily dedicated to clinical pediatrics and advocacy for children's health. He wrote the standard textbook of pediatrics of that era and served as Chief of Pediatrics at Bellevue Hospital. In Boston between 1870 and 1900, Charles Minot and Charles Putnam established academic pediatric courses at Harvard Medical School. In 1893, Thomas Rotch became the first Professor and Chair of Pediatrics with full faculty privileges at Harvard Medical School, the first chair of pediatrics in the nation.

L. Emmett Holt (1855–1924), a brilliant physician and scientist, pioneered basic science investigations and clinical research into a variety of disorders of children. In 1899, he succeeded Jacobi as Professor of Pediatrics at Columbia University. He also authored a classic textbook of pediatrics that went through many editions and profoundly influenced and guided the development of modern pediatrics.

Origins of Children's Hospitals—1855 to 1900

Children's hospitals had evolved from foundling homes in Europe in the 19th century [26]. The first modern hospital devoted to children, the 300-bed Hôpital des Enfants Maladies, was established in Paris in 1802 by the French government and became the leading center in Europe for the study of pediatric disorders and the training of physicians in the care of children. Over the next 50 years, modern children's hospitals were developed in St. Petersburg, Vienna, Prague, Turin, and the major cities of Germany. In 1852, London's Hospital for Sick Children in Great Ormond Street opened—the first children's hospital in England. Using this hospital as a model, in 1855 three Philadelphia physicians committed to the care of children, *Drs. Lewis, Bache,* and *Penrose*, and various charitable supporters established the first children's hospital in North America, The Children's Hospital of Philadelphia. The hospital had 12 beds for *children of the poor* plus a large outpatient clinic. The hospital moved in 1867 to a 70-bed facility (Figure 1.4) and in 1916 to a 120-bed hospital with adjacent research and outpatient buildings. In 1974, the hospital moved to its current location adjacent to the University of Pennsylvania as a 310-bed comprehensive pediatric medical center. The next children's hospital in the United States was founded in Boston in 1869 with 20 beds, growing over the following century into the nation's leading pediatric center for training and research in the 20th century. Children's hospitals were founded in New York City and Washington, DC, in 1870, in Toronto in 1875, and in many other North American cities in the late 19th and early 20th centuries.

The Twentieth Century

Following upon the productivity of late 19th century medicine and public health, at the outset of the 20th century confidence in scientific medicine generated a fervent commitment by scientists and health professionals to find the causes and effective treatments for presumably incurable diseases and to rescue those with life-threatening disorders.

Landmark Advances Related to Critical Care Medicine—1900 to 1960

The foundations of critical care medicine in the first half of the 20th century in large measure depended on the innovative and prodigious accomplishments of physiologists and biochemists from Europe and North America. The major foci of these investigators concerned ventilation and circulation, tissue and cellular respira-

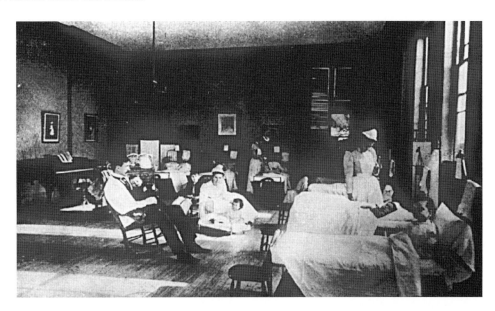

FIGURE 1.4. Surgical ward of the Children's Hospital of Philadelphia about 1880. Note the presence of three nurses for six patients as well as a young physician rocking a toddler. For entertainment of the children there is a piano rather than a television set. (From the archives of The Children's Hospital of Philadelphia, courtesy of Shirley Bonnem.)

tion, and blood pH, oxygen, and carbon dioxide levels and transport. In 1902, *Joseph Barcroft* (1872–1947), professor of physiology at Cambridge University, in collaboration with Oxford physiologist *John Scott Haldane* (1860–1936), developed a method for measuring oxygen and carbon dioxide content in 1.0 mL of blood. Barcroft also further defined the shape and shifts of the oxyhemoglobin dissociation curve, including the effects of pH and temperature on the release of oxygen in man and other species [27]. This and numerous other investigations culminated in his 1928 classic publication *The Respiratory Function of Blood*. Barcroft's other contributions to physiology are discussed later. In 1903, *Willem Einthoven* (1860–1927), professor of physiology at the University of Leyden in the Netherlands, improved on earlier string galvanometers to devise the first practical electrocardiograph. For this he received the Novel Prize in 1924. *John Haldane* in 1905 also discovered a practical way to measure oxygen and carbon dioxide tensions in small samples of end-expired gas and correctly determined the alveolar PCO_2 in normal adults to be approximately 40 mm Hg. Haldane, an avid mountaineer, is best known as the father of high altitude medicine, along with Barcroft, his friend and mountaineering colleague. Together they performed pioneering respiratory studies at altitude in the Alps and the Andes, and Barcroft also in California's High Sierras, where a mountain has been named for him. *August Krough* (1874–1949), perhaps Denmark's greatest physiologist, in 1910, while a young investigator at the University of Copenhagen, proved for the first time that gas exchange in the lung occurs by simple diffusion. Later work on the control of blood flow through arterioles and capillaries explained the variations in tissue blood flow at rest and under other conditions. This particular work won him the Nobel Prize in 1920. He is also considered the father of exercise physiology.

To prevent needless deaths of mothers and infants required changes in social attitudes, including those of the medical profession, government support and intervention, and dedicated leadership. Two individuals stand out as exemplary leaders in maternal and child health during the first two decades of the 20th century—Sara Josephine Baker and Julia Lathrop. These two women estab-

lished the relationship between social conditions such as poverty and the health status of individuals, especially pregnant women, infants, and young children. *Sara Josephine Baker* (1873–1945), an 1898 graduate of The Women's Medical College of New York, interned in Boston where she came to appreciate the close correlation between poverty and infant and maternal morbidity and mortality. In 1907, she became Assistant Commissioner of Health of New York City and led various public health efforts. Most notable was the identification of *Typhoid Mary* (Mary Mallon), a private household cook, as the source case for a small epidemic of typhoid fever in the city. The following year Baker was appointed Director of the city's new Bureau of Child Hygiene, the first such agency in the nation [28]. In this post she developed innovative programs aimed at lowering maternal and infant mortality, especially among poor immigrants. These included midwife training, basic hygiene in homes and child care centers, and training girls of 12 years and older how to properly care for infants and toddlers in order to help their working mothers. She also created a school health program that was replicated in 35 states. At the time of her retirement in 1923, New York City had the lowest infant mortality rate of any major city in the United States.

Julia Lathrop (1858–1932), a pioneering social worker and epidemiologist who trained with Jane Addams, the founder of modern social work, at Hull House in Chicago, from 1893 to 1909 gained public health and social advocacy experience as a member of the Illinois Board of Charities, which governed the state's mental institutions and infirmaries. Extensive personal inspection of chaotic facilities under their jurisdiction combined with her powerful ability to garner data and persist in her agenda led in 1909 to the adoption of statewide reform of these institutions. In 1903 she cofounded and later directed the Chicago Institute of Social Science, which eventually became the School of Social Service Administration of the University of Chicago. With these and many other achievements, and vigorous support from fellow social workers and nurses in the reform movement, she became the choice of President William Howard Taft in 1912 to be the first woman appointed to a major federal administrative position, Director of the new U.S.

Children's Bureau of the Department of Commerce and Labor [29]. This Bureau was modeled after the New York City agency headed by Dr. S. Josephine Baker. As a savvy administrator, Lathrop did not tackle the contentious issue of child labor at first but concentrated her energy on the appalling maternal and infant mortality rates among industrial laborers' families. Lathrop and her small staff, on a bureau annual budget of $25,000, carried out a landmark 1913 epidemiological study of maternal and infant mortality in Johnstown, Pennsylvania, then a highly industrialized city in the middle of the state. She demonstrated statistically for the first time that infant mortality was inversely related to the father's income; infant mortality rate was 197 per 1,000 live births whose fathers earned $1,200 or more per year. Lathrop also proved that babies delivered by physicians had a much lower mortality. She followed up these studies with a model program for maternal prenatal and postnatal education of young women in and infant care, nutrition, and general hygiene that later became replicated in many states by their departments of health. Lathrop's early leadership set the mission for the bureau that persists to this day, serving mothers and children of all socioeconomic classes as well as health professionals through research, advocacy, and education [29,30].

Joseph Barcroft, upon retirement from the Chair in Physiology at Cambridge University in 1932, at age 60 years began his second highly productive career as an investigator, teacher, and mentor by establishing and directing a new laboratory at Cambridge dedicated to maternal–fetal physiology. Their studies, conducted in the pregnant ewe, focused on distribution of blood flow, the left-shift of the oxyhemoglobin dissociation curve, and fetal circulation with the new technique of cine-radiography. Upon determining the low oxygen tension of fetal arterial blood, approximately 40 mm Hg, Barcroft described the condition as *Everest-in-utero*, an oft quoted description of fetal blood and tissue oxygen levels. One of Barcroft's most apt students was American *Donald H. Barron*, later professor of physiology at Yale where he initiated seminal studies in maternal and fetal physiology and trained some of America's leading physiologists.

The performance of cardiac catheterization by Forssmann in 1929 (see later) and its clinical application by Cournand and Richards in 1940 launched the fields of modern clinical cardiovascular physiology and cardiology. Other extraordinary achievements exemplifying this period include the discovery and typing of red blood cell surface antigens and their categorization as blood groups by Karl Landsteiner in the early 1900s, the discovery of insulin and its use in treating diabetes by Macleod, Best, and Banting in 1921, and the discovery of the antibacterial properties of the mold *Penicillium* by Fleming in 1929 followed by its production and clinical use in 1940 by Florey and Chain. Each of these investigators except Best became Nobel laureates for their discoveries.

Origins of Critical Care Medicine—1900 to 1960

During the first half of the 20th century, the acute care of the critically ill and injured, especially children, advanced at a relatively slow pace despite advances resulting from the management of the wounded in World War I. Yet certain accomplishments before 1960 provided the foundation for the astounding achievements of the following 40 years in the acute care of critically ill children. Four fields emerging in Western Europe and North America between 1900 and 1960 set the stage for the evolution of pediatric critical

care medicine: (1) adult respiratory intensive care, (2) neonatology and newborn intensive care, (3) pediatric general and cardiac surgery, and (4) pediatric anesthesiology. A brief consideration of each of these clinical fields follows, including the emergence of PICUs in Sweden and France, which led the way for the development of PICUs elsewhere in Europe and North America in the 1960s and 1970s, and eventually to the subspecialty of pediatric critical care medicine.

Adult Intensive Care

The concept of frequent assessment of respiratory rate and breathing patterns, as well as skin color, heart rate, and body temperature, in patients undergoing anesthesia and after operations evolved in Germany and the United States between 1890 and 1910. When ventilation appeared to be failing, mechanical assistance to breathing was occasionally attempted but with limited success. One exception occurred in 1910 in the Trendelenburg Clinic of Leipzig. Two thoracic surgeons, A. Lawen and R. Sievers, developed a volume pre-set, electrically powered piston-cylinder ventilator with a draw-over humidifier [31]. They reported using the ventilator, always with a tracheostomy tube, during ether anesthesia for thoracic operations and in postoperative ventilatory support. Also, they ventilated older children and adults with acute respiratory failure caused by narcotic or strychnine overdose, toxic gas inhalation, or status seizures caused by epilepsy or tetanus. For the latter patients they used curare to relax muscles for adequate ventilation. Unfortunately they published their work in a single paper in a journal that lacked a wide international readership, so their remarkable achievements went virtually unnoticed for over 40 years. Similarly, advances in airway management with flexible metal or coated fibrous orotracheal tubes inserted with digital guidance during anesthesia or for upper airway obstruction did not become standard practice, and few physicians acquired the requisite skills.

An organized protocol for airway diagnosis and management, including laryngoscopy, bronchoscopy, and tracheostomy, was first developed in the early 1900s in the United States by *Chevalier Jackson* (1858–1955). A surgeon at Temple University in Philadelphia, Jackson's system, for infants, children, and adults, utilized a series of endoscopes and tracheostomy tubes with specified sizes that were manufactured by the Pilling Company of Philadelphia. Jackson also led a large surgical training program in the emerging field of otorhinolaryngology. This equipment and the Jackson precepts of endoscopy and airway management became the standard practice throughout the United States for the next 50 years. Despite numerous adaptations in practice and equipment, Jackson's principles still serve as the foundation of modern surgical airway management.

As mentioned earlier, cardiovascular physiology and cardiology took a great leap forward in 1929 when *Werner Forssmann*, a young German surgeon from Berlin, performed cardiac catheterization on himself. His report caused some scorn from certain medical authorities, resulting in a 10-year delay in clinical exploitation of the procedure. In 1940, *Andre Cournand* and *Dickinson Richards* resurrected the technique to study traumatic shock in patients at Bellevue Hospital in New York City. Forssmann, Cournand, and Richards received the Nobel Prize for Physiology and Medicine in 1956.

The poliomyelitis epidemics of the 1920s through the mid-1950s in Europe and the United States provided the impetus for the development of modern respiratory care and for intensive care medicine. Although tuberculosis wreaked far more death and disability worldwide, the public's fear of paralysis, inability to breathe, and long-term crippling effects, especially in children of all social classes, made polio the number one dreaded disease. Various attempts to treat ventilatory failure caused by bulbar polio proved futile until the late 1920s, when a unique collaboration between an engineer and two physicians at the Children's Hospital of Boston and Harvard Medical School resulted in an effective solution. After several years of development and trials in animals, in 1929 *Philip Drinker*, an engineer, and physicians *Louis Shaw* and *Charles McKhann* introduced the first mechanical ventilator that would have widespread application and be mass produced [32]. This electrically powered negative pressure body tank (with head exposed to the room) became known as the *iron lung*. In 1932, pediatrician *James Wilson*, also at the Children's Hospital of Boston, established a four-bed large box ventilator that functioned as an intermittent negative pressure room resulting in ventilation of the four child occupants; a nurse cared for the children from inside the box while others attended their airways and heads outside, thus obviating the difficulty of patient access through the side portholes of the iron lung, but creating other problems with individual ventilatory requirements (Figure 1.5). Over the subsequent 15 years, thousands of infants, children, and adults with bulbar polio received ventilatory support with iron lungs throughout the developed world. In the United States during the 1930s and 1940s, despite the severe economic depression and World War II, dedicated physicians and nurses created numerous discrete units to care for polio patients of all ages suffering from respiratory failure and supported with a tracheostomy and the iron lung ventilator.

These polio units represent the first respiratory intensive care units with specialized nursing and medical staffs providing 24-hour care for patients with organ-system failure (Figure 1.5). These units operated continuously until the late 1950s, when acute bulbar polio became a rarity in the United States and Western Europe as a result of the Salk and Sabin polio vaccines. However, a major step forward in the development of critical care medicine occurred earlier in Europe. The polio epidemics in Scandinavia in the summers of 1950 through 1952 proved devastating in scope and severity and created a health care crisis in 1952, especially in Denmark. The number of polio patients in respiratory failure flooding into Copenhagen's main communicable disease hospital exceeded the number of available iron lung ventilators, and the anesthesiologists were sought to aid in management. *Dr. Bjorn Ibsen* (Figure 1.6) and his department of anesthesia physician and nurses employed orotracheal intubation with sedation, manual positive pressure ventilation with an anesthesia bag-valve system to restore proper ventilation, and tracheal suctioning and chest percussion to control secretions [33]. This was followed after hours or days by tracheostomy and longer term manual ventilation provided by rotating teams of nurses, medical students, residents, and staff physicians. Ibsen worked closely with internist *H.C.P. Lassen* and clinical biochemist *Poul Astrup*, the inventor of the first blood gas analyzing technique using ultramicro volumes of blood, to achieve astounding success. Their management reduced the mortality rate of bulbar polio from 90% to 47%. This experience [34], and the continued leadership of Ibsen in developing critical care, set the stage for the imminent development of respiratory intensive care units elsewhere in Europe and later in the decade in the United States. Eventually the Engstrom volume pre-set positive pressure mechanical ventilators from Sweden [35] and similar intermittent

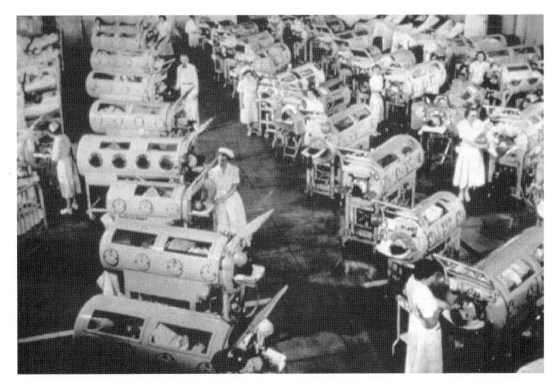

FIGURE 1.5. The polio unit of the Los Angeles County Hospital in early 1950's. Note that 37 or more patients are cared for by only 6 nursing staff. (From Warren E. Collins, Inc., Cambridge. MA as reproduced in Landmark Perspective: The Iron Lung. JAMA 1986;255:1476–1481.

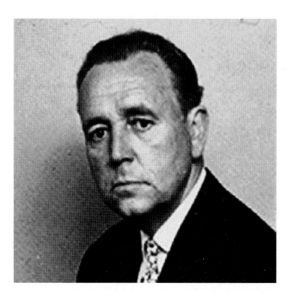

FIGURE 1.6. Bjorn Ibsen, MD, the father of modern critical care medicine, in Copenhagen in 1952. His advocacy and persistence in establishing and staffing specialized units for the care of critically ill and injured patients throughout Scandinavia led to similar units in Great Britain and throughout Europe in the 1950s and in the United States in 1959. (Photograph provided to the author by Peter Safar, MD.)

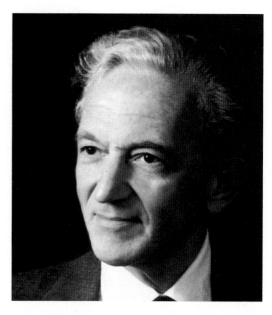

FIGURE 1.7. Peter Safar, MD, the father of critical care medicine in North America and one of the originators of modern cardiopulmonary resuscitation. (Courtesy of Peter Safar, MD.)

positive pressure ventilators (IPPV) relieved the human ventilators in those patients who developed chronic respiratory failure.

The demonstrated need to cohort patients in respiratory failure and to provide geographic full-time physicians and nurses for their care, as well as the proven superiority of tracheal intubation and IPPV, led to the creation of respiratory and general medical–surgical intensive care units in Denmark, Sweden, and Great Britain. *Dr. Alex Crampton-Smith*, a professor of anesthesia, established a neurologic and a respiratory intensive care unit at the Oxford University's Churchill Hospital where he trained some of the pioneers in critical care medicine and conducted research. This respiratory unit and similar units founded in Cardiff, Copenhagen, and Stockholm served as prototypes for future critical care units throughout the world [36]. Although children occasionally received care in these early units, only one pediatric intensive care unit, of which we are aware, opened before 1960 (see below).

In the 1950s in North America, postanesthesia recovery rooms served as the locus for most patients requiring acute life support, although some hospitals created special nursing units for certain categories of medical or surgical patients. In 1958, the first physician-directed intensive care units in North America opened at the Baltimore City Hospital under the leadership of *Peter Safar* (Figures 1.7 and 1.8) [37] and at the Toronto General Hospital led by *Barrie Fairley*. The respiratory intensive care unit at the Massachusetts General Hospital opened in 1962 and set the standard for academic critical care medicine for the next 40 years through its excellence in clinical care, training of physicians, nurses, and other professionals, and research into the fundamental causes of respiratory failure in adults [38]. The staff of this unit became prominent leaders in academic anesthesiology and critical care medicine over the next 20 years, including *Myron Laver, John Hedley-White, Henning Pontoppidan,* and *Henrik Bendixen*, the last two being Danish trained physicians who emigrated to the United States. This group conducted landmark research into acute respiratory failure in the adult with results being published in eminent journals. These culminated in a

review that established the standards for respiratory intensive care and an excellent, succinct book that remains pertinent today. This group also trained numerous future leaders in adult critical care in the United States, Europe, and Japan over the next 30 years.

Peter Safar, in the late 1950s, as mentioned above, inaugurated a revolution in the techniques of cardiopulmonary resuscitation through his clinical studies at Baltimore City Hospital, proving that the long-held techniques for airway maintenance and *artificial respiration* taught to generations of physicians and lifeguards to be virtually worthless [14]. Instead, the ancient method of mouth-to-mouth ventilation with forward jaw thrust and cervical extension provided a clear airway and effective gas exchange. Across town at Johns Hopkins Hospital, surgeon *J. Jude* and engineer *C.W. Kouwenhoven*, through studies in dogs and later in anesthetized humans, proved the efficacy of closed chest cardiac massage in restoring circulation to the brain and central circulation. Although *Beck* and co-workers in 1946 demonstrated electrical defibrillation of the heart through thoracotomy, and *Zoll* and colleagues proved the efficacy of external defibrillation in 1952 and external cardiac pacing in 1956, these techniques did not come into common practice in resuscitation until the late 1950s along with positive pressure ventilation and closed cardiac massage. In 1963, *Bernard Lown* and his team achieved successful external cardioversion of atrial fibrillation. Safar has written a brief but quite comprehensive history of modern resuscitation [39].

Peter Safar moved to the University of Pittsburgh in 1960 to assume the chairmanship of anesthesiology and quickly established a large multidisciplinary adult intensive care unit and academic program directed by a Swedish surgeon and anesthesiologist, *Ake Grenvick*. This program developed the concept and eventually the practice in Pittsburgh of care for the critically ill or injured patient to receive resuscitation and stabilization from trained paramedics, to be transported in a mobile intensive care unit by that team, to be further treated by full-time emergency medicine physicians, nurses, and respiratory therapists, and then to be transferred to the multidisciplinary general intensive care unit with continuing

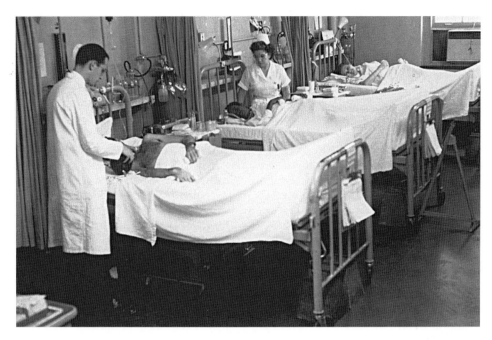

FIGURE 1.8. The intensive care unit at Baltimore City Hospital in 1959, the first intensive care unit in the United States established and directed by Peter Safar, MD. (Courtesy of Peter Safar, MD.)

care by trained critical care physicians, nurses, and other professionals. Concurrently, cardiologists *Harry Weill* and *Herbert Shubin* established a cardiovascular intensive care unit at the University of Southern California focusing on shock and cardiopulmonary failure with state-of-the art electronic monitoring, and surgeon *William Shoemaker* at UCLA developed an early version of today's shock-trauma emergency and intensive care facility. Both of these groups did extensive clinical research that helped broaden the foundation of critical care medicine from its singular focus on resuscitation and respiratory failure.

The field of critical care medicine became formally organized when 26 physicians representing anesthesiology, internal medicine, surgery, and pediatrics met in 1970 and founded the Society of Critical Care Medicine (SCCM) [40]. Drs. Weill, Shubin, Safar, and Shoemaker and other pioneers in critical care from the United States and Canada focused the mission of SCCM, which it retains to this day, on education of health care professionals and the public, on establishing guidelines for intensive care units, and on the training of subspecialists in critical care medicine. Early on critical care nurses were integrated into the society. The recognition of critical care fellowships by the Accreditation Council on Graduate Medical Education and sub-board certification in critical care medicine followed in the 1980s (see later).

Neonatal Intensive Care and Perinatology

The French obstetricians *Ettiene Stephane Tarnier* (1828–1897), inventor of the first practical infant incubator, and *Pierre Constant Budin* (1846–1907) inaugurated newborn pediatrics and intensive care of the premature infant with their creation of a special nursery and department for premature babies at the Hôpital la Charitre in Paris in the 1880s and 1890s [41,42]. With their dedicated full-time medical and nursing staff, they developed improved incubators with controlled heat, gavage feeding of breast milk from the mother or a staff of wet nurses, and strict sanitary practices. They set their

weight limit for premature infants at less than 2,500 g, and trained both physicians and nurses in the care of small infants. Emphasis on breast feeding as soon as feasible, maternal and infant hygiene, and maternal education, in addition to intensive care in the special nursery, resulted in a reduction of infant mortality at that institution from 197 before this program to 46 per 1,000 births by 1900. This success inspired others in Europe before World War I such as *Heinrich Finkelstein* in Berlin and *Arvo Yllpo* in Helsinki, the latter pioneering research on prenatal and postnatal growth as well as the pathology found in premature infants. *Albrecht Peiper* of Leipzig dedicated his career to the care of preterm infants, describing early neurologic development in 1924 and, in 1937 pulmonary disorders including hyaline membrane disease (referred to as *infant respiratory distress syndrome* since the early 1960s).

In the United States, premature infants in incubators were part of public exhibitions, such as the Chicago Exhibition of 1914, the Chicago World's Fair of 1933, and the Coney Island boardwalk from 1903 until the early 1940s. Following the display of infants under his care at the Chicago Exhibition of 1914, *Julius Hess* (1876–1955) founded the nation's first premature infant center at Michael Reese Hospital in that city. Also in 1914 he designed a more reliable incubator that became the standard for the next 25 years. In 1922, he wrote the first book focused on the premature infant and those with congenital anomalies. He also cared for the two smallest infants (birth weights 690 and 740 g) before 1925 to survive beyond 1 month; both died at 2 ½ months of apparent aspiration caused by overfeeding.

The merger of basic science, clinical understanding, and technical proficiency in acute newborn care emerged in an important way in the 1930s and 1940s. Exchange transfusion in the newborn with severe jaundice and anemia was first successfully achieved by *Alfred Hart* of Canada in 1928 and subsequently by others using the sagittal sinus or saphenous vein or radial artery for vascular access. In 1932, *Louis Diamond, Kenneth Blackfan,* and *James Baty* at Children's Hospital of Boston correctly described the hemolytic anemia and jaundice of the newborn as one disorder that they named *erythroblastosis fetalis*. After *Levine* and *Stetson* identified blood group incompatibility as the cause (1938), and *Landsteiner* and *Weiner* discovered the Rhesus (Rh) system of antigens and antibodies (1939), Diamond and his colleagues in 1946 provided the definitive therapy. With compatible donor blood, and using a plastic feeding tube, they cannulated the umbilical vein, permitting facile flow of the blood being exchanged. This highly effective technique soon became the standard practice, remaining so to this day.

Another important contribution of this period to survival of preterm newborns was the development of the modern incubator, the *isolette*, in 1938, by *Charles Chappel*, a pediatrician at the Children's Hospital of Philadelphia, and the Air Shields Company (personal communication, S. Bonnem). This early Isolette provided excellent caretaker visibility through the Plexiglas cover, a consistent thermal environment, a fresh supply of humidified air or supplemental oxygen, and minimal exposure to external contamination except through portholes closed with rubber or plastic on the sides. Chappel conducted lengthy clinical trials in the hospital's nursery but never published the design or the successful results of the trials. Regardless, this device with some modifications became the standard incubator for the next 40 years.

The concepts underlying the current methods of neonatal cardiopulmonary resuscitation and management of respiratory failure in the newborn emanated from the original studies of Barcroft and his colleagues at Cambridge and from the brilliant work of *Geoffrey Dawes* and his collaborators and fellows at the Nuffield Institute for Medical Research at Oxford University. During the 1950s and 1960s, through a long series of exceptional studies in fetal and newborn lambs and other animals, they defined mammalian fetal and transitional newborn circulation and metabolism. *McCance* and *Widdowson* in England and *Friis-Hansen* in Finland conducted classic clinical studies in newborn fluid balance. At Oxford, *K. Cross* studied newborn respiratory control and *Hill* investigated infant thermal control and lipid metabolism. At the Children's Hospital of Boston between 1930 and 1960, *James Gamble* created the analytic approach to fluid and electrolyte management of infants and children, and *Richard Day* studied thermal regulation in infants and defined clinical practices to minimize thermal stress. *Fritz Talbott* at the Massachusetts General Hospital performed definitive investigations of basal metabolism in infants and children. At the Boston Lying-In Hospital, *Clement Smith*, the father of American neonatology, conducted extensive clinical studies that, combined with the work and writings of others, enabled him to produce his textbook on physiology of the newborn, the first edition in 1945 and the fourth and final edition in 1976 [43].

In 1959 at Harvard, *Mary Ellen Avery*, a pediatric research fellow, and *Jere Mead*, a pulmonary physiologist, reported their discovery of a deficiency of alveolar surfactant in the lungs of newborns dying from respiratory distress syndrome (RDS) [44]. This etiologic assumption proved correct, allowed for rational and effective supportive respiratory care, and led to effective therapy with insufflated surfactant some 20 years later. Concurrently, *L. Stanley James* of New Zealand was recruited to Columbia University by *Virginia Apgar*, creator of the Apgar score and first Chair of Anesthesiology at that university, to establish a neonatal research center with both basic science and clinical research. James and others, including South African cardiologist *Abraham Rudolph*, then also in New York City, through investigations in newborn monkeys and human neonates confirmed the prior work of Dawes in lambs. They established the physiologic basis underlying current clinical principles

for supporting the normal and treating the abnormal adaptation of the newborn to extrauterine life. These talented scientists and clinicians thus laid the scientific and clinical foundation for modern neonatology and neonatal intensive care that would follow in the 1960s and beyond.

From 1960 onward, pediatricians specializing in newborn care, as well as pediatric surgeons and anesthesiologists in major North American pediatric centers, advocated for and created special newborn units in which they could cohort infants with a variety of life-threatening conditions, including severe birth asphyxia, prematurity, congenital anomalies, pneumonia, and erythroblastosis. In these units the focus shifted from merely supportive care, such as warmth, fluids, and nutrition, to more invasive measures directed at treating respiratory and other vital system failure. Some of these early neonatal intensive care units were established in Boston at the Lying-In Hospital by Clement Smith; New York City at Columbia University by *William Silverman*; Philadelphia by *Thomas Boggs* at Pennsylvania Hospital and by surgeon *C. Everett Koop* at Children's Hospital; Toronto at the Hospital for Sick Children by *Paul Swyer*; Baltimore by *Alexander Schaffer* and Mary Ellen Avery at Johns Hopkins Hospital; Nashville at Vanderbilt University by *Mildred Stahlman*; Cleveland by *Marshall Klaus* at Case-Western Reserve University; Denver at Children's Hospital by *Joseph Butterfield*; and San Francisco at the University of California by *John Clements* and *William Tooley*.

However, the challenge of treating respiratory failure in the neonate initially met with little success despite occasional case reports of infants surviving with mechanical ventilation. The first breakthrough occurred with a report in 1959 from Capetown, South Africa, where pediatrician *Peter Smythe*, and anesthesiologist *Arthur Bull* cared for infants with neonatal tetanus. Because of a native Bantu practice of covering the newborn's umbilical stump with cow dung, the condition was fairly common, and the affected infant's tetanic muscle seizures caused respiratory failure. Using a tracheostomy, intramuscular injections of curare, and an adapted Radcliffe adult ventilator, Smythe and Bull and their team ventilated 10 infants (ages 4 to 14 days) for up to 10 days with three long-term intact survivors [45]. This experience proved, for the first time, that neonates could survive mechanical ventilation for more than a week. Subsequently this team achieved better survivals, and in the 1960s neonatologists in South Africa, such as *H. deV. Heese* and *A.F. Malan*, realized remarkable gains in the management of critically ill newborns. An interesting historical note is that *I. David Todres*, pediatric anesthesiologist, neonatologist, and intensivist at the Massachusetts General Hospital for the past 30 years (and one of the contributors to this textbook), was a medical student at Capetown at this time and participated with Smythe and Bull in the care of their infants, thus stimulating his interest in intensive care of the newborn (I. David Todres, personal communication).

The next significant achievement in the treatment of neonatal respiratory failure occurred in 1963–1964 at Toronto's Hospital for Sick Children under the leadership of Paul Swyer and two fellows, *Maria Delivoria-Papadopoulos* and *Henry Levison* [46] (Figure 1.9). This group treated 20 preterm infants suffering extreme asphyxia caused by RDS (apnea, bradycardia, or cardiac arrest, pH less than 7.0, $PaCO_2$ over 80 mm Hg, and PaO_2 less than 40 mm Hg in 100% oxygen) with positive pressure mechanical ventilation and other supportive care. Seven infants survived intact, thus vindicating earlier anecdotal reports of the efficacy of this approach for neonates with respiratory failure. The group then undertook mecha-

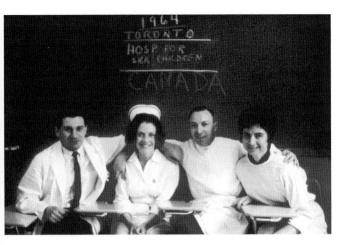

FIGURE 1.9. The leaders of the team from Toronto's Hospital for Sick Children that in 1964 first proved the efficacy of mechanical ventilation in a series of patients by saving 7 of 20 severely asphyxiated preterm infants with respiratory failure caused by respiratory distress syndrome. Director of Neonatology Paul Swyer, MD, is second from the right, flanked by Maria Delivoria-Papadopoulos, MD (far right), Head Nurse Lynn Schoemaker, and Henry Levison, MD (far left). (Courtesy of Dr. Maria Delivoria-Papadopoulos.)

nical ventilation earlier in the course of respiratory failure with remarkably improved outcomes. In their papers and lectures they emphasized the need for a full-time team of physicians, nurses, and therapists working in a fully equipped intensive care unit.

The Toronto experience gave justification to other neonatologists as well as pediatric anesthesiologists and surgeons who were aggressively treating neonatal respiratory failure and encouraged others to begin such a program. Shortly thereafter, positive end-expiratory pressure (PEEP) during mechanical ventilation, proven effective in raising blood oxygen levels and treating atelectasis in adults, became integral to the respiratory care of neonates. Throughout the remainder of the decade all of the neonatal centers mentioned earlier developed similar respiratory support capabilities, as did Stanford University with *Phillip Sunshine* and *Penelope Cave*, Children's Hospital of Pittsburgh with *Timothy Oliver*, Montreal with *Leo Stern*, Winnipeg Children's Hospital with *Victor Chernick*, and numerous others.

Although intermittent or continuous raised expiratory airway pressure had been used for treating pulmonary edema and atelectasis in adults, these methods had not been tried in infants with similar conditions. In 1968, *George Gregory*, a pediatric anesthesiologist and neonatologist at the University of California in San Francisco, applied the technique of continuous positive airway pressure (CPAP) with tracheal intubation to preterm newborns with RDS with considerable success [47]. Many infants experienced improved blood oxygen levels at lower inspired oxygen concentrations as well as improved spontaneous ventilation, obviating the need for mechanical ventilation. Subsequent studies in the 1970s by Gregory and others showed that similar benefits occurred in infants with less severe respiratory insufficiency treated with CPAP by facial mask or nasal cannulas.

In the latter 1960s Paul Swyer, Leo Stern, and others advocated strongly for regional organization of perinatal care centers providing specialized obstetric services and neonatal intensive care units throughout Canada, with transport of the woman with a high-risk pregnancy to such centers for delivery. This approach indeed

lowered neonatal mortality, as demonstrated in a classic epidemiologic study in Quebec Province and in Nova Scotia during 1967 and 1968. Similar regional organization for perinatal care slowly evolved in the United States over the next three decades.

As consistent a phenomenon as any in medicine, progress in treating a disorder invariably leads to unforeseen complications and new disorders. So it was with these early advances in treating life-threatening conditions in the neonate such as RDS and birth asphyxia. Paramount among the complications associated with survival were neonatal brain injury and chronic lung disease. The former condition resulted in the need for and creation of multidisciplinary interventional programs to minimize long-term adverse effects and facilitate childhood development. Chronic lung disease began as diffuse infiltrates on chest radiographs of infants with RDS who usually required mechanical ventilation and inspired oxygen concentrations over 40% beyond 7 to 10 days. This was noted by our neonatology group at Pennsylvania Hospital and The Children's Hospital of Philadelphia (CHOP) in several infants surviving RDS with short-term or no mechanical ventilation who required supplemental oxygen beyond 3 weeks of age. In May 1967 we encountered our first case of prolonged mechanical ventilation in a newborn with severe RDS and multiple pneumothoraces who developed diffuse infiltrates suggestive of fibrosis on chest radiograph. He required mechanical ventilation for 6 weeks and a tracheostomy for subglottic granulomas and narrowing. By age 3 months he did well without supplemental inspired oxygen and was discharged to home care by a devoted family. At age 18 months his chest radiograph had almost cleared, and he was decannulated after surgical removal of subglottic granulomas. He grew and developed normally, graduating from college in 1988. This one case convinced our group to not withdraw mechanical ventilation from an infant because of any preconceived time limit, but to plan support based on the infant's overall prognosis for survival, other medical issues, and the parents' viewpoint. In that same year of 1967, neonatologists at Stanford University observed this chronic lung disorder in a number of infants with RDS, which their radiologist *W.H. Northway* and pathologist *R.C. Rosan* termed *bronchopulmonary dysplasia*, or BPD [48]. Also in 1967, at University College Hospital in London, *Hawker, Reynolds,* and *Taghidzadih* independently described the same clinical, radiographic, and pathologic findings of BPD, a disorder that would become familiar to all who treat respiratory failure in neonates.

Pediatric General and Cardiac Surgery

The development of an organized body of knowledge and skills addressing surgical care of infants and children in North America began with *William E. Ladd (1880–1967)* of Boston. Educated and trained in surgery at Harvard University, Ladd joined the staff of the Children's Hospital of Boston in 1910, and after World War I he devoted his career exclusively to children's surgery, becoming the first full-time surgeon at a children's hospital. Ladd devised effective operative procedures for a wide variety of noncardiac congenital anomalies in the neonate including inguinal and diaphragmatic hernias, intestinal atresias and malrotation, and esophageal atresia, as well as conditions such as intussusception and Wilm's tumor. He trained the founding generation of pediatric surgeons in North America and elsewhere in the world, including *Robert Gross*, his successor as chair in 1945, and the father of pediatric cardiovascular surgery. Ladd and Gross authored the first comprehensive American textbook of pediatric surgery and wrote numerous papers that formed the foundation of pediatric surgical literature. The next generation of pediatric surgeons in this country can trace their heritage back to Robert Gross and those he trained. In 1946, one of his first and most prominent fellows, *C. Everett Koop*, came to Boston from the University of Pennsylvania for 6 months. Koop returned to Philadelphia to become the first specially trained and full-time Surgeon-in-Chief at CHOP.

Over the following decade, advances in newborn care coupled with progress in pediatric surgery and anesthesia led to significant reductions in the mortality associated with life-threatening anomalies and disorders. However, by 1956, Koop found that open infant ward nursing and house staff care no longer met the needs of infants surviving anesthesia and operations despite complex and often multiple lesions. With funding from the Pennsylvania Department of Health, he and the nursing staff created the nation's first neonatal intensive care unit for postoperative care, a unit with only three isolettes, a dedicated nursing team, and minimal monitoring equipment. The new Director of Anesthesiology, *Leonard Bachman*, and his staff provided respiratory care that by 1960 included tracheal intubation and mechanical ventilation. This unit expanded in 1962, again with state support, into a modern 12-bed infant intensive care unit with bedside electronic monitoring. To my knowledge, this facility represented the first intensive care unit for neonatal surgical patients in the United States. Similar facilities soon emerged in other pediatric surgical centers. Mortality rates for congenital lesions such as esophageal atresia with tracheoesophageal fistula continued to decline, due in great measure to their improved postoperative care in these units.

The era of pediatric cardiovascular surgery began when Robert Gross at the Children's Hospital of Boston ligated the patent ductus of a 7-year-old girl named Lorraine, who was in profound cardiac failure on August 26, 1938 [49]. The girl recovered and thrived, fortunately for all concerned, especially Gross, who had performed the operation against the orders of his chief, Dr. Ladd, who was away. As Dr. Gross said decades later to 50-year-old Lorraine, "It is a good thing you lived, or I would have been a farmer!" The first successful repair of coarctation of the aorta was independently described by *C. Crafoord* in Sweden and Gross in 1945. Also in that year, *Alfred Blalock* (surgeon), *Helen Taussig* (cardiologist), and *Vivien Thomas* (an extraordinary African-American laboratory assistant) created the subclavian-to-pulmonary artery shunt for tetralogy of Fallot at Johns Hopkins Hospital. The successful operations led to the need for specialized postoperative nursing and medical care for these patients. Initially the locus of this care was often in the postanesthetic recovery room with readily available anesthesiologists and a nursing staff familiar with airway and cardiopulmonary management. Once the children's condition stabilized, they would be transferred to a surgical ward where the cardiac patients were grouped together for specialized nursing care. This was the model used at CHOP (L. Bachman, personal communication) and at the Hospital for Sick Children in Toronto (A. Conn, personal communication) throughout the 1950s up to the late 1960s.

John Gibbon at Jefferson Medical College Hospital of Philadelphia in 1953 performed the first successful open cardiac operation using cardiopulmonary bypass to close an atrial septal defect in an adolescent girl who recovered and thrived. Shortly thereafter, *John Kirklin* and his colleagues at the Mayo Clinic in Rochester, Minnesota, using cardiopulmonary bypass with the Mayo-Gibbon machine, achieved astounding success for that time in repairing a variety of congenital cardiac lesions, including ventricular septal defects and tetralogy of Fallot. The era of definitive correction of these lesions had begun. A recent succinct chapter by Carol Lake reviews these and related events [50].

Throughout the 1960s, pediatric general, cardiac, and neurologic surgeons expanded the scope of operations in older infants and children as well as neonates. They became more skilled at treating trauma victims, resulting in increasing survival of children with complex problems demanding more sophisticated surveillance and management. This provided a powerful impetus for development of multidisciplinary pediatric intensive care units in major pediatric centers.

Pediatric Anesthesiology

Anesthesiologists have played a vital role in the development of critical care medicine from its inception during the polio epidemics of the 1950s through the 1980s. As mentioned earlier, the first adult intensive care units usually were established and at least partly staffed by anesthesiologists because of their knowledge and skills in airway and ventilatory management, circulatory monitoring and support, and vascular access abilities. This represented a logical and natural extension of their expertise from the operating room and recovery room. Thus, pediatric anesthesiologists led the initial development of pediatric critical care.

Pediatric anesthesiology evolved slowly as a clinical subspecialty in the early 20th century [51], beginning in 1919 with *Charles Robson* at Toronto's Hospital for Sick Children. He founded the first full-time department of pediatric anesthesia in North America. Some 27 years elapsed before *Robert Smith* established the next influential department at Children's Hospital of Boston in 1946. He joined Robert Gross who had just succeeded Ladd as the Chief of Surgery and the first Ladd Professor of Pediatric Surgery at Harvard Medical School. During the 1950s similar departments became established at the children's hospitals of Philadelphia, Pittsburgh, Montreal, Detroit, and Los Angeles, as well as in Western Europe, especially in England and Sweden. There followed vigorous expansion of the subspecialty in the 1960s, with recognition as a special clinical field by the American Academy of Pediatrics.

As noted, pediatric anesthesiologists assumed leadership of pediatric respiratory care services and intensive care units in North America and Europe between 1955 and 1972 [52]. Their knowledge and skills in acute emergency care in the operating room, their full-time presence in the hospital, and the confidence of their pediatric and surgical colleagues in their ability to provide surveillance and life support to children with organ failure gave the impetus to their role as leaders in establishing many of the original PICUs.

The Original Pediatric Intensive Care Units—1955 to 1971

Goran Haglund, a Swedish pediatric anesthesiologist, established the first multidisciplinary pediatric intensive unit on record in 1955 at the Children's Hospital of Goteborg, the major pediatric medical and surgical center for western Sweden (Barbro Ekstrom-Jodal, personal communication). Since 1951, Haglund and his colleagues had used the knowledge and skills acquired in managing polio patients to provide intensive care services, including mechanical ventilation, to newborns with RDS, postoperative children with sepsis, and cases of severe pneumonia. On September 7, 1955, they opened the *Pediatric Emergency Ward*, their term for an intensive care unit for inpatients. This original PICU consisted of seven acute care beds divided among four rooms as well as a small operating room equipped with anesthesia apparatus for minor operations and endoscopic procedures. The medical staff consisted of Dr. Haglund, the unit's director and also Chief of Anesthesiology, two of his staff anesthesiologists who rotated on the service, plus a staff surgeon, a staff pediatrician, and a full panel of consultants. Six full-time nurses and 15 nurse assistants provided 24-hour intensive nursing coverage. In the first 5 years the unit's staff provided 10,688 patient days of care to 1,183 infants and children, of whom 161 (13.6%) died. Haglund reported on his initial concepts and experience at the 1956 meeting of the Scandinavian Society of Anesthesiologists, and a lengthy abstract was published in the society's journal in 1957. Unfortunately, he did not publish a further report of his innovative accomplishment until 1976 in a chapter of proceedings of a neonatology conference [53]. His chapter makes fascinating reading as he recalls the development of intensive care of infants and children in his hospital from 1951 to 1971; he discusses dealing with appropriate staffing for the volume of patients, maintaining morale of the medical and nursing staff, managing the dying child, and other problems quite familiar to critical care physicians and nurses today.

There appears to be no record of another PICU until 1961 when *Hans Feychting*, also a pediatric anesthesiologist, established a unit at St. Goran's Children's Hospital in Stockholm (B. Ekstrom-Jodal, personal communication). In 1963, neonatologists *J.B. Joly* and *G. Huault* founded the Centre du Reanimation at Hôpital St. Vincent de Paul, the oldest existing children's hospital in Paris. Here they provided care for critically ill children of all ages, especially those in respiratory failure [54]. About this same time, Australian pediatric anesthesiologists *Ian H. McDonald* and *John Stocks* developed the PICU at the Royal Melbourne Children's Hospital, also focusing

on acute respiratory failure and the new technique of prolonged nasotracheal intubation in its management [55]. These were followed by the intensive therapy unit at the Alder Hey Children's Hospital in Liverpool that opened on September 1, 1964 under the leadership of *G. Jackson Rees*, the chief of anesthesia and a world-renowned pediatric anesthesiologist. The newly constructed unit accommodated 13 nonsurgical patients, including neonates, most of whom had acute respiratory failure or severe airway obstruction. The unit included a minor operating room with anesthesia equipment, a small chemistry laboratory, offices, and storage space. Rees has described the unit and the management of respiratory failure at that time in considerable detail [56]. Similar units undoubtedly developed elsewhere in Europe, which was well ahead of North America in critical care at the time, but they do not appear to be documented in the English language literature.

On this side of the Atlantic, the recovery room (Figure 1.10) remained the most common site for intensive care of children. Occasionally, special rooms on a medical or surgical ward would be designated for intensive nursing care. Such arrangements, however, usually lacked a full-time medical and nursing staff and the organizational structure of a PICU. To my knowledge, the first physician-directed multidisciplinary PICU in North America was established at CHOP in January 1967 as an outgrowth of a hospital-wide respiratory intensive care service [57]. The unit consisted of an open ward of six beds equipped with bedside electronic monitoring (electrocardiography, impedance pneumographic respiratory rate, and two direct blood pressure channels) and respiratory support capabilities. An adjacent procedure room could serve as an isolated seventh bed. An intensive care chemistry laboratory, manned 24 hours per day by a technician, was located next to the

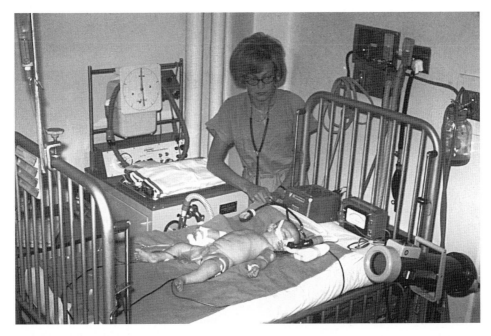

FIGURE 1.10. Five-month-old infant in 1965 with acute respiratory failure caused by severe bronchiolitis receiving mechanical ventilation with neuromuscular blockade (curare) and a nasotracheal tube in the recovery room (postanesthetic care unit) of the Children's Hospital of Philadelphia. The ventilator is a pediatric modified Emerson PV-1. Monitoring consists of an Electronics for Medicine ECG oscilloscope (lower right), a Yellow Springs thermistor rectal thermometer, a Beckman polarographic oxygen analyzer to measure inspired oxygen concentration, and a Tycos infant blood pressure cuff and aneroid manometer. Not seen is the warming blanket unit under the patient. Sterile suction catheters are kept in trays on the top of the ventilator. The nurse is checking the infant's arterial pressure. This infant recovered intact after 3 days' mechanical ventilation and supportive therapy. The care by dedicated and skilled nurses, then as now, provided the key to a successful outcome for this baby, and numerous others, before pediatric intensive care units were established. (Photograph by the author.)

unit with a pass-through window for handing blood samples and receiving written reports. The nursing staff were full time in the unit, and most had previously served in the recovery room or the infant intensive care unit or cared for patients on the cardiac surgery or respiratory intensive care services. I was the medical director and worked closely with two other anesthesiology staff, Leonard Bachman (Chief of Anesthesiology) and *Charles Richards*, and an allergist/pulmonologist, *David Wood* to share duties and call. One of four pediatric anesthesiology/critical care fellows was in or immediately available to the PICU on a 24-hour per day basis. Rounds with the nurses, fellows, and the anesthesiology staff physician on service were conducted each morning and late afternoon. We were most fortunate to have close relationships with C. Everett Koop (Chief of Surgery and a strong supporter of critical care), *William Rashkind* (the father of interventional pediatric cardiology), *John Waldhausen* (one of the nation's few full-time pediatric cardiac surgeons and a creative thinker), and *Sylvan Stool* (a pioneer in pediatric otolaryngology), as well as the support of numerous pediatric and surgical consulting staff and house officers. We also hosted many visiting physicians from all over the world for periods of 1 day to several weeks (Figure 1.11). In the first 3 years we cared for over 600 critically ill infants and children annually, many requiring mechanical ventilation for acute respiratory failure caused by asthma, bronchiolitis, or pneumonia or following complex cardiovascular surgery. The ventilators used most were the adult or pediatric Emerson PV-1, a volume pre-set piston/cylinder machine powered by an electric motor, with simplicity of operation and repair, low cost, and exceptional durability. A simple water column attached to the expiratory valve provided PEEP when that modality came into common use around 1967. We employed these ventilators in their various upgraded models from 1964 until the early 1980s when the more sophisticated and versatile microprocessor machines, such as the Siemens 900 series, became available.

Having learned of the experience in Australia, we were among the first in North America to employ nasotracheal intubation for longer term airway management in the treatment of acute respiratory failure in newborns as well as older infants and children [58].

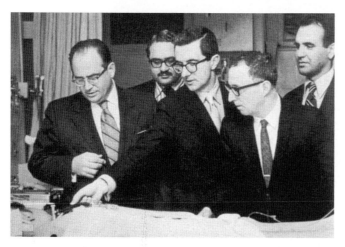

FIGURE 1.11. In the new six-bed PICU at the Children's Hospital of Philadelphia in 1967, Drs. John Downes (center), Director of the Unit, Leonard Bachman (second from right), Director of Anesthesiology, and Sylvan Stool (second from left), Director of Otolaryngology, discuss a patient with two visiting pediatric cardiologists from the Soviet Union. (Photograph by the author.)

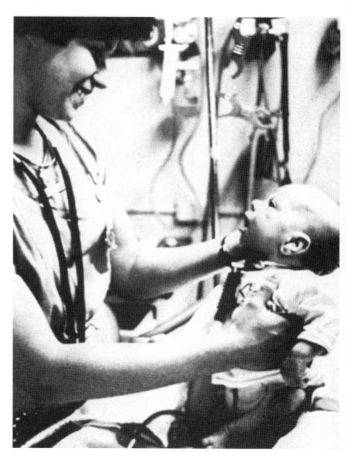

FIGURE 1.12. An infant with chronic respiratory failure from bronchopulmonary dysplasia requiring a tracheostomy and long-term mechanical ventilation in the PICU at the Children's Hospital of Philadelphia in 1967. Note the baby's response to the nurse who is playing with her patient and providing normal mother–infant interactions. (Photograph by the author.)

Dr. Theodore Striker, our first critical care fellow, and the pediatric surgical fellows worked closely with Sylvan Stool in developing new techniques for tracheostomy care with plastic tubes rather than the traditional silver metal tubes [59], ultimately creating guidelines for the use of endotracheal tubes versus tracheostomy [60]. Although 52% of our patients with acute respiratory failure recovered within 2 to 30 days, a small number neither died nor were able to be liberated from mechanical ventilation. These infants with chronic respiratory failure (ventilated over 30 days) because of bronchopulmonary dysplasia or congenital anomalies required assisted ventilation for up to a year but usually recovered (Figure 1.12). Our group also helped to train some of the early leaders in pediatric critical care, including *Russell Raphaely* and *Stephan Kampschulte* (see later). Dr. Raphaely joined our staff after fellowship in 1968 and became director of the PICU from 1972 to 1996, as well as President of the Society of Critical Care Medicine from 1992 to 1994.

By the early 1970s, nursing care as well as monitoring and life support equipment had become quite sophisticated for that time in the few PICUs that were operating (Figure 1.13). The major emphasis remained on respiratory and circulatory support and surveillance, along with temperature control, fluid and acid–base balance, and sedation and analgesia. Respiratory therapists became better trained and proved to be exceptionally helpful over the succeeding

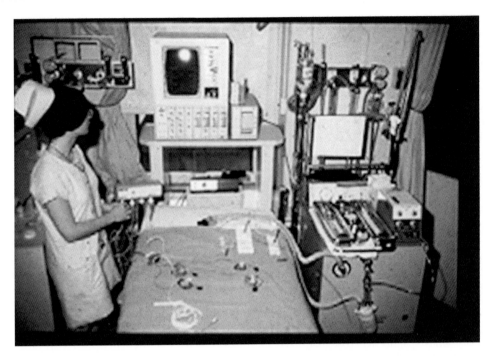

FIGURE 1.13. In 1971, a bed with technological support awaiting the arrival of a postoperative cardiac surgical patient in the PICU of the Children's Hospital of Philadelphia. Equipment consists of an Emerson PV-1 ventilator, a Statham monitoring console with ECG and four vascular pressure channels with miniature strain gauges (on bed) and infusion pump (below monitoring console). Not shown are an overhead warmer and the warming/cooling blanket unit. (Photograph by the author.)

decades. Clinical research in the 1960s and early 1970s at CHOP focused on the pathogenesis, diagnostic criteria, and management of acute respiratory failure from a variety of causes, including pneumonia and bronchiolitis, status asthmaticus, and postoperative cardiac surgery in infants with complex cardiopulmonary defects. Guidelines for the clinical diagnosis and treatment of respiratory failure evolved from these studies and those of others in North America and Europe.

In 1969, Stephan Kampschulte, an anesthesiologist from Munich who had trained in anesthesia and adult critical care with Peter Safar and Ake Grenvik at the University of Pittsburgh and in pediatric critical care at CHOP, became director of the second multidisciplinary PICU in North America at the Children's Hospital of Pittsburgh [61]. This 10-bed unit, fully equipped for its time, accepted pediatric patients of all ages, including neonates with RDS or post-repair of anomalies, as well as the whole range of critical disorders of older infants and children. Kampschulte also had a full range of subspecialists cooperating and a vigorous training program. One of his fellows was *Peter Holbrook* who became the first director of the PICU at the Children's Hospital National Medical Center in Washington, DC, and a President of the Society of Critical Care Medicine. Also in 1969, *James Gilman*, a pediatric anesthesiologist and *Norman Talner*, a pediatric cardiologist, established a six-bed multidisciplinary PICU at the Yale New Haven Medical Center.

Pediatric Critical Care Medicine—1970 to 1979

In 1971, at the Hospital for Sick Children in Toronto, *Alan Conn* resigned as director of the department of anesthesiology to become director of a new multidisciplinary 20-bed PICU, by far the largest and most sophisticated unit in North America (Alan Conn, personal communication). The establishment of this unit and a critical

care service culminated a decade of efforts by Conn and his associates to cohort critically ill older infants and children in one geographic area other than the postanesthesia recovery area. This advanced complex was the forerunner of units developed in major pediatric centers throughout North America over the following decade. Also in 1971, *David Todres*, the anesthesiologist and neonatologist mentioned previously and *Daniel Shannon*, a pediatric pulmonologist, founded a 16-bed multidisciplinary unit for pediatric patients of all ages at the Massachusetts General Hospital (D. Todres, personal communication). Both of these units also established vibrant training programs in critical care medicine and conducted clinical research. Among their numerous accomplishments, Conn became a noted authority on the management of near-drowning victims, and Todres pioneered long-term mechanical ventilation for children at home with chronic respiratory failure. These early PICUs and their training programs had an apparently favorable impact on mortality and morbidity rates—particularly those associated with acute respiratory failure. Units and programs similar to those described earlier were developed in most major pediatric centers in North America and Western Europe during the 1970s and early 1980s.

Certain programs were particularly notable for their large volume of patients, numbers of physicians trained in pediatric critical care, and research contributions. Included among these were those mentioned above as well as certain ones established between 1971 and 1980. These include the program at the Children's Hospital National Medical Center under *Peter Holbrook* and the program at the Children's Hospital of Dallas under *Daniel Levin*, The Johns Hopkins Hospital under *Mark Rogers* and *Steve Nugent*, and the Children's Hospital of Boston under *Robert Crone*. In addition, several PICUs with a medical director were established in smaller children's hospitals and in a few large community hospitals with a sizeable pediatric service.

In Europe, numerous PICUs were created during this period, but I am aware of several that appeared to have influenced pediatric critical care in their home country and beyond. *Francois Beaufil*, a pediatrician, inaugurated a PICU and program at Hôpital Breton-neau in Paris; *Jean Laugier*, a neonatologist, founded a PICU at the University Hospital in Tours; *Didiere Moulin*, a general pediatri-cian, became the first director of the new PICU at Louvain Univer-sity near Brussels; and *David Hatch,* a pediatric anesthesiologist, and his colleagues established the first multidisciplinary PICU at the Hospital for Sick Children in Great Ormond Street, London. As one would expect, during the 1970s and 1980s, a frequent and stimu-lating exchange of fellows and staff occurred among these pro-grams and the programs in Europe, Australia, and North America, resulting in rapid dissemination of progressive ideas in clinical care, education, and research.

Pediatric Critical Care—1980 to 1989

The decade of the 1980s brought many innovations in care and the development of critical care units in virtually every tertiary pediatric center. According to a 1979 Ross Planning Associates nationwide survey, 152 PICUs of four beds or more were identified among respondents, and another 42 units were thought to exist, for a total of 194 PICUs [62]. Only 40% had a pediatric intensivist avail-able at all times, the physician attending staff averaged 1.6, only 31% had critical care fellows in training although 91% had rotating pediatric residents in the unit, and over 40% consisted of fewer than seven beds. Only half of the units stated they had an affiliated transport system, and few had a *stepdown* unit for transitioning patients to the hospital ward or home. Over the next 10 years the average bed capacity of units increased as did their fulltime critical care physician staffs, the presence of critical care fellows, and access to a pediatric transport system and a stepdown unit. By 1990, some 235 PICUs existed across the nation [62].

Although the major PICUs of the 1970s had multidisciplinary staffs, the decade of the 1980s witnessed the widespread inclusion of full-time critical care and consulting physicians and allied health professional staff immediately available for care in the PICU. The consultants included a full range of pediatric medical and surgical subspecialists. The allied health professionals consisted of respiratory therapists, developmental and child life therapists, social workers, and chaplains. Availability of separate rooms for parents to rest, consultation rooms for families, and adequate space for nursing and physician staff to work and confer became the norm for new or renovated PICUs. In the early 1980s new or expanded units opened at the Children's Hospitals of Cincinnati, Seattle, St. Louis, Milwaukee, Atlanta (Eggleston Children's), Denver, Salt Lake, Montreal, and London, Ontario. Also units and programs opened in Houston (Texas Children's), at the University of California at San Francisco (Moffitt Hospital), Stanford Univer-sity, and in many other locations across North America.

The decade of the 1980s also will be remembered as the time when pediatric critical care medicine became a defined, recognized subspecialty. The growing need for critical care services for chil-dren in tertiary centers, the increasing number of pediatricians and pediatrician-anesthesiologists devoted to critical care, and the expanding body of knowledge about life-threatening conditions in children called for formal recognition of an emerging specialty. This also required its integration into organized medicine, stan-dards for training, and methods for reimbursement and funding. An important step toward those ends occurred in 1981 with the founding of the Section on Pediatric Critical Care of the Society of Critical Care Medicine (SCCM) by Peter Holbrook, Russell Rapha-ely, and others, this being the first section within the society. In 1983, a joint proposal of the Committee on Hospital Care of the American Academy of Pediatrics and the Pediatric Section of SCCM provided published guidelines for organizing, staffing, and equip-ping a pediatric intensive care unit, thereby establishing an author-itative consensus on the requirements a hospital should meet in order to declare that it had a PICU and critical care services [63]. The following year, 1984, the American Academy of Pediatrics formed a Section on Critical Care Medicine.

During the same period, the American Council on Graduate Medical Education (the body approving all residency and fellow-ship programs in the United States), the American Boards of Anes-thesiology, Medicine, Pediatrics, and Surgery, and leadership of SCCM representing the four specialties (anesthesiologist Peter Safar, internist William Grace, surgeon William Shoemaker, and pediatrician Peter Holbrook) conducted long and intense negotia-tions. They set out to resolve whether critical care medicine should be an independent specialty with adult and pediatric divisions or a subspecialty of the each of the four major boards. In 1986, the latter view prevailed, and, in 1987, the American Board of Pediat-rics created a sub-board in Critical Care Medicine, which required a 3-year fellowship with 1 year of research training, and offered a certifying exam. Pediatric intensivists seeking certification who trained in anesthesiology or surgery without a formal pediatric residency and who could demonstrate extensive pediatric critical care experience took the sub-board examination in critical care of their primary board. Also during this decade, three pediatric intensivists became the President of SCCM: *George Gregory* (1982), *Dharampuri Vidyasagar* (1984), and *Peter Holbrook* (1988). In 1987, Mark Rogers, then Chair of Anesthesiology and Critical Care Medi-cine, and his colleagues at the Johns Hopkins Hospital published the first major textbook in pediatric critical care, an important achievement in defining the new subspecialty's body of knowledge [64]. Daniel Levin and *Frances Morriss* at the Children's Hospital of Dallas edited the next comprehensive text in 1990 [65], soon fol-lowed by several others [66–68].

Throughout the decade advances in pediatric medicine and especially in pediatric general surgery and the surgical subspecial-ties influenced the content and styles of pediatric critical care prac-tice, education, and research. For example, pediatric emergency medicine emerged in the early 1980s as a distinct discipline [69], quickly becoming an essential component of an effective system of care for the critically ill and injured child. By the end of the decade it developed a Section in the American Academy of Pediatrics, had an American Council on Graduate Medical Education–approved 3-year subspecialty fellowship, and soon thereafter sub-board certification under the American Board of Pediatrics. Emergency medicine staff and fellows usually rotated through the PICU as part of their training, thereby establishing a close working relationship between the two disciplines.

The focus on cardiopulmonary resuscitation (CPR) of children and adults, stimulated by the research and advocacy of Peter Safar at the University of Pittsburgh since the 1960s, expanded to include cerebral resuscitation leading to techniques that could enhance brain recovery [70]. Adult and *pediatric trauma* received attention long delayed, with collaboration among emergency medicine and transport, critical care, and trauma surgeons to create statewide systems for care of victims and designated regional pediatric trauma centers in children's hospitals [71,72].

Pediatric cardiac critical care emerged as a distinct discipline during the early and middle 1980s in response to the exceptional clinical requirements of newborns and infants under 3 months of age with complex congenital cardiovascular lesions. These infants usually had lesions diagnosed in utero by the newly developed modality of fetal echocardiography. They would be stabilized for hours to weeks and then undergo palliation or correction with cardiopulmonary bypass and deep hypothermic cardiac arrest for periods up to 1 hour [73]. Over 90% of the infants survived the procedures with variable neurologic and cardiopulmonary outcomes [74], which improved considerably throughout the next two decades. Separate cardiac PICUs with full-time physician and nursing teams were created at the Children's Hospitals of Boston, Philadelphia, Los Angeles, and at the University of Michigan (C.S. Mott Children's Hospital) to care for cardiac medical and surgical patients and to train pediatric intensivists and cardiologists in the intricacies of their care. Such units existed in nearly every major pediatric cardiac center by the mid-1990s (Figure 1.14). This evolution of modern pediatric cardiology, cardiac surgery, and anesthesia has recently been succinctly described [75].

Although not initially required by the American Council on Graduate Medical Education, pediatric second- and third-year residents in most programs rotated through the PICU for several weeks to 3 months of training in the fundamentals of pediatric critical care medicine. Such rotations had begun in the 1960s and 1970s in those hospitals with PICUs and became the norm in the 1980s. These rotations enhanced the knowledge and technical skills of future general pediatricians in the stabilization and early care of the critically ill child and provided a fertile ground for recruitment of young talented physicians into the new subspecialty.

Among the many technological advances of this decade, the widespread introduction and use of pulse oximetry probably ranks as the most important for patient safety [76,77]. Microprocessor

controlled ventilators represented another significant improvement in the support of children [78], with versatility for virtually all modes of assisted and/or controlled ventilation for a wide range of ages and body sizes. These ventilators and the use of lower inspiratory pressures with permissive mild hypercapnia appeared to reduce the incidence and severity of lung injury associated mechanical ventilation in infants. The introduction of the pressure support mode of assisted ventilation in the mid-1980s and the considerably improved synchronization of an infant or child's spontaneous inspiratory effort with initiation of the ventilator's tidal breath both improved the patient's comfort while being ventilated and facilitated liberation from assisted ventilation [79]. Extracorporeal membrane oxygenation (ECMO), introduced in the 1970s in adults, using greatly improved gas exchange membranes and safer mechanisms proved life-saving for newborn infants with persistent pulmonary hypertension and severe hypoxemia. This laid the foundation for successful use in the 1990s of this complex modality in the treatment of infants with congenital diaphragmatic hernia before and after operation and in life support of infants and children with intractable respiratory failure caused by acute respiratory distress syndrome (ARDS) [80].

Beginning in the early 1980s, the assessment and management of both acute and chronic pain in infants and children, for the first time in modern medical history, began to receive dedicated attention by groups of pediatric anesthesiologists, neurologists, and others [81]. Over the next two decades considerable progress has been made in quantifying pain, defining mechanisms, utilizing specific drugs other than opiates, and educating physicians, nurses, and parents in pain control. Most children's hospitals now have pain teams with a small, dedicated staff of physicians and nurse practitioners who provide full-time consultant coverage to inpatients and frequently offer outpatient pain clinics. The knowledge and skills of these teams has greatly reduced the suffering of

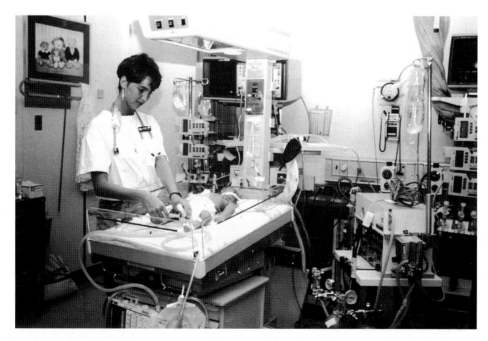

FIGURE 1.14. In 1992, an infant after cardiac surgery in the 20-bed cardiac ICU of the Children's Hospital of Philadelphia. Equipment in addition to the infant warmer-bed consists of a Siemens ventilator, Hewlett-Packard multichannel monitoring console and pressure transducers (to the rear of the bed), multiple infusion pumps on an IV pole, thoracic drainage pumps (not seen), and multiple gas mixtures of CO_2 and O_2 (in front of ventilator) for regulation of pulmonary vascular pressures and flows. Again, the bedside nurse remains essential to the infant's recovery. (Photograph by the author.)

critically ill neonates, older infants, and children. Solid organ transplantation made a quantum advance in the early 1980s with the introduction of cyclosporine for immunosuppression [82]. The numbers of children undergoing liver, heart, and kidney transplantation with long-term survival increased dramatically over the decade as a result, although the problems of rejection and opportunistic infection continued to require lengthy stays in the PICU for many patients.

The numbers of children with severe, disabling conditions requiring long-term technological support increased steadily throughout the decade [82a]. In 1983, Surgeon General C. Everett Koop convened a workshop on this issue in Philadelphia that concluded with strong recommendations for allocation of greater resources to these patients and assessment of outcomes as well as support of families, especially those caring for these children at home [83]. Subsequently the federal Bureau of Maternal and Child Health provided grant funding for five state programs across the nation to address some of the issues, especially for children with chronic respiratory failure. In 1987, the U.S. Congress Office of Technology Assessment defined the *technology-dependent child* as *one who needs both a medical device to compensate for the loss of a vital body function and substantial and ongoing nursing care to avert death or further disability* (Publication No.OTA-TM-H-38, May, 1987). All these programs quickly reached their maximum enrollment. The previously existing program for home care of ventilator-assisted children in Pennsylvania (based at CHOP) began the decade with 5 children enrolled, and had 65 enrollees statewide by 1989. Outcomes varied in this heterogenous population of chronically ill children, with liberation from mechanical ventilation being achieved eventually in nearly all children with BPD or other forms of chronic lung disease in infants, whereas those with nervous system or muscular disorders usually survived only with continuing ventilatory support. Overall long-term survival rates varied from 65% to 75% in series of 50 to 100 patients [84]. Deaths of these children at home in approximately 20% to 25% of instances were caused by preventable technical accidents, including airway occlusion and ventilator disconnection.

Organized study of the short-term outcomes of patients admitted to PICUs began in the early 1980s with *Timothy Yeh* and *Murray Pollack's* adaptation of a severity of illness scoring system used for critically ill adults, the therapeutic intervention scoring system (TISS). This focused on the major life support and other therapies being employed as markers of severity of the patient's condition. Although useful for billing purposes, TISS seemed less valuable as a true indicator of the patient's condition. Murray Pollack and his colleagues at The Children's Hospital National Medical Center then developed a system to estimate the degree of physiologic instability and impairment, the physiologic stability index (PSI) [85]. They subsequently proved the validity of the PSI as a predictor of morbidity and survival, demonstrating the close conformity of the predicted and observed mortality rates over nine diverse institutions with acute PICUs. This group then developed the more advanced pediatric risk of mortality score (PRISM) [86]. Despite the usefulness of the PSI and PRISM, widely varying admission practices and patient conditions, the number of long-stay patients (over 12 days), and the availability of stepdown or long-term care units make assessment of the quality of care in a specific acute PICU in comparison to other PICUs exceptionally complex. Adrienne Randolph of the Hospital for Sick Children, Toronto, and the Evidence Based Medicine in Critical Care Group recently described the difficulties in achieving valid comparisons of outcome performances of pedi-

atric and adult intensive care units and proposed guidelines for remedying the problem [87].

Pediatric Critical Care—1990 to 1999

During the decade of the 1990s pediatric critical care medicine grew and matured into a recognized subspecialty that faced new challenges and opportunities. As the decade began, 313 hospitals had PICUs with an average of 8 beds per unit [88]. The major children's hospitals had much larger PICUs, ranging from 12 to 30 acute beds; the largest was the 30-bed acute unit, with 20 general and 10 cardiac beds, and a 12-bed respiratory rehabilitation unit comprising the critical care complex at CHOP. In the early 1990's, the American Council on Graduate Medical Education approved 26 (of approximately 50) pediatric critical care training programs for a 3-year subspecialty fellowship consisting of 2 years of clinical training and 1 year of research. These initial programs trained many of today's leaders in pediatric critical care. Throughout the decade a gradual increase in the number of PICUs and training programs resulted from the increasing demand for specialized care of critically ill and injured infants and children.

The Pediatric Section of SCCM and the Committee on Hospital Care of the American Academy of Pediatrics in 1993 revised their guidelines on organization and levels of care for PICUs and updated this document in 2004 [89]. Pollack and his colleagues conducted several landmark studies demonstrating the effectiveness of pediatric intensive care provided in tertiary hospitals on improving survival and other outcomes that helped to inform these national guidelines [90,91].

The subspecialty of pediatric critical care nursing evolved during the 1970s and 1980s, in concert with that of their adult counterpart. Critical care nurses (adult and pediatric) were admitted to the SCCM from its inception. Pediatric critical care nurses founded their own society in the mid-1990s with a journal and became recognized as a vital subspecialty of pediatric nursing. Subsequently in the early 1990s advanced practice nurses and pediatric nurse practitioners began to specialize in pediatric critical care, assuming important collaborative roles with physicians and other nurses in clinical care and research. Respiratory therapy technologists (now with college degrees and certification) not only helped regulate mechanical ventilation but also performed bedside pulmonary function tests and assisted with respiratory monitoring. Yet as the nationwide shortage of registered nurses worsened during this decade, the availability of experienced pediatric critical care nurses became severely limited in some hospitals, an experience that had periodically occurred during the previous 25 years. As the demands for more complex and diverse pediatric critical care services grew, nurses in the PICUs of major centers worked longer hours covering more patients, often affecting their personal lives and limiting career development.

Pediatric critical care staff physicians frequently experienced similar stresses of staff shortfalls, increased clinical and teaching demands, and stringent research and publication requirements for faculty promotion. Some of these physicians and nurses experienced *burnout*, characterized by feelings of fatigue, being undervalued by medical colleagues and administrators, lack of professional success and satisfaction, inadequate personal time, and no end in sight. They either changed careers or considerably curtailed their critical care activities. In 1995, *Alan Fields* and colleagues published the results of a nationwide survey of 474 board-certified pediatric critical care physicians using a questionnaire and a validated burnout scale [92]. They reported a disturbing finding that 50% of those surveyed were at risk of or actually were experiencing burnout. This phenomenon was observed occasionally in the medical and nursing staff and trainees in PICUs in the 1970s and 1980s as the patient census often stretched resources to their limits or even exceeded them. With the nursing shortages and inordinate limitations on reimbursement experienced by many centers in the early and mid-1990s, recruitment into pediatric critical care medicine and nursing lagged behind demands, and burnout became a more pressing issue.

Resolution to a considerable extent followed when critical care physicians and nurses collaborated in advocating vigorously for limiting PICU admissions to levels compatible with appropriate care, increasing funding for PICU nurses' salaries and adequate staffing, and creating consensus guidelines for personnel requirements to achieve optimal care [93]. Another significant advance was the development of master's level programs for pediatric critical care nurse practitioners to complement the physician staff in the clinical care of patients and in clinical investigation. The first such program originated in the early 1990s at the School of Nursing of the University of Pennsylvania in collaboration with CHOP and was soon emulated by several other academic nursing centers. Burnout continues to be a risk for physicians and nurses in any critical care setting and in other clinical services with a significant incidence of severe patient impairment or death. Clinical leaders need to identify those with the condition and to provide effective remedies [94].

Regionalization of pediatric critical care evolved in a fragmented manner during the 1970s and 1980s, although the requirements for an optimally effective system for adults and children were laid out by Safar in the late 1960s. Models for such a system also were developed in the early 1970s for perinatal intensive care [95], as well as for trauma victims and patients with acute coronary insufficiency. It became evident in the 1980s, based on experience with regionalization of adult and pediatric emergency trauma care, that an effective system for children must include ground and air emergency transport with paramedics trained in pediatric acute care, emergency departments with pediatric emergency medicine physicians, and a well-staffed and equipped PICU in each demographic region. Yeh in 1992 reviewed existing guidelines and described a model for a pediatric critical care regional system developed by the SCCM and the American Academy of Pediatrics for northern California [96].

According to outcome studies in the 1980s and early 1990s, cardiopulmonary–cerebral resuscitation in infants and children outside of intensive care or operating room settings seems to have made little progress over prior decades in achieving greater survival and better neurologic outcomes [97]. Whether this is due to delayed diagnosis, improper CPR, or the actual inadequacy of *proper* CPR is nearly impossible to determine. The application of pediatric CPR guidelines developed in the 1980s, simulation training of physicians, nurses, and others in Pediatric Advanced Life Support (PALS) courses (initiated in 1988), the widespread use of *mock codes* in hospitals, appropriate limitation of the duration of CPR and the knowledge gained from basic science and laboratory animal research should result in better outcomes in the future.

Throughout the 1980s and 1990s, pediatric head trauma from vehicular causes declined significantly because of the acceptance and routine use of infant car seats, child restraints and seat belts, and bicycle and other sport helmets. Unfortunately, in large urban areas some of this progress has been offset by (1) an alarming increase since 1985 in child abuse and domestic violence resulting in the *shaken baby syndrome* and (2) an epidemic of handgun violence in which children were caught in the line of fire related to neighborhood drug trafficking and the socially deprived adolescent's inability to peacefully resolve conflict. These etiologies of critical injuries and death lie at the intersection of clinical medicine, public health, and social policy [98,99]. Since the 1960s, leaders in pediatrics and public health and other children's advocates have sought our national government's firm and long-term commitment to innovative and inevitably complex solutions; sadly, the government's response has been tepid at best, and thousands of preventable deaths of children and adolescents continue to occur [100]. Although the incidences of these forms of trauma and related mortality appear to have declined somewhat from the middle 1990s onward, they still represent a significant public health problem. For example, over 20,000 children and adolescents are killed or injured by guns annually in the United States [100]. A nationwide failure of an integrated social, educational, and economic policy, coupled with poor access of most Americans to effective mental health care and counseling, as well as our lack of will to remedy disgraceful federal and state gun control laws, portend continued excessive mortality in young Americans.

The prevalence of severe chronic diseases and disabling disorders among infants and children increased steadily over the previous two decades but in the 1990s became a focus of attention by child health professionals. This phenomenon resulted from many factors, including (1) continued decline in infant mortality rate with improved perinatal and neonatal care and increased survival of extremely premature newborns (less than 1,000 g birth weight), (2) advances in pediatric anesthesia and surgery, and (3) commitment by neonatologists, pediatric intensivists, pulmonologists, and neurologists to offer ventilatory support and extend the lives of infants and children with severe central nervous system and neuromuscular disorders. Advances in pediatric oncology also increased substantially the numbers of children surviving with cancer but also children with varying degrees of immunosuppression, those undergoing bone marrow transplantation and its sequelae, and the need for critical care to cope with opportunistic infections.

The prevalence of chronic respiratory failure increased in most PICUs, putting pressure on acute and intermediate stepdown care beds and creating greater demand for high technology home care [101]. The decade of the 1990s also saw an increased focus on the ethical and psychosocial issues confronting health professionals and families in the PICU. Since the development of modern neonatology and CPR in the early 1960s, physicians, nurses, and sick children and their families faced concerns regarding futility of care and withdrawal of support, persistent vegetative state, do-not-resuscitate orders, and end-of-life relief of pain and anxiety. Consensus agreements that served as guidelines applicable to both adults and children were developed in the 1980s and especially in the 1990s by various professional organizations [102–105]. Ruth Purtilo and David Todres have provided an excellent summary of ethical principles and their application in pediatric critical care [106]. Although recognition of the terrible stresses faced by parents and families of children in the PICU dates from the 1970s [107,108], a family-centered orientation to adult and pediatric critical care became the standard of care in the late 1980s and 1990s. Todres, Earle, and Jellinek have effectively summarized the principles for empowering parents and communicating with families of children in the PICU [108].

From the 1960s onward, the cost of critical care of neonates, infants, and children, as well as that of adults, has been questioned and debated, yet seldom accurately assessed, especially in terms of outcomes. Total health care costs rose steadily at annual rates of 9% to 12% from 1960 through 1991, exceeding the cost of living, inflation and growth of the gross domestic product [109]. Many critics pointed to excessive use of unproven technology, such as computed tomography scans in the early 1970s, and intensive care for aged or terminally patients, disregarding their complex and compelling needs, and the wishes of their families. In fact, the rising expenses appeared to derive more from significant improvement of survival at both ends of the age spectrum, causing a greater prevalence of chronic disorders, as well as inefficient regionalization of resources and a private health care insurance system with excessive administrative overhead [110,111]. The complicated financial and administrative implications for adult critical care medicine of so-called health care economic reforms imposed by federal law for Medicare and Medicaid throughout the 1980s have been ably summarized by Augenstein and Peterson [112] and by Rosen and Bone [113]. Fortunately, neonatal and pediatric critical care experienced somewhat less stringent and complex burdens until the imposition of the managed care policies of the 1990s. These policies resulted in instances of denial of appropriate services and potential deterioration in the quality of children's health care. In 1995 the American Academy of Pediatrics issued its statement on principles to be followed in the managed care of all pediatric and young adult patients and updated this document in 2000 and 2003 [114,115]. This gave pediatricians and pediatric hospital services a solid basis for appealing adverse judgments and policies by insurance organizations.

Accurate analysis of actual costs, as opposed to charges, of care in the PICU is difficult to obtain but was accomplished by Chalom and colleagues for the acute PICU at CHOP during the year 1994 [116]. They determined the median daily cost per patient, except for attending physician's fees, to be $2,600, with a median total cost of $7,900 for the PICU stay. However, these figures ranged widely with a standard deviation of $23,900 in total costs. The costs of home care of both adults and children with chronic respiratory failure and other severe disabilities are substantially less than those of inpatient care but still pose a formidable financial burden to insurers and to families confronted with out-of-pocket expenses [117].

Before 1970, physicians rendering critical care services seldom billed for these services other than for emergency care, resuscitation, or tracheal intubation for which their department might receive $50.00 or less. At the time, departments of anesthesiology usually underwrote the funding for the intensivists' services in children's hospitals or large academic centers. Beginning in the mid-1970s, with the inclusion of pediatric and neonatal services and procedures in the Current Procedural Terminology (CPT) terms and codes for billing, pediatric intensivists or their departments began to bill more consistently and to receive reimbursement for the complex services being provided by attending physicians. In the 1980s, Russell C. Raphaely, MD, and other leaders from SCCM, in the face of the new Resource-Based Relative Value Scale (RBRVS), advocated long and hard with the federal Health Care Finance Administration (which controlled Medicare and Medicaid) and commercial insurance corporations. They struggled with considerable success for improved reimbursement commensurate with the complexity of care provided by pediatric and adult intensive care physicians. These efforts for adequate reimbursement have continued up to the present time.

The Twenty-First Century: Pediatric Critical Care in the Current Era—2000 and Beyond

As the new century opens, pediatric critical care medicine has become a mature medical discipline, well recognized for its services and expertise by health care professionals and an increasing proportion of the public. A recent nationwide survey indicated the existence of 337 PICUs with medical directors [118]. In the United States by 2003, the American Board of Pediatrics had certified 1,134 physicians in pediatric critical care medicine, and there were 59 American Council on Graduate Medical Education–approved pediatric critical care fellowship programs (2005 website data from the American Board of Pediatrics and SCCM). However, the workforce requirements nationwide for pediatric critical care continued to exceed the supply, in great measure because of two developments: (1) the remarkable shift toward selection of a career in general pediatrics by graduating residents throughout the 1990s (from 57% in 1990 to 73% in 1998) and (2) the perception of many residents that shortages of critical care physicians and nurses often creates an extremely stressful working environment without ample time for one's family and for the scholarly activities necessary for career advancement in academic centers. In 1996, 103 residents entered PCCM fellowships, but this dropped to 72 in 1997. Since 1998, a shift back to more subspecialty selection by graduating residents has occurred. By the year 2000 recruitment into PCCM had almost recovered, with 99 pediatricians entering first year fellowships and a total of 262 fellows in training. This number of additional physicians in the subspecialty, with fewer than 100 completing a fellowship each year, will likely prove to be insufficient to meet the future clinical, educational, and research demands of the field and to replace the natural attrition caused by career changes, illness, and retirement. The solution to this workforce shortage will require intensive, ongoing study and planning that is integrated with overall planning for future acute and chronic child health care.

As pediatric critical care has matured over the past 25 years, the issues of patient safety, continuous quality improvement (CQI), and immediate as well as long-term patient outcomes came to the forefront. These are reviewed and addressed elsewhere in this textbook. Research on a broad front, including outcomes analyses from individual hospitals and coalitions of institutions, bedside clinical investigation, and basic science laboratory studies related to critical care conditions will continue to define the body of knowledge that constitutes *pediatric critical care medicine*.

Many of the advances in managing critical conditions achieved over the past two decades, as well as the leading issues confronting pediatric critical care today, have been recently described in concise, authoritative reviews [119–121]. Among the leading issues are (1) improving outcomes in cardiopulmonary–cerebral resuscitation and brain injury, (2) developing postintensive care rehabilitation from severe illness and injury, (2) ensuring adequacy of pediatric advance directives and palliative care, (3) ensuring compassionate and effective end-of-life care in the intensive care unit, and (4) integrating home care of children requiring long-term technological support with relevant hospital and community services before and after discharge from the PICU. The American Academy of Pediatrics has issued useful guidelines on bioethics, including support for individualized decisions involving the parents regarding the use of life-sustaining treatment [122], and the SCCM has published guidelines on non-heart-eating organ donation [123].

Regional disparities in the availability and quality of pediatric emergency and critical care services also continues to be an important cause of adverse outcomes in critically ill and injured children. A recent review reveals a growing body of evidence suggesting that many hospitalized children with critical illnesses who die never received the highest level of care [124]. According to a recent survey of 101 hospital emergency departments, a majority of hospitals without a designated inpatient pediatric department will still admit critically ill children, although 90% of these facilities will transfer severely injured children to a hospital with pediatric trauma services [125]. Emergency medical services for children are still a relatively underdeveloped component of most state and local emergency medical system programs [126]. Also, children with severe chronic disorders and disabilities requiring acute emergent care present an especially difficult array of problems for the nonpediatric hospital [127]. The American Academy of Pediatrics and the SCCM have published a joint consensus report on regionalization of services for critically ill and injured children with recommendations by physicians with expertise in emergency medicine and transport, trauma care, and critical care of infants and children [128]. The need for regional organization of critical medical services and disaster planning, and our nation's failure to accomplish this, was clearly demonstrated by the 2005 catastrophe in New Orleans and the Gulf Coast caused by hurricane Katrina and its aftermath. Effective regional planning and elimination of regional disparities in services will require steadfast commitment by leaders in pediatric emergency and critical care medicine.

The greatest obstacles to better health for our nation's children lie not within the immediate purview of the health care professions but within our society at large. Poverty is a central issue and remains a pervasive cause of poor health and adverse outcomes in millions of American children. Significant disparities in children's access to comprehensive health care remain despite 40 years of Medicaid insurance and endless discussions and debates. These disparities stem mainly from two sources: (1) lack of continuous private or public health insurance (usually associated with family incomes near the federal poverty levels) and (2) lack of regional and national planning for distribution of health services, including pediatric emergency transportation, emergency departments, and critical care facilities. There have been occasional progressive accomplishments such as state Children's Health Insurance Programs (CHIPs) for uninsured children whose families do not qualify for Medicaid and lack health insurance. Nonetheless, a study of nearly 27,000 children in 2000 and 2001 revealed that 6.6% of those under 18 years of age lacked health insurance for the entire year and 7.7% for part of the year [129]. Of the nation's 72 million children, 14.3%, or approximately 10 million children, did not have regular access to primary or subspecialty care and often had incomplete immunizations. If suffering from a major chronic condition, they were likely to have inadequate care and unfilled prescriptions [129,130]. Such disparities appear to extend to intensive care of children according to a recent study of 5,700 PICU admissions in multiple children's hospitals; uninsured children suffered a higher degree of physiologic derangement on admission with a

higher hospital mortality rate, yet survivors had a shorter length of stay [131].

The only solution to this nationwide blight is national legislation ensuring universal access for every person to comprehensive, high-quality, and humane health care. The American Academy of Pediatrics has long advocated for such legislation, as have many other health care professional organizations. Surveys indicate that the majority of Americans regard health care as a right and universal access as necessary for a healthy nation. However, the political will of both major national parties to begin designing and implementing the required legislation is sadly lacking at this time. Achieving elimination of regional and economic disparities in care, and the more difficult goal of universal access to health care for all Americans, requires the persistent and coordinated efforts of health care professional organizations, hospital associations, insurers, our elected representatives, government agencies, and especially concerned parents and families. If we emulate our predecessors, such as Abraham Jacobi, Josephine Baker, and Peter Safar, and strive persistently against all odds to achieve these goals step by step, the results will be greatly improved children's health status, improved outcomes from severe illnesses and trauma, and longer, healthier lives for all our children.

References

1. Second Book of Kings 4:29–37. The Jerusalem Bible. New York: Doubleday Co.; 1968:396–397.
2. Antyllus (117 AD) as cited by Paulus Aegenita (625–690 AD). In: Adams F. The Seven Books of Paulus Aegenita, vol 2, book 6. London: Syndemah Society; 1846:301.
3. Desault PJ. Oeuvre Chirurgicales. Expose de la Doctrine et de la Pratique de Desault; par Bichat. Paris; 1801:266–267
4. Herholdt JD, Rafn CE. Life Saving Measures for Drowning Persons. Copenhagen: H. Tikiob; 1796:52, as cited by Gillespie NA. Endotracheal Anesthesia. Madison: University of Wisconsin Press; 1963:6.
5. Todres ID. History of pediatric critical care. In Fuhrman BP, Zimmerman JJ, eds. Pediatric Critical Care, 3rd ed. St. Louis: Mosby; 2005:7–14.
6. Porter R. The Greatest Benefit to Mankind. New York: WW Norton, 1997:178–461.
7. Major RH. A History of Medicine, vol 1. Springfield, IL: Charles C. Thomas; 1954:404–550.
8. Major RH. A History of Medicine, vol 2. Springfield, IL: Charles C. Thomas; 1954:565–878.
9. Garrison FH. An Introduction to the History of Medicine. Philadelphia: WB Saunders; 1929:217–793.
10. Osler W. The Evolution of Modern Medicine. The Silliman Lectures of April 1913. New Haven: Yale University Press; 1921. (The Classics of Medicine Library, Gryphon Editions, Birmingham, AL, pp 146–233.)
11. Vesalius A. De Humani Corporis Fabrica. Basel: Libri Septum; 1543.
12. Harvey W. Exercitatio Anatomica de Motu Cordis et Sanguinis in Animalibus. English translation by G. Keynes, 1928. The Classics of Medicine Library. London: Nonesuch Press; 1978.
13. Zimmer C. The Soul Made Flesh. New York: Free Press; 2004: 117–260.
14. Safar P. Ventilatory efficacy of mouth-to-mouth artificial respiration. JAMA 1958;167:335–341.
15. Long CW. An account of the first use of sulfuric ether by inhalation as an anesthetic in surgical operations. South Med J 1849;5:705–713.

16. Bigelow HJ. Insensibility during surgical operations produced by inhalation. Boston Med Surg J 1846;35:309–317.

17. Gill G. Nightingales. New York: Ballantine Books; 2004:313–434.

18. Lister J. On the antiseptic principle of the practice of surgery. Lancet, 1867. Reprinted in Rapport S, Wright H, eds. Great Adventures in Medicine. New York: Dial Press; 1952:256–262.

19. Astrup P, Severinghaus JW. The History of Blood Gases, Acids and Bases. Copenhagen: Munksgaard International; 1986:113–256.

20. Porter R. The Greatest Benefit to Mankind. New York: WW Norton; 1997:338–340.

21. Cone TE. History of American Pediatrics. Boston: Little Brown Co.; 1979:102–103.

22. Haggerty RJ. Abraham Jacobi, MD, Respectable rebel. Pediatrics 1997;99:462–466.

23. Burke EC. Abraham Jacobi, MD: The man and his legacy. Pediatrics 1998;101:309–312.

24. O'Dwyer J. Fifty cases of croup in private practice treated by intubation of the larynx. Med Rec 1887;32:557.

25. Cone TE. History of American Pediatrics. Boston: Little Brown Co.; 1979:109.

26. Radbill SX. A history of children's hospitals. Am J Dis Child 1955;109: 411–416.

27. Astrup P, Severinghaus JW. The History of Blood Gases, Acids and Bases. Copenhagen: Munksgaard International; 1986:143–150.

28. Cone TE. History of American Pediatrics. Boston: Little Brown Co.; 1979:154–155.

29. Cone TE. History of American Pediatrics. Boston: Little Brown Co.; 1979:156–157.

30. Child Health in America. DHEW Publication No. (HSA) 76-5015. 1976:25–31.

31. Lawen A, Sievers R. Zur praktischer awendung der intrumentallen kunstilchen respiration am menschen. Munch Med Wochenschr 1910; 57:2221–2225.

32. Drinker P, McKhann CF. The use of a new apparatus for the prolonged administration of artificial ventilation. JAMA 1929;92:1658–1660 (reprinted in JAMA 1986;255:1473–1480).

33. Astrup P, Severinghaus JW. The History of Blood Gases, Acids and Bases. Copenhagen: Munksgaard International; 1986:257–258.

34. Lassen HCA. A preliminary report on the 1952 epidemic of poliomyelitis in Copenhagen. Lancet 1953;1:37–41.

35. Engstrom CG. Treatment of severe cases of respiratory paralysis by the Engstrom universal ventilator. BMJ 1954;2:666–669.

36. Pontoppidan H, Wilson RS, Rie MA, Schneider RC. Respiratory intensive care. Anesthesiology 1977;47:96–116.

37. Safar P, DeKornfeld TJ, Pearson JW, Redding JS. The intensive care unit—a three year experience at Baltimore City Hospitals. Anesthesia 1961;16:275–284.

38. Bendixen HH, Egbert LD, Hedley-Whyte J, Laver MB, Pontoppidan H. Respiratory Care. St. Louis: Mosby Co.; 1965.

39. Safar P. On the history of modern resuscitation. Crit Care Med 1996;24(2)(Suppl):S3–S11.

40. Hoyt JW, Grenvik A, Ayers SM, Greenbaum DM, Safar P. History of the Society of Critical Care Medicine. Crit Care Med 1996;24(1)(Suppl): P3–P9.

41. Lussky RC. A century of neonatal medicine. Minn Med. 1999;82:1–12 (MMA internet edition).

42. Cone TE. Perspectives in neonatology. In Smith GF, Vidyasagar D, eds. Historical Review and Recent Advances in Perinatal Medicine—Neonatology on the Web. 1980:5–18.

43. Smith CA, Nelson NM (eds): The Physiology of the Newborn Infant, 4th ed. Springfield, IL: Charles C. Thomas; 1976.

44. Avery ME, Mead J. Surface properties in relation to atelectasis and hyaline membrane disease. Am J Dis Child 1959;97:517–522.

45. Smythe PM, Bull A. Treatment of tetanus neonatorum with intermittent positive-pressure respiration. Br Med Bull 1959;2:107–113.

46. Delivoria-Papadopoulos M, Swyer PR. Assisted ventilation in terminal hyaline membrane disease. Arch Dis Child 1964;39:481–484.

47. Gregory G, Kitterman J, Phibbs R. Treatment of the idiopathic respiratory distress syndrome with continuous positive airway pressure. N Engl J Med 1971;284:1333–1340.

48. Northway WH, Rosan RC, Proter DY. Pulmonary disease following respiratory therapy of hyaline membrane disease. N Engl J Med 1967;276:357–362.

49. Gross RE, Hubbard JP. First surgical ligation of a patent ductus arteriosus. JAMA 1939;112:729–731.

50. Lake CL. History of pediatric anesthesia. In: Lake CL, ed. Pediatric Cardiac Anesthesia, 3rd ed. Stamford, CT: Appleton and Lange; 1998: 1–5.

51. Costarino AT, Downes JJ. Pediatric anesthesia—historical perspective. Anesthesiol Clin North Am 2005;23:573–595.

52. Downes JJ. The historical evolution, current status, and prospective development of pediatric critical care. Crit Care Clin 1992;8:1–22.

53. Haglund G, Werkmaster K, Ekstrom-Jodal B, McDougall DH. The pediatric emergency ward—principles and practice after 20 years. In: Stetson JB, Swyer PR, eds. Neonatal Intensive Care. St. Louis: WH Green; 1976:73–87.

54. Joly JB, H'uault G, Amsili J. Place de l'intubaton et de ventilation artificialle dans le traitment des bronchioalveolites graves du nourisson. Arch Fr Pediatr 1967;24:303–311.

55. McDonald IH, Stocks JG. Prolonged nasotracheal intubation. Br J Anaesth 1965;37:161–167.

56. Rees GJ. Intensive therapy in paediatrics. BMJ 1966;2:1611–1616.

57. Bachman L, Downes JJ, Richards CC, Coyle D, May E. Organization and function of an intensive care unit in a children's hospital. Anesth Analg 1967;45:570–574.

58. Striker TW, Stool S, Downes JJ. Prolonged nasotracheal intubation in infants and children. Arch Otolaryngol 1967;85:106–109.

59. Stool SE, Groff DB. Disposable plastic tracheostomy tubes. Laryngoscope 1969;79:1088–1094.

60. Downes JJ, Fulgencio T, Raphaely RC. Acute respiratory failure in infants and children. Pediatr Clin North Am 1972;19:423–443.

61. Kampschulte S, Safar P. Development of a multidisciplinary pediatric intensive care unit. Crit Care Med 1973;1:308–315.

62. Yeh TS. Regionalization of pediatric critical care. Crit Care Clin 1992;8:23–35.

63. Committee on Hospital Care of the American Academy of Pediatrics and the Pediatric Section of the Society of Critical Care Medicine. Guidelines for pediatric intensive care units. Crit Care Med 1983; 11:753–761.

64. Rogers MC, ed. Textbook of Pediatric Intensive Care, two volumes. Baltimore: Williams & Wilkins; 1987.

65. Levin DL, Morriss FC, eds. Essentials of Pediatric Intensive Care. St. Louis: Quality Medical Publishing; 1990.

66. Fuhrman BP, Zimmerman JJ, eds. Pediatric Critical Care. St. Louis: Mosby Year Book; 1992.

67. Holbrook PR, ed. Textbook of Pediatric Critical Care. Philadelphia: WB Saunders; 1993.

68. Todres ID, Fugate JH, eds. Critical Care of Infants and Children. Boston: Little Brown & Co.; 1996.

69. Ludwig S, Fleischer GR, eds. Textbook of Pediatric Emergency Medicine. Philadelphia: Lippincott-Williams & Wilkins Co.; 1983.

70. Safar P. History of cardiopulmonary–cerebral resuscitation. In: Kaye W, Bircher N, eds. Cardiopulmonary Resuscitation. New York: Churchill Livingston; 1989:1–53.

71. Ramonofski ML, Morse TS. Standards of care for the critically injured pediatric patient. J Trauma 1982;22:921–933.

72. Colombani PM, Buck JR, Dudgeon DL, Miller D, Haller JA. One-year experience in a regional pediatric trauma center. J Pediatr Surg 1985;20:8–13.

73. Norwood WI, Lang P, Hansen DD. Physiologic repair of aortic atresia–hypoplastic left heart syndrome. N Engl J Med 1983;308: 23–26.

74. Newberger JW, Jonas RA, Wernowski G. A comparison of the perioperative neurological effects of hypothermic circulatory arrest versus low-flow cardiopulmonary bypass in infant heart surgery. N Engl J Med 1993;329:1057–1064.

75. Lake CL. History of pediatric cardiac anesthesia. In: Lake CL, ed. Pediatric Cardiac Anesthesia, 3rd ed. Stamford, CT: Appleton and Lange; 1998:1–5.

76. Cohen DE, Downes JJ, Raphaely RC: What difference does pulse oximetry make? Anesthesiology 1988;68:181–184.

77. Fanconi S, Doherty P, Edmunds J. Pulse oximetry in pediatric intensive care: comparison with measured saturations and transcutaneous oxygen tension. J Pediatr 1985;107:362.

78. Miyasaka K. Mechanical ventilation. In: Holbrook PR, ed. Textbook of Pediatric Critical Care. Philadelphia: WB Saunders Co.; 1993.

79. Bohn D. Lung salvage and protection ventilatory techniques. Pediatr Clin North Am 2001;48:553–572.

80. Fuhrman BP, Dalton HJ. Progress in pediatric extracorporeal oxygenation. Crit Care Clin 1992;8:191–202.

81. Brill JE. Control of pain. Crit Care Clin 1992;8:203–218.

82. Guzzetta PC. Renal transplantation. In: Holbrook PR, ed. Textbook of Pediatric Critical Care. Philadelphia: WB Saunders Co.; 1993:613–620.

82a. Schreiner MS, Downes JJ, Kettrick RG, Ise C, Voit R. Chronic respiratory failure in infancy with prolonged ventilator dependency. JAMA 1987;258:3398–3404.

83. Report of the Surgeon General's Workshop on Children with Handicaps and Their Families. Washington, DC: DHHS, publication 83-50194; 1983.

84. Frates RC, Splaingard ML, Smith EO. Outcomes of home mechanical ventilation in children. J Pediatr 1985;106:850–857.

85. Pollack MM, Ruttimann UE, Getson PR. Accurate prediction of the outcome of pediatric intensive care. N Engl J Med 1987;316:134–139.

86. Pollack MM, Ruttimann, Getson PR. Pediatric risk of mortality (PRISM) score. Crit Care Med 1988;16:1110–1116.

87. Randolph AG, Guyatt GH, Carlet J. Understanding articles comparing outcomes among intensive care units to rate quality of care. Crit Care Med 1998;26:773–781.

88. Zechman EK, Reynolds SJ. Socioeconomics of pediatric critical care. In: Fuhrman BP, Zimmerman JJ, eds. Pediatric Critical Care. St. Louis: Mosby Year Book; 1992:23–33.

89. Rosenberg DI, Moss MM, and the AAP Section on Critical Care and Committee on Hospital Care. Guidelines and levels of care for pediatric intensive care units. Pediatrics 2004;114:1114–1125.

90. Pollack MM, Alexander SR, Clarke N, Ruttimann UE, Tesselaar HM, Bachulis AC. Improved outcomes from tertiary center pediatric intensive care: a statewide comparison of tertiary and non-tertiary facilities. Crit Care Med 1991;19:150–159.

91. Pollack MM, Cuerdon TT, Patel KM, Ruittimann UE, Getson PR, Levetown M. Impact of quality-of-care factors on pediatric intensive care unit mortality. JAMA 1994;272:941–946.

92. Fields AI, Cuerdon TT, Brasseux CO, Getson PR, Thompson AE, Orlowski JP, Youngner SJ. Physician burnout in pediatric critical care medicine. Crit Care Med 1995;23:1425–1429.

93. American College of Critical Care Medicine, Society of Critical Care Medicine. Critical care services and personnel recommendations based on a system of categorization into two levels of care. Crit Care Med 1999;97:422–426.

94. Kennedy D, Barloon LF. Managing burnout in pediatric critical care: the human care commitment. Crit Care Nurs Q 1997;20:63–71.

95. Swyer PR. The regional organization for special care of the neonate. Pediatr Clin North Am 1970;17:761–776.

96. Yeh TS. Regionalization of pediatric critical care. Crit Care Clin 1992;8:23–35.

97. Goetting MG. Mastering pediatric cardiopulmonary resuscitation. Pediatr Clin North Am 1994;41:1147–1182.

98. Spivak H, Prothrow-Stith D, Hausman AJ. Adolescents, violence and intentional injury. Pediatr Clin North Am 1988;35:1339–1348.

99. Wise PH, Meyers A. Poverty and child health. Pediatr Clin North Am 1988;35:1169–1186.

100. Reich K Culross PL, Behrman RE. Children, youth and gun violence: analysis and recommendations. Future Children 2002;12:5–23 (see www.futureofchildren.org).

101. Davidson Ward SL, Keens T. Home mechanical ventilators and equipment. In: McConnell MS, Imaizumi SO, eds. Guidelines for Pediatric Home Health Care. Elk Grove Village, IL: American Academy of Pediatrics; 2002:177–186.

102. Luce JM. Ethical principles in critical care. JAMA 1990;263:696–700.

103. Council on Scientific Affairs and Council on Ethical and Judicial Affairs (AMA). Persistent vegetative state and the decision to withdraw or withhold life support. JAMA 1990;263:426–430.

104. Truog RD, Brett AS, Frader J. The problem with futility. N Engl J Med 1992;326:1560–1564.

105. Lantos JD, Berger AC, Zucker AR. Do-not-resuscitate orders in a children's hospital. Crit Care Med 1993;21:52–55.

106. Purtilo R, Todres ID. Ethical aspects of pediatric intensive care. In: Todres ID, Fugate JH, eds. Critical Care of Infants and Children. Boston: Little Brown and Co.; 1996.

107. Green M. Parent care in the intensive care unit. Am J Dis Child 1979;133:119–120.

107a. Rothstein P. Psychological stress in families of children in a pediatric intensive care unit. Pediatr Clin North Am 1980;27:613–620.

108. Todres ID, Earle M, Jellinek MS. Communicating with families in the pediatric intensive care unit. In: Todres ID, Fugate JH, eds. Critical Care of Infants and Children. Boston: Little Brown and Co.; 1996:679–683.

109. Ayers SM. The promise of critical care: effective and humane care in an era of cost containment. In: Shoemaker WC, Ayers SM, Grenvik A, Holbrook PR, eds. Textbook of Critical Care, 3rd ed. Philadelphia: WB Saunders; 1995:1–7.

110. Ginzberg E. High-tech medicine and rising health care costs. JAMA 1990;263:1820–1822.

111. Woolhandler S, Himmelstein DU. The deteriorating administrative efficiency of the U.S. health care system. N Engl J Med 1991;324:1253–1258.

112. Augenstein JS, Peterson EA. Economic considerations in critical care. In: Shoemaker WC, Ayers SM, Grenvik A, Holbrook PR, eds. Textbook of Critical Care, 2nd ed. Philadelphia: WB Saunders; 1987:1465–1474.

113. Rosen RL, Bone RC. Financial implications of ventilator care. Crit Care Clin 1990;6:797–805.

114. American Academy of Pediatrics, Committee on Health Financing. Guiding principles for managed care arrangements for health care of newborns, infants, children, adolescents and young adults. Pediatrics 2000;105:132–135.

115. American Academy of Pediatrics, Committee on Health Financing. Principles of child health care financing. Pediatrics 2003;122:997–999.

116. Chalom R, Raphaely RC, Costarino AT. Hospital costs of pediatric intensive care. Crit Care Med 1999;27:2079–2085.

117. Downes JJ, Parra MM. Costs and reimbursement issues in long-term mechanical ventilation. In: Hill NS, ed. Long Term Mechanical Ventilation. New York: Marcel Decker; 2001:353–374.

118. Odetola FO, Clark SJ, Freed GL, Bratton SL, Davis MM. A national survey of pediatric critical care resources in the United States. Pediatrics 2005;116:1059.

119. Vidyasagar D, ed. Progress in Pediatric Critical Care. Critical Care Clinics 1992;8:1–228.

120. Orlowski JP. Pediatric Critical Care. Pediatr Clin No Amer 1994;41:1147–1438.

121. Orlowski JP, ed. Pediatric Critical Care—A New Millennium. Pediatr Clin No Amer 2001;48:553–814.

122. American Academy of Pediatrics Committee on Bioethics. Ethics and the care of critically ill infants and children. Pediatrics 1996;98:149–152.
123. American College of Critical Care Medicine, SCCM, Ethics Committee. Recommendations for nonheartbeating organ donation. Crit Care Med 2001;29:1826–1831.
124. Watson RS. Location, location, location: regionalization and outcome in pediatric critical care. Curr Opin Crit Care 2002;8:344–348.
125. Athey J, Dean JM, Ball J, Wiebe R, Melese-d'Hopital I. Ability of hospitals to care for pediatric emergency patients. Pediatr Emerg Care 2001;17:170–174.
126. Dieckmann RA, Athey J, Bailey B, Michael J. A pediatric survey for the National Highway Safety Administration: emergency medical services system reassessments. Prehosp Emerg Care 2001;5:231–236.

127. American Academy of Pediatrics Committee on Pediatric Emergency Medicine. Emergency preparedness for children with special health care needs. Pediatrics 1999;104:e53.
128. American Academy of Pediatrics and Society of Critical Care Medicine. Consensus report for regionalization of services for critically ill or injured children. Pediatrics 2000;105:152–155.
129. Olson LM, Tang SS, Newacheck PW. Children in the United States with discontinuous health insurance coverage. N Engl J Med 2005;353:382–391.
130. Starfield B. Insurance and the U.S. health care system. N Engl J Med 2005;353:418–419.
131. Lopez AM, Tilford JM, Anand KJS, Chan-Hee J, Green JW, Aitken ME, Fiser DH. Variation in pediatric intensive care therapies and outcomes by race, gender and insurance status. Pediatr Crit Care Med 2006;7:2–6.

2
Epidemiology of Critical Illness

R. Scott Watson and Mary E. Hartman

Introduction

Since the first intensive care units (ICUs) were established in the United States in the 1960s, there has been a gradual growth in the appreciation of the importance and magnitude of critical illness. In the 1980s, Jacobs and Noseworthy [1] reported that ICU expenditures in the United States accounted for 1% of the gross domestic product, and similar findings were reported more recently [2]. The frequency of critical illness and the provision of critical care services have now reached what can be considered epidemic proportions. Of the 38 million annual U.S. hospital admissions of children and adults [3], nearly 6 million, or 2% of the U.S. population, are admitted to an ICU [4]. The disease burden of the myriad disorders and conditions that constitute critical illness is of sufficient scale that efforts to prevent and treat critical illness have implications for overall public health.

The clinical epidemiology of critical illness is vital to inform clinical care, meaningful patient-oriented research, and health policy in critical care. Describing the natural history of disease informs the development of treatments to improve outcomes and the care delivered at the bedside. Understanding the burden of disease influences the prioritization of research efforts and the allocation of health care resources. Knowledge of risk factors for disease aids in prevention of disease, timely intervention to treat it, and selection of study populations. However, there are a number of challenges in performing clinical epidemiologic research in critical care, not the least of which is related to a core principle of epidemiology. Delineating the epidemiology of a disease or condition starts with the ability to identify it, both reliably (different clinicians classify a patient in the same way as each other and over time) and validly (the classification distinguishes people with the disease from those without it). In critical care, this may be conceptually straightforward but is operationally challenging. In this chapter, we discuss several issues related to clinical epidemiology in critical care and summarize some of the large-scale work that has been done examining the epidemiology of critical illnesses in children.

Challenges of Defining a Population in Critical Care

Critical illness is made up of a heterogeneous group of conditions and disorders that share a risk of organ dysfunction, long-term morbidity, and mortality. However, definitions of the syndromes that most consider quintessential critical care *diseases* (sepsis, acute respiratory distress syndrome [ARDS] / acute lung injury [ALI], and even organ failure) lack gold standard tests by which to identify them. By necessity, then, definitions have been developed by consensus and expert opinion. Although these definitions represent a substantial improvement over the prior state of phenomenologic disarray, they still suffer from limitations in reliability and validity [5,6]. Even the minimum degree of organ dysfunction, or risk thereof, that suggests that a patient is *critically* ill is often debated.

Another challenge to identifying patients with critical illness is that critical illness is often defined by where care takes place (i.e., the ICU) and the interventions used to treat it (e.g., mechanical ventilation, infusions of medications to support hemodynamics, continuous renal replacement therapy). Although convenient, these definitions are significantly limited. The definition of an illness cannot rely on the availability of an ICU bed. Care that is provided in an ICU in one country or region may be provided on the ward in another (and even in a given hospital, the availability of ICU beds may change with hospital and ICU census). Critical illness often begins before ICU admission and can last beyond ICU discharge. The use of many interventions varies by provider, even when controlling for patient factors, such as severity of illness, so it is much easier to determine which patients received an intervention than it is to determine which patients actually needed it [7–11]. Nonetheless, with the increasing availability of large-scale databases and increasing numbers of large-scale epidemiologic studies of prospectively collected data, the size and scope of pediatric critical illness are beginning to be characterized.

D.S. Wheeler et al. (eds.), *Science and Practice of Pediatric Critical Care Medicine*,
DOI 10.1007/978-1-84800-921-9_2, © Springer-Verlag London Limited 2009

Epidemiology of Children Receiving Critical Care Services

National estimates of the overall use of ICU services for children are limited. Extrapolating from a survey conducted in 2001 by Randolph and colleagues [12] for which pediatric ICU (PICU) directors were asked to report their annual number of PICU admissions, over 230,000 children are admitted to PICUs annually. In preliminary work, Garber et al. [13] estimated that 480,000 infants and children less than 20 years old received intensive care services in the United States in 2001 (in neonatal ICUs [NICUs], PICUs, and pediatric beds in adult ICUs). These patients represented 6.6% of pediatric hospitalizations. The population-based incidence of ICU care for infants was 10 to 25 times that for older children. Hospital mortality rate was 2.4% (or over 11,000 deaths nationally), was similar across age groups, and was consistent with that reported in Randolph and colleagues' survey (2.9%) [12]. Mean hospital costs were $19,000 per patient, and total ICU costs were nearly $8 billion nationally (30% of all hospital costs for children) [13].

Angus et al. [14] performed a study of the use of ICU services at the end of life for children and adults and found that one in five Americans overall died while using ICU services in the United States in 1999. Although many more adults than children died, children were more likely than adults to receive ICU services at the end of life. Nearly half of infants and one third of older children who died in 1999 received ICU care. Subsequent preliminary analyses of the pediatric sample from this population found that 29% of children aged 1 to 19 years who died did so after receiving ICU care, and, among hospitalized children who died, ICU care was much more common for those without a history of chronic illness [15].

Despite the limitations of a geographic definition of critical illness, our understanding of the magnitude of critical illness among children is enhanced by information about the provision of pediatric critical care services [16]. Only 9% of counties in the United States have PICUs, and 99% of the PICUs are located in urban counties [17]. The number of hospital beds overall for children has been decreasing since the 1980s in the United States, but ICU beds for children have been increasing. In 1989, Pollack and others identified 276 pediatric-specific ICUs in the United States, with an average of 528 admissions per year [18]. Pediatric intensivists were available to 73% of the units, and reported mortality rate was 5.5%. In 2001, Randolph and colleagues found 349 PICUs, with an average of 672 admissions per year [12]. Pediatric intensivists were available to 94% of the units, and reported mortality rate was 2.9%. The number of available PICU beds between 1995 and 2001 increased by 24% and outpaced population growth of children by 17.5%. The number of beds per child varied substantially by region—from 1 per 15,250 children in Arkansas, Louisiana, and Texas to 1 per 27,440 in New England. Whether this variation reflects different regional pediatric critical care needs is unknown.

The reason for the increasing numbers of PICU beds is also unclear and likely multifactorial. It may reflect changes in referral patterns, with an increasing number of smaller hospitals providing care for patients previously transferred to larger units. Although this would be somewhat surprising in light of increasing evidence that higher volume units have better severity-adjusted outcomes than their smaller counterparts [19–21], health care financing affords incentives to provide intensive care services even at smaller hospitals. On the other hand, patients who remain at smaller hospitals may be less severely ill than those who are transferred to tertiary care and may merely require additional monitoring that is not available on the wards of many hospitals.

Perhaps the most important factor in the increasing demand for PICU services is an increasing number of children in the population living with chronic medical conditions. Success in the treatment of extremely low-birth-weight babies, children with neurodevelopmental abnormalities, cancer, or cystic fibrosis, and organ transplant recipients has lead to longer life expectancies and decreased mortality rates. These successes have also led to an increased number of children living at increased risk of critical illness [22–26]. In a population-based study at a tertiary PICU in New York, almost half (45%) of all unscheduled admissions to the PICU were for patients with chronic health conditions, 32% of whom received technology-assisted care (such as mechanical ventilation, oxygen, tracheostomies, and intravenous therapies) [27]. Children with chronic conditions were 3.3 times more likely than healthy children to have an unscheduled PICU admission, and those receiving technology-assisted care were 373 times more likely. The most common conditions were neurologic, accounting for 15% of all unscheduled admissions. Similarly, 23% of all admissions (both scheduled and unscheduled) to a large, tertiary PICU had preexisting neurodevelopmental disorders [28]. Although hospital mortality rate was only 3%, patients were discharged with significantly greater needs for ventilatory and nutritional technology support than they had on admission. In addition to increasing the number of PICU admissions, children with chronic illness may require lengthy PICU stays. Indeed, former premature babies admitted to the PICU consumed more health care resources than their nonpremature counterparts, including longer lengths of stay and higher rates of mechanical ventilation [29].

Epidemiology of Mechanical Ventilation and Acute Respiratory Distress Syndrome/Acute Lung Injury

The provision of mechanical ventilation (MV) for acute respiratory failure was a major motivating factor in the development of ICUs and is one of the hallmarks of critical care. National estimates of respiratory failure among infants and children have been derived from analyses of administrative records of patients receiving mechanical ventilation. Of course, some patients are ventilated in the ICU for reasons other than respiratory failure (such as extreme hemodynamic instability or after prolonged surgery). Therefore, the incidence of MV is higher than the incidence of respiratory failure. Rates of mechanical ventilation were higher in neonates than in any other age group (80,000 babies per year, or 1.8 % of U.S. neonates) [30]. Although very-low-birth weight babies had extremely high rates of MV (52%/year), one third of ventilated neonates were of normal birth weight. Hospital mortality rate was 11.1%, and total U.S. hospital costs were $4.4 billion in 1994. Preliminary work examining older children found that 35,000 children aged 1 to 19 years were ventilated in the United States in 1999 [31]. Duration of MV was 4 or more days for over one third of patients. Most were ventilated for medical (as opposed to surgical) reasons, and the most common associated condition was severe sepsis (in 35%). Hospital mortality rate (13.8%) was higher than that of neonates, and estimated national hospital costs were lower ($1 billion).

The epidemiology of ARDS and ALI is being systematically assessed in adults. A recent study found that the age-adjusted incidence in patients 15 years and older in King County, Washington, was 86.2/100,000/year (which projects to 190,600 cases per year nationally) in 1999–2000 [5]. Hospital mortality rate was 38.5%, and both incidence and mortality rate increased with age. The most common risk factor for development of ALI was severe sepsis (present in 79% of cases of ALI). Efforts to understand the epidemiology of pediatric ARDS are hampered by a lower incidence in children and challenges in defining ARDS in infants and very young children. The only prospective population-based study of ARDS in children found only 7 new cases of ARDS in 3 months (February, April, and June) in 94 ICUs in Germany. These cases represented 1.5% of ventilated children and a population-based prevalence of 5.5/100,000 children (with an incidence of 3.1/100,000/year) [32]. Based on this incidence, the authors estimated that 500 children develop ARDS in Germany annually.

Epidemiology of Sepsis

Not only is the treatment of sepsis an integral component of critical care, but sepsis also provides a good example of how defining a syndrome, even broadly, facilitates its study and determines its characteristics. In 1992, the American College of Chest Physicians/Society of Critical Care Medicine Consensus Conference met to standardize the definitions of sepsis and severe sepsis so that they might be more clearly applied in research and clinical practice [33]. The group defined *sepsis* as a systemic inflammatory response syndrome resulting from infection, *severe sepsis* as sepsis associated with organ dysfunction, hypoperfusion, or hypotension, and *septic shock* as sepsis with arterial hypotension despite adequate fluid resuscitation [33]. These definitions now frequently serve as criteria for inclusion in randomized, controlled trials for sepsis therapies [34–40] and are increasingly employed by medical practitioners around the world. One of the significant advantages of this standard terminology is that it has allowed us to begin to understand the magnitude of sepsis. Sepsis and severe sepsis are much more common than previously realized, and they are important causes of serious morbidity and mortality in both children and adults.

The U.S. Centers for Disease Control and Prevention (CDC) lists septicemia (*a systemic disease associated with organisms or their toxins in the blood*) as the seventh leading cause of death for children aged 1–4 years and eighth for children aged 5–9 years [41]. Other investigators have examined severe sepsis specifically, applying consensus definitions to large administrative datasets containing records of U.S. hospitalizations. In 1995, over 42,000 children younger than 20 years old were hospitalized with severe sepsis in the United States, and 4,400 of them died (for a hospital mortality rate of 10.3%) [42]. Compared with other conditions in the CDC's list of leading causes of death, severe sepsis deaths exceeded all but three among infants and all but one among older children. Almost half of children with severe sepsis (48%) were less than 1 year old. Severe sepsis was more common among boys than girls and more common in children with underlying illness. In preliminary analyses of data from 1999, incidence rates of severe sepsis increased by 11% over the 4-year period, and hospital mortality rate decreased [43]. The increased incidence was secondary to increased numbers of very-low-birth-weight babies in the United States and an increased rate of sepsis among those babies. Although hospital mortality rate from 1995 to 1999 was unchanged among previously healthy children, it decreased to 9.0% overall in 1999 because of lower mortality among children with underlying illness. The three most common pathogens for children with severe sepsis in the United States were *Staphylococcus* (all types), *Streptococcus* (all types), and fungus, although viral etiologies were not examined [42].

In a single-center study in Montreal, Proulx et al. [44] examined the incidence of sepsis and related conditions in a university pediatric intensive care unit. This group examined 1,058 admissions to their PICU between 1991 and 1992 and identified 245 cases of sepsis (23% of all PICU admissions), 46 cases of severe sepsis (4%), and 25 cases of septic shock (2%). Mortality rate among the children with sepsis was 6% [44].

Multiple organ dysfunction (MOD) is often associated with severe sepsis. Details about its pathophysiology are poorly understood, and its effects on mortality are still being studied [45,46]. Kutko et al. [47] studied 96 cases of septic shock in 80 patients at a large academic PICU over 2 years to determine the impact of MOD on mortality in septic shock. Over 70% of sepsis cases occurred in patients with cancer (19% of whom had undergone a bone marrow transplant), and half occurred in patients with neutropenia. Indwelling catheters were present in over 58% of cases. Multiple organ dysfunction was present in almost 73% of cases at some point in time during the PICU course, and the mortality rate for this group was 36%. In Proulx's sepsis cohort, discussed above, 29% developed MOD, with a mortality rate of 32% [44]. A finding common among these studies is that there were few or no deaths among children who were previously healthy and no deaths among patients without MOD.

Epidemiology of Status Asthmaticus

As the most common chronic disease among children, asthma's epidemiology has been extensively studied, and increasing numbers of investigators have examined the epidemiology of status asthmaticus. Asthma affects 5% to 7% of U.S. children. Its prevalence increased from 1980 to 1996 and leveled off between 1997 and 2000. It is one of the most common reasons for pediatric hospitalization in the United States [48], and hospitalization rates increased between 1980 and the mid-1990s [49,50]. In 2000, there were 152,000 pediatric hospital admissions for asthma, which generated total U.S. hospital charges of $835 million (2% of U.S. health care charges for children) [51]. Although status asthmaticus is a common reason for ICU admission, an average of only 8% of children hospitalized with asthma at pediatric centers require PICU care [52]. The use of invasive MV varies substantially by center (from 3% to 47% of PICU patients [7]), by region of the United States (from 6% to 27% of PICU patients at pediatric centers [52]), and by year (from 8% to 18% of ICU patients between 1992 and 2001 in a single state [53]). This variation persists even when controlling for severity of illness [7], and children with Medicaid insurance have higher rates of tracheal intubation and longer lengths of stay than patients with commercial insurance, even when controlling for severity of illness [54].

Mortality rates for children with asthma are increasing [49,50,55,56], but death is still uncommon after patients are admitted to the hospital. Two recent, large studies found 0.3%–0.4% hospital mortality rate among patients admitted to tertiary PICUs [7,52] and a 2.8% mortality rate among tracheally intubated patients [7]. Mortality is highest for adolescents (twice that of younger children), and children of African American decent are more than four times as likely to die from asthma as white children [49]. Risk factors for asthma-related death include previous life-threatening attacks, severe disease, recent hospital admission or emergency room visit, poor adherence to medical regimens [57,58], and prior history of asthma-induced respiratory failure requiring mechanical ventilation [59]. Some patients with near-fatal asthma (requiring mechanical ventilation or resulting in unconsciousness) have been found to have decreased sensitivity to hypoxia and blunted perception of dyspnea [60].

Conclusion

Improving definitions of the syndromes that characterize critical illness, the development of efficient information technology, and the creation of extensive databases that include PICU patients have enabled large-scale epidemiologic research to be conducted in critical care. As evident from the discussion, however, this work is incomplete. We need better estimates of basic critical care syndromes and interventions, such as ARDS and continuous renal replacement therapy. We also need to examine further reasons for variation in care, the relationship between risk factors of disease, hospital course, and postdischarge outcome, and how public health and medical interventions affect the incidences and outcomes of critical illnesses in children.

Recent and impending developments in the health care of children will affect the epidemiology of pediatric critical illness. Populations of children known to be at high risk for critical illness (e.g., premature babies, technology-dependent or immunosuppressed children) continue to grow. New vaccines may decrease the rate of severe sepsis in previously healthy children. Genetic and immunologic analyses will identify children at high or low risk of severe illness and sequelae. They will enhance our therapeutic effectiveness by allowing us to provide specific treatments to children based on more robust information regarding the likelihood of responsiveness [61]. The success of pediatric critical care study networks will increase our knowledge about the efficacy and effectiveness of interventions for critical illness and will enhance our understanding of the natural history of critical illness. The thoughtful use of the tools of clinical epidemiology can facilitate these advances, help us refine application, and let us understand their ramifications.

References

1. Jacobs P, Noseworthy TW. National estimates of intensive care utilization and costs: Canada and the United States. Crit Care Med 1990; 18:1282–1286.
2. Cowan CA, Lazenby HC, Martin AB, et al. National health expenditures, 1999. Health Care Finance Rev 2001;22:77–110.
3. Merrill CT, Elixhauser A. Hospitalization in the United States, 2002. HCUP Fact Book No. 6. Report No. AHRQ, Publication No. 05-0056. Rockville, MD: AHRQ; 2005.
4. Kersten A, Milbrandt EB, Rahim MT, et al. How big is critical care in the US? Crit Care Med 2003;31(Suppl):A8.
5. Rubenfeld GD, Caldwell E, Peabody E, et al. Incidence and outcomes of acute lung injury. N Engl J Med 2005;353:1685–1693.
6. Goss CH, Brower RG, Hudson LD, Rubenfeld GD. Incidence of acute lung injury in the United States. Crit Care Med 2003;31:1607–1611.
7. Roberts JS, Bratton SL, Brogan TV. Acute severe asthma: differences in therapies and outcomes among pediatric intensive care units. Crit Care Med 2002;30:581–585.
8. Bungard TJ, Ghali WA, Teo KK, McAlister FA, Tsuyuki RT. Why do patients with atrial fibrillation not receive warfarin? Arch Intern Med 2000;160:41–46.
9. Bungard TJ, McAlister FA, Johnson JA, Tsuyuki RT. Underutilisation of ACE inhibitors in patients with congestive heart failure. Drugs 2001;61:2021–2033.
10. Sim I, Cummings SR. A new framework for describing and quantifying the gap between proof and practice. Med Care 2003;41: 874–881.
11. Bickell NA, McEvoy MD. Physicians' reasons for failing to deliver effective breast cancer care: a framework for underuse. Med Care 2003;41:442–446.
12. Randolph AG, Gonzales CA, Cortellini L, Yeh TS. Growth of pediatric intensive care units in the United States from 1995 to 2001. J Pediatr 2004;144:792–798.
13. Garber N, Watson RS, Linde-Zwirble WT, et al. The size and scope of intensive care for children in the US. Crit Care Med 2003;31(Suppl): A78.
14. Angus DC, Barnato AE, Linde-Zwirble WT, et al. Use of intensive care at the end of life in the United States: an epidemiologic study. Crit Care Med 2004;32:638–643.
15. Watson RS, Linde-Zwirble WT, Hartman ME, et al. ICU use at the end-of-life in US children. Crit Care Med 2002;30(Suppl):A147.
16. Odetola FO, Clark SJ, Freed GL, Bratton SL, Davis MM. A national survey of pediatric critical care resources in the United States. Pediatrics 2005;115:e382–e386.
17. Odetola FO, Miller WC, Davis MM, Bratton SL. The relationship between the location of pediatric intensive care unit facilities and child death from trauma: a county-level ecologic study. J Pediatr 2005; 147:74–77.
18. Pollack MM, Cuerdon TC, Getson PR. Pediatric intensive care units: results of a national survey. Crit Care Med 1993;21:607–614.
19. Tilford JM, Simpson PM, Green JW, Lensing S, Fiser DH. Volume-outcome relationships in pediatric intensive care units. Pediatrics 2000;106:289–294.
20. Birkmeyer JD, Siewers AE, Finlayson EVA, et al. Hospital volume and surgical mortality in the United States. N Engl J Med 2002;346: 1128–1137.
21. Dudley RA, Johansen KL, Brand R, Rennie DJ, Milstein A. Selective referral to high-volume hospitals: estimating potentially avoidable deaths. JAMA 2000;283:1159–1166.
22. Newacheck PW, Taylor WR. Childhood chronic illness: prevalence, severity, and impact. Am J Public Health 1992;82:364–371.
23. Reiss J, Gibson R. Health care transition: destinations unknown. Pediatrics 2002;110:1307–1314.
24. Feudtner C, Hays RM, Haynes G, Geyer JR, Neff JM, Koepsell TD. Deaths attributed to pediatric complex chronic conditions: national trends and implications for supportive care services. Pediatrics 2001; 107:e99.
25. Hack M. Consideration of the use of health status, functional outcome, and quality-of-life to monitor neonatal intensive care practice. Pediatrics 1999;103:319–328.
26. Noble L. Developments in neonatal technology continue to improve infant outcomes. Pediatr Ann 2003;32:595–603.
27. Dosa NP, Boeing NM, Ms N, Kanter RK. Excess risk of severe acute illness in children with chronic health conditions. Pediatrics 2001; 107:499–504.
28. Graham RJ, Dumas HM, O'Brien JE, Burns JP. Congenital neurodevelopmental diagnoses and an intensive care unit: defining a population. Pediatr Crit Care Med 2004;5:321–328.
29. Slonim AD, Patel KM, Ruttimann UE, Pollack MM. The impact of prematurity: a perspective of pediatric intensive care units. Crit Care Med 2000;28:848–853.
30. Angus DC, Linde-Zwirble WT, Griffin M, Clermont G, Clark RH. Epidemiology of neonatal respiratory failure in the US: projections from California and New York. Am J Respir Crit Care Med 2001;164: 1154–1160.

31. Watson RS, Linde-Zwirble WT, Hartman ME, Clermont G, Angus DC. Epidemiology of mechanical ventilation in non-infant US children. Crit Care Med 2002;30(Suppl):A131.

32. Bindl L, Dresbach K, Lentze MJ. Incidence of acute respiratory distress syndrome in German children and adolescents: a population-based study. Crit Care Med 2005;33:209–212.

33. American College of Chest Physicians/Society of Critical Care Medicine Consensus Conference. Definitions for sepsis and organ failure and guidelines for the use of innovative therapies in sepsis. Crit Care Med 1992;20:864–874.

34. Annane D, Sebille V, Charpentier C, et al. Effect of treatment with low doses of hydrocortisone and fludrocortisone on mortality in patients with septic shock. JAMA 2002;288:862–871.

35. Rivers E, Nguyen B, Havstad S, et al. Early goal-directed therapy in the treatment of severe sepsis and septic shock. N Engl J Med 2001; 345:1368–1377.

36. Briegel J, Forst H, Haller M, et al. Stress doses of hydrocortisone reverse hyperdynamic septic shock: a prospective, randomized, double-blind, single-center study. Crit Care Med 1999;27:723–732.

37. Reinhart K, Meier-Hellmann A, Beale R, et al. Open randomized phase II trial of an extracorporeal endotoxin adsorber in suspected Gram-negative sepsis. Crit Care Med 2004;32:1662–1668.

38. Molnar Z, Mikor A, Leiner T, Szakmany T. Fluid resuscitation with colloids of different molecular weight in septic shock. Intensive Care Med 2004;30:1356–1360.

39. Bertolini G, Iapichino G, Radrizzani D, et al. Early enteral immunonutrition in patients with severe sepsis: results of an interim analysis of a randomized multicentre clinical trial. Intensive Care Med 2003;29: 834–840.

40. Busund R, Koukline V, Utrobin U, Nedashkovsky E. Plasmapheresis in severe sepsis and septic shock: a prospective, randomised, controlled trial. Intensive Care Med 2002;28:1434–1439.

41. Center for Disease Control and Prevention. National Vital Statistics Report, vol 50, no. 16. Atlanta, GA: CDC; 2002:1–36.

42. Watson RS, Carcillo JA, Linde-Zwirble WT, Clermont G, Lidicker J, Angus DC. The epidemiology of severe sepsis in children in the United States. Am J Respir Crit Care Med 2003;167:695–701.

43. Watson RS, Linde-Zwirble WT, Lidicker J, et al. The increasing burden of severe sepsis in U.S. children. Crit Care Med 2001;29(Suppl):A8.

44. Proulx F, Fayon M, Farrell CA, Lacroix J, Gauthier M. Epidemiology of sepsis and multiple organ dysfunction syndrome in children. Chest 1996;109:1033–1037.

45. Al Zwaini EJ. Neonatal septicaemia in the neonatal care unit, Al-Anbar governorate, Iraq. East Mediterr Health J 2002;8:509–514.

46. Ali Z. Neonatal bacterial septicaemia at the Mount Hope Women's Hospital, Trinidad. Ann Trop Paediatr 2004;24:41–44.

47. Kutko MC, Calarco MP, Flaherty MB, et al. Mortality rates in pediatric septic shock with and without multiple organ system failure. Pediatr Crit Care Med 2003;4:333–337.

48. McCormick MC, Kass B, Elixhauser A, Thompson J, Simpson L. Annual report on access to and utilization of health care for children and youth in the United States—1999. Pediatrics 2000;105:219–230.

49. Akinbami LJ, Schoendorf KC. Trends in childhood asthma: prevalence, health care utilization, and mortality. Pediatrics 2002;110:315–322.

50. Fulwood R, Parker S, Hurd SS. Asthma—United States, 1980–1987. MMWR Morbid Mortal Weekly Rep 1990;39:493–497.

51. Owens PL, Thompson J, Elixhauser A, Ryan K. Care of Children and Adolescents in U.S. Hospitals. Report No. AHRQ Publication No. 04-0004. Rockville, MD: AHRQ; 2003.

52. Bratton SL, Odetola FO, McCollegan J, Cabana MD, Levy FH, Keenan HT. Regional variation in ICU care for pediatric patients with asthma. J Pediatr 2005;147:355–361.

53. Hartman ME, Linde-Zwirble WT, Watson RS, Angus DC. Changes in incidence, management, and care of pediatric status asthmaticus over the last decade. Crit Care Med 2005;33(Suppl):A4.

54. Bratton SL, Roberts JS, Watson RS, Cabana M. Intensive care of pediatric asthma: differences in outcome and Medicaid insurance. Pediatr Crit Care Med 2002;3:234–238.

55. Centers for Disease Control and Prevention. Asthma mortality and hospitalization among children and young adults, United States, 1980–1993. MMWR CDC Surveill Summ 1996;45(17):350–353.

56. Serafini U. Can fatal asthma be prevented? A personal view. Clin Exp Allergy 1992;22:576–588.

57. Greenberger PA, Patterson R. The diagnosis of potentially fatal asthma. N Engl Reg Allergy Proc 1988;9:147–152.

58. Lowenthal M, Patterson R, Greenberger PA, Grammer LC. The application of an asthma severity index in patients with potentially fatal asthma. Chest 1993;104:1329–1331.

59. Rea HH, Scragg R, Jackson R, Beaglehole R, Fenwick J, Sutherland DC. A case–control study of deaths from asthma. Thorax 1986;41: 833–839.

60. Kikuchi Y, Okabe S, Tamura G, et al. Chemosensitivity and perception of dyspnea in patients with a history of near-fatal asthma. N Engl J Med 1994;330:1329–1334.

61. Israel E, Chinchilli VM, Ford JG, et al. Use of regularly scheduled albuterol treatment in asthma: genotype-stratified, randomised, placebo-controlled cross-over trial. Lancet 2004;364:1505–1512.

3
Ethics in the Pediatric Intensive Care Unit

K. Sarah Hoehn and Robert M. Nelson

Introduction

The pediatric intensive care unit (PICU) is a complex and often intense environment where a multidisciplinary group of clinicians apply a diverse range of cognitive and technical skills and resources in hopes of returning a critically ill child to an acceptable level of functioning or health. Fortunately, the vast majority of these efforts are successful. At other times, doubts can arise concerning the appropriate use of PICU technology given, for example, diagnostic or prognostic uncertainty, differing judgments about the acceptability of an outcome, or a perception of limited resources. Simply because we can intervene, should we? Such doubts when expressed can lead to disagreement and perhaps conflict among clinicians and family members. The potential for conflict, whether apparent or real, can be exacerbated by a compressed time frame, individual stress, the involvement of multiple clinical services, and so forth. At such times, careful ethical analysis combined with respectful listening and collegial communication is essential to help resolve the issues. This chapter discusses the ethical issues involved in setting limits on the use of technology in the PICU, including the use of medications and artificially provided hydration and nutrition. These issues are then set within the broader context of communication and conflict resolution. The chapter ends by highlighting several ethical issues raised in the context of organ procurement and research with critically ill children.

Setting Limits

Forgoing Life-Sustaining Medical Treatment

Most critically ill children recover and return to an acceptable quality of life. Some children either respond partially or fail to respond to life-sustaining medical treatment (LSMT), leading to death within minutes to years. In fact, most children who die in the PICU do so after a decision has been made to either limit or withdraw (i.e., forgo) some form of LSMT [1]. The use of LSMT assumes that the burden of treatment is justified by the anticipated outcome of an acceptable quality of life. As the anticipated quality of life deteriorates or becomes increasingly unlikely, or as the burden of treatment becomes intolerable, continued LSMT may not make sense. Decisions to limit LSMT may include not attempting resuscitation, not escalating inotropic or ventilator support, or not starting new treatments (such as endotracheal intubation or new modes of ventilation). Decisions to withdraw LSMT may include stopping inotropic support, decreasing or stopping ventilator support, stopping endotracheal intubation, or stopping artificially provided hydration and nutrition.

The reasons for forgoing LSMT can be grouped into two broad categories: the intervention either (1) does not or will not work (i.e., futility) or (2) is not worth doing as the burden of treatment outweighs any expected or actual benefit (i.e., disproportionate burden) [2]. For example, performing a tracheotomy and instituting long-term ventilation for a child in a persistent vegetative state who aspirates and develops respiratory failure may be disproportionately burdensome, but it is not futile. The majority of decisions to forgo LSMT in the PICU are based on the judgment of disproportionate burden rather than on the more limited concept of futility.

The judgment that continued LSMT presents a disproportionate burden involves a complex and value-laden balancing between the burden of intervention and the benefit of the anticipated outcome for the child. In striking this balance, the focus should be on the quality of the child's experience and not on the worth of that child's life to others. Although pain and agitation can be minimized through medication, caregivers and parents may perceive differently the degree to which a child is suffering and to what purpose. The loss of interaction with a child who is on extracorporeal membrane oxygenation (ECMO) or nonconventional forms of mechanical ventilation because of the need for sedating medication may be especially difficult for parents. In conversation, clinicians should seek to understand the parents' perspective and the role of factors such as tolerance for disability, hope for recovery, religious faith, views of other family members, and so forth.

Clinicians often use the term *futility* broadly and thus obscure the fact that the assessment of disproportionate burden rests on a value judgment about the anticipated outcome that the family may not share. As futility may be used to justify a decision to forgo

D.S. Wheeler et al. (eds.), *Science and Practice of Pediatric Critical Care Medicine*,
DOI 10.1007/978-1-84800-921-9_3, © Springer-Verlag London Limited 2009

LSMT absent parental agreement, an overly broad interpretation of futility inappropriately privileges clinicians' values over those of the parents and family. The concept of futility should refer to only those interventions that will not in fact achieve a given physiologic outcome. An appeal to futility should not short-circuit the process of communication by which medical interventions are determined to be disproportionately burdensome [3].

Disclosing "Bad News"

Approaching a child's parents to initiate a discussion about forgoing LSMT can be difficult. The perceived futility of a given treatment, which would otherwise be provided (e.g., attempted resuscitation) or is underway (e.g., prolonged ECMO for respiratory failure) argues in favor of initiating such a conversation. A reasonable starting point is to explore a parent's hopes and expectations about possible outcomes, the anticipated burden of treatment in attempting to achieve an acceptable outcome, and the degree of uncertainty in predicting a child's response to treatment. However, a recommendation to forgo LSMT before a family is ready to consider the options risks a loss of trust, a hardening of viewpoints, and thus damaging the working relationship with a child's parents so necessary for shared decision making. Parents often prefer to hear difficult information from a clinician who knows the family and can communicate truthfully, clearly, and compassionately. Parents also may be more comfortable exploring initial doubts about on-going LSMT with someone other than the responsible physician [4].

The disclosure of *bad news* is often poorly handled. Parents may perceive a clinician to be indifferent and inconsiderate, resulting in emotional distress. Lack of training, inexperience, and feelings of inadequacy about communicating with parents over end-of-life issues may distress clinicians and impact negatively on the quality of care. Clinicians who feel less competent and inadequately supported may distance themselves emotionally in stressful situations, perhaps leading to depression and other symptoms [4,5].

Do Not Attempt Resuscitation Orders

The discussion of options for resuscitation in the event of either a respiratory or a cardiac arrest may be the first time that a parent has considered forgoing LSMT. The limitation of resuscitation efforts occurs in at least four broad contexts: (1) a decision to not attempt resuscitation (DNAR) is a necessary component of forgoing other LSMT (e.g., endotracheal extubation); (2) the patient is currently stable, but the future need for resuscitation would indicate that other interventions have failed; (3) the patient is currently stable, but the patient's condition would make future resuscitation disproportionately burdensome; or (4) the patient is deteriorating and there are no other available interventions to reverse the process, including resuscitation.

Although DNAR orders are often discussed as part of a broader palliative care plan, the continued provision of all appropriate curative interventions is consistent with deciding to forego resuscitation in the future should these efforts fail. Health care providers often assume that the presence of a DNAR order indicates the desire to not pursue other interventions to forestall death. This assumption is inappropriate absent an explicit decision to this effect. Health care providers may also assume that the absence of a DNAR order obligates them to performing a prolonged resuscitation in a *one size fits all* manner. As long as the futility of initiating or continuing resuscitative efforts does not cloak a unilateral judgment about the moral value of a child's outcome, a physician should tailor resuscitative efforts to the clinical condition of the child (including the possibility of not initiating resuscitation at all). Finally, the effectiveness and/or acceptable burden of specific resuscitative interventions may vary depending on the patient's clinical condition and anticipated outcome. Thus, DNAR orders should address separately the provision of mechanical ventilation with or without endotracheal intubation, the use of cardiac medications, chest compressions, and cardioversion. A parent may want a focused resuscitation in hopes of sustaining a child's life while acknowledging the unacceptable burden of more *invasive* interventions such as endotracheal intubation or cardioversion.

Time-Limited Trials

The widespread use of innovative treatments, the pace of technological change, and the lack of appropriately controlled clinical studies render uncertain many if not most predictions of patient outcome absent severe multiorgan system failure. Under such circumstances, the concept of a *time-limited trial* offers the advantage of assessing individual response to treatment and then withdrawing LSMT in the face of either disproportionate burden or futility. The time frame for evaluating the success or failure of such an intervention (e.g., ECMO for non-neonatal respiratory failure or following cardiac arrest) should be stated from the outset. Even so, parents may find it difficult to agree to the withdrawal of LSMT as this time limit approaches. For many clinicians, the continued provision of burdensome or futile treatment to a dying child may be difficult to tolerate. An important first step in trying to resolve such a situation is to negotiate with parents a limited time period for making a decision about withdrawing LSMT. The negotiation process will involve a difficult balancing of the patient's best interest, the perceived burden of ongoing pain and suffering, and the parents' hopes and fears for the life of their child. The clinician should strive for a mutually respectful and supportive relationship with the parents while maintaining open communication about these difficult issues.

The use of *time-limited trials* has been supported by the prevailing view that there are no moral or legal differences between withholding or withdrawing interventions that are not medically indicated. The perceived reluctance to withdraw interventions once started has often been attributed to emotional or psychological difficulties. The alleged symmetry between the application and removal of technology assumes that the technology itself is *value neutral* and that any other changes that may occur over time apart from the presence or absence of the medical indication for that technology are not morally relevant. Both assumptions may not be appropriate, especially when transitioning from an acute to a chronic technology [6]. If uncertainty remains about the ongoing provision of LSMT, one should exercise caution when transitioning to a surgically placed tracheostomy and/or gastrostomy tube. The transition to more intense forms of technological support such as ECMO following cardiac arrest usually occurs under great duress, limited time, and uncertainty. However, the ability of a child to survive for prolonged periods is limited under these conditions, and the pain and agitation of the child can be effectively managed with appropriate use of medications. As such, when escalating technological support, the consequences of a wrong decision, while difficult and troubling, are usually more contained.

Medication Use When Forgoing Life-Sustaining Medical Treatment

Narcotics and sedatives should be used appropriately to treat pain and/or anxiety associated with forgoing LSMT. Children already may be receiving one or more of these medications, and clinicians should then anticipate changes in the need for medication depending on the LSMT being withdrawn. Withdrawal of inotropic medications, or artificially provided hydration and nutrition, is not associated with increased pain or anxiety. Removal of an endotracheal tube and mechanical ventilation may result in decreased pain yet increased anxiety depending on the level of consciousness of the child. Anxiety as a result of "air hunger" marked by tachypnea and a variable level of consciousness may require treatment with higher doses of medications such as barbiturates or benzodiazepines or the introduction of a new medication involving a different mechanism of action (such as ketamine). Parents (and others) are often distressed by a child's *agonal breathing* marked by slow gasping breaths and a depressed level of consciousness. In this case, anticipatory education about the process of dying is important because the administration of sedatives and narcotics will not eliminate such breathing.

The use of medication when withdrawing LSMT has generated controversy over the years. When directed toward the relief of pain and anxiety, there are no data supporting the view that the use of medications hastens death. Even if such data existed, the primary relief of pain and agitation under these circumstances is considered to be a moral good of such magnitude that the secondary effect of hastening death would be an acceptable (albeit unintended) consequence. Two key features of this so-called *doctrine of double effect* (DDE) are worth noting: (1) the unintended outcome (e.g., death) should not be the means of achieving the intended outcome (i.e., relief of pain); and (2) intentionality is not a psychological state, but an objective feature of the act itself (i.e., choice of medication, dose, timing, route of administration, and so forth reveal the agent's intent). In effect, the DDE provides a moral framework for a single action to be the cause of an intended good outcome and an unintended (but foreseeable) bad outcome. In a related argument, the cause of death after endotracheal extubation of a child with progressive and unresponsive respiratory failure is the disease process and not the act of extubation—an interpretation upheld by the U.S. Supreme Court [7]. However brief the time between extubation and death, the choice is not *death* but *how to live while dying* [8]. The DDE provides an important moral framework for those clinicians who desire to provide compassionate end-of-life care without intending or causing the death of their patients.

Medications that produce neuromuscular blockade (NMB) should never be initiated for the purposes of withdrawing LSMT. As patients have been known to survive the withdrawal of mechanical ventilation, the effects of NMB should be reversed if feasible. If the degree of NMB is such that reversal is not possible within a reasonable time, some argue that the ongoing burden of treatment absent an acceptable outcome argues in favor of withdrawing LSMT despite the presence of NMB. The moral acceptability of this approach depends on at least two factors: (1) the certainty of death from the underlying disease process and (2) the provision of adequate analgesia and anxiolysis while under NMB. This situation is best avoided through the judicious use of NMB, combined with monitoring techniques that would allow for the reversal of NMB before withdrawing mechanical ventilation.

Artificial Hydration and Nutrition

The forgoing of artificially provided hydration and nutrition (APHN) is an emotionally and politically charged issue. Artificially provided hydration and nutrition is a medical procedure (i.e., equivalent to endotracheal intubation and mechanical ventilation) and includes the administration of water and nutrients through devices such as peripheral or central intravenous catheters or tubes inserted into the stomach or small intestine through the nose, mouth, or abdominal wall. As such, forgoing APHN should be evaluated using the same criteria as any other form of LSMT [9]. In light of the diversity of opinion about the ethical acceptability of forgoing APHN, such a request should be initiated by the child's parents and not by health care providers. Some argue that such an approach may discriminate against those parents who are unaware of the option to forgo APHN. Others argue that such an approach minimizes the imposition of a professional bias against disability and the appearance of institutional discrimination in the provision of necessary medical services.

When presented with such a request, clinicians need to be aware of any applicable institutional policy and state and federal laws and advise parents accordingly (perhaps in consultation with the institutional ethics committee or independent legal counsel). There may be specific state statutes defining the *clear and convincing evidence* required to determine the prior expressed wishes of the patient (usually an adult) and permitting a *substituted judgment* to withdraw APHN. This *substituted judgment* is not possible by young children or by patients who became incompetent before expressing such wishes. Alternatively, there may be case law and/or state statutes that allow a surrogate decision to withdraw APHN based on the patient's *best interests*. However, the rulings are generally in regard to adult patients and are thus of uncertain pediatric applicability. Although forgoing APHN under the appropriate circumstances may be ethically defensible, such a decision should be made by a child's parents after due consideration of the moral and legal implications.

Individuals who argue that APHN should never be withdrawn even if a patient is in a persistent vegetative state (PVS) may inadvertently encourage surrogate decision makers to withdraw prematurely other forms of LSMT. For example, patients who experience a prolonged asphyxial event (e.g., from cardiac arrest) often are dependent initially on both cardiac and ventilatory support. Fearing the outcome of PVS, and the future inability to withdraw APHN, surrogate decision makers may decide to withdraw inotropic support and/or mechanical ventilation before the diagnosis of PVS has been confirmed.

The Role of Palliative Care in the Pediatric Intensive Care Unit

Many children admitted to the PICU are facing a life-threatening or terminal condition. As such, the child and family may benefit from integrating palliative care principles and practices into the routine provision of LSMT. Life-sustaining medical treatment can be broadly defined as any intervention that may prolong the life of a patient or alter substantially the expected progression toward death. Palliative care interventions focus on the relief of symptoms and conditions that may detract from a child's (and family's) quality of life regardless of the impact on a child's underlying disease process. For example, parents may need to grieve the loss of their previously normal child following a severe traumatic brain injury before being able to make decisions about ongoing treatment. Also, adequate symptom relief (such as pain and anxiety) should be provided independent of the impact on *curative* interventions. The focus should be on the quality of the child's overall experience, with the goal of adding *life to the child's years, not simply years to the child's life* [10]. A palliative care plan involves the assessment of available diagnostic and therapeutic interventions based on the goal of improving a child's quality of life while living with a life-threatening or terminal disease. At times, surgical procedures such as placement of central intravenous access (i.e., a port) or a tracheostomy tube may be justified to improve a child's quality of life.

Advance Directives

The 1991 federal Patient Self-Determination Act requires that health care institutions ask adult patients whether they have completed an advance directive (AD) and, if not, of their right to do so. An adult (i.e., over 18 years of age) who is admitted to a PICU must be asked about and informed of the availability of an AD. The use of an AD in pediatrics has generally been limited to inpatient settings for at least two reasons: (1) the availability of parents and (2) the lack of a standardized process to facilitate the identification, validation, and interpretation of an outpatient AD. An adolescent with a chronic and/or life-threatening condition should be supported in developing an AD as part of a comprehensive plan for end-of-life care [5].

Triage

At times, the resources available to patients in the PICU (e.g., ECMO circuits) or the available PICU beds for admitting new patients may be limited. As a general rule, a clinician owes a *duty to care* to one's current patients. This duty obligates one to have a clear plan for dealing with limited resources, such as diverting or transferring patients to other facilities or staffing critical care beds in other areas of the hospital such as the postanesthetic recovery room. If available resources truly remain limited, a process of triage may be appropriate. Patients who are critically ill and need intensive care services, yet have a good likelihood of recovery, should receive highest priority. Patients with a terminal and irreversible illness who would not benefit from intensive care services should be given lower priority [11].

The Process of Delivering Care

The delivery of patient care in the PICU involves a multidisciplinary team approach, which requires good communication and collaboration among team members (including other responsible and consulting services). Close attending physician supervision of critical care fellows and residents rotating through the PICU is essential to quality patient care and safety. The opportunity to develop cognitive and procedural skills under such supervision should be consistent with the educational objectives for each level of training. Limitations in work hours for fellows and residents require systems of communication for ensuring the continuity of patient care across transitions in personnel. Finally, there should be a robust, easily accessible, and collaborative process of continuous quality improvement in the PICU involving representatives of the entire multidisciplinary team. In addition to reducing the possibility of future errors, the presence of such a process can be reassuring to parents when they are told (as they should be) about errors that have occurred that impact on the care of their child.

Moral Distress

Moral distress, as a general term, refers to the distress an individual who is working within a hierarchy may feel when asked to perform tasks about which one has a deeply felt moral objection. Moral distress has been used to describe the experience of nurses who must continue to treat a patient despite the personal conviction that LSMT should be withdrawn. However, moral distress may describe the experience of anyone (e.g., resident, fellow, or attending physician) who lacks the authority to act on a personal moral conviction. In fact, this feeling of disempowerment may involve the entire multidisciplinary PICU team in the face of parental refusal to authorize the withdrawal of LSMT. The solution is not to take unilateral action, but to have a process of open and respectful communication that allows for the expression of the different points of view. For those whose moral distress is not assuaged by such a process, there should be a mechanism in place by which they can remove themselves from the distressing situation (e.g., reassignment to another patient, transfer to another physician).

Communication with Parents

Informed consent in pediatrics involves a combination of parental permission and child assent, when appropriate [12]. Before being performed, necessary procedures should be discussed with parents, if reasonably available. The discussion should include the reasons for the procedure, complications, any alternatives, timing, and consequences. Procedures that are necessary to ensure the ongoing health and welfare of the child should be performed without delay. This approach is consistent with the ethical focus on the child's best interest and on the accepted legal precedent that even nonemergent procedures (such as suturing of minor lacerations) should take place without delay even absent parental permission.

Parents (and others) are morally and legally obligated to act in a child's best interest when making decisions about medical care. Given the diversity of religious and cultural values concerning child rearing in the United States, parents are granted wide discretion in determining which actions contribute to a child's health and well being. There are, however, limits on parental discretion. Thus, critical care providers should seek legal intervention when parents refuse to authorize *effective medical treatment that is likely to prevent substantial harm or suffering or death*. In fact, clinicians should provide such medical care while waiting for such an authorization, even over the objections of parents [13]. In addition, a parent of a child who has been critically injured by physical abuse has a conflict of interest when a decision to withdraw LSMT may change a legal charge faced by a parent, guardian, relative, or acquaintance from assault to manslaughter or homicide. When a physician suspects such a conflict, a court-appointed guardian ad litem should be sought who will represent the child's interests [14].

Communication with Children and Adolescents

Parents have the authority and responsibility to make decisions concerning a child's medical care, even over a child's objections. Nevertheless, a child (if capable) may benefit from exercising some control over his or her environment, such as the timing or location of a procedure (e.g., where to place an intravenous line). Many if not most adolescents are competent to make decisions about their medical treatment. The legal extent to which an adolescent can make health care decisions varies according to state law. An adolescent (i.e., person under the age of majority) may be considered *emancipated* and thus granted adult rights through court action or as a result of marriage, military enlistment, or being self-supporting and living independently. In effect, the *emancipated* adolescent should be treated in all aspects as an adult. A *mature minor* is a more narrow concept, focused on whether an adolescent is capable of and has the authority to give informed consent for certain forms of medical treatment [15]. Both legal concepts have limited application in the PICU, although we often justify adolescent involvement in decision making based on psychological maturity. Children and adolescents with chronic and life-limiting conditions often are (and should be, if capable) involved in decisions about their medical treatment. When an adolescent becomes an adult, hospitals are required to provide information about an AD and durable power of attorney for health care (DPHCA). A young adult living with a life-threatening illness may designate one parent as his or her DPHCA, which can be quite useful to resolve conflict in the event of parental conflict, separation, or divorce.

Decisions by Terminally Ill Adolescents

Normal adolescent development involves a gradual separation from parents, the development of self-confidence and individuality, and the ability to function independently. The process by which an adolescent takes on increasing autonomy in health care decisions may be accelerated for children with chronic disease. However, a chronically ill and/or dying adolescent may fail to reach other normal developmental milestones because of a lack of peer interaction or a need for ongoing parental support. While maintaining parental involvement, an adolescent should be supported in expressing his or her wishes about medical treatment [5].

An adolescent over the age of 14 years is presumed to have the capacity to make binding medical decisions, including the provision of LSMT for a dying adolescent. Most adolescents want to share decision making with other family members, stressing the importance of open communication and flexibility about treatment preferences apart from legal status. The preparation of an AD may clarify the wishes of a dying adolescent and garner the support of responsible parents (and others) for the adolescent's insights, values, and autonomy. From the time of diagnosis, clinicians should include a child in medical decisions in a developmentally appropriate manner with an increasing level of involvement. The mutual respect and trust that evolves from such an approach will minimize future conflict as the adolescent's condition deteriorates [5].

Conflict Resolution

A culture of open and respectful communication, including differences of opinion about difficult and complex treatment decisions, will minimize conflict. Conversations should be held in a private location with sufficient family support available, such as a social worker or chaplain. Individuals, including family members, whose behavior is disruptive or threatening should be invited to leave with a security escort to ensure the safety of staff and other family members. Hospitals are required to have a mechanism for conflict resolution, which often involves the institutional ethics committee. The membership, policies, and procedures of an institutional ethics committee should conform to accepted professional standards, especially if it is involved in consultation over difficult ethical issues in the PICU [16].

Declaring Death and Organ Transplantation

Organ donation can occur after a patient is declared dead after either irreversible cessation of neurologic function (i.e., *brain death*) or cardiac asystole (i.e., *non-heart-beating donor* [NHBD]) [17–19]. The request for organ donation should be separated from the clinical discussion of brain death or withdrawal of LSMT. Parents and other family members may ask questions of the clinicians, but the in-depth discussion of organ donation should be done by other persons specifically trained for this purpose [20]. This decoupling approach improves donation rates and avoids an apparent conflict of interest between caring for the patient before death and organ procurement after death.

Brain Death

Guidelines for determining brain death in children have been established, combining clinical examination over differing periods of time depending on the child's age with confirmatory tests such as an electroencephalogram (demonstrating electrical cerebral silence) or cerebral perfusion study (demonstrating absent blood flow to the whole brain). Many institutions (and some states) have established policies stipulating the required examinations, tests, and observation periods to reduce variability in adhering to the guidelines [18]. Parents who are struggling with the reality of a child's death under these circumstances may be helped by observing a skilled clinician perform a complete *brain death* examination, including an apnea test. The clinician should have performed the complete examination previously so as not to be surprised by unexpected findings, such as vigorous spinal reflexes.

Two states (New York and New Jersey) allow families to object on religious grounds to the declaration of death using *brain death* criteria [18]. Under such circumstances, parents still may be receptive to forgoing LSMT. A unilateral decision by clinicians not to start new or escalate existing interventions is reasonable. However, a unilateral decision to withdraw existing interventions may be inappropriate absent the need to triage scarce PICU resources. Institutional processes for conflict resolution, including legal involvement if necessary, should be followed. Absent pertinent state law, third party reimbursement for the cost of continued LSMT for a *brain dead* patient may need to be addressed.

Cardiac Death

Recently protocols have been developed to allow for organ procurement after cardiac asystole (i.e., NHBD), under either controlled (i.e., after planned withdrawal of LSMT) or uncontrolled (i.e., after failed cardiopulmonary resuscitation [CPR]) circumstances [17]. The use of NHBD protocols in pediatrics following planned withdrawal of LSMT may increase significantly the number of transplantable organs [20]. The number of available organs somewhat depends on the choice of an acceptable time period for asystole to occur after the withdrawal of LSMT and before organ procurement (generally 1 to 2 hours).

Ethical concerns about NHBD protocols center on two principles that have served as the basis for organ donation: (1) the *dead donor rule,* limiting donation of vital organs to the irreversibly dead, and (2) the absence of conflict of interest between clinical care and organ procurement. With NHBD protocols, irreversibility means no spontaneous return of circulation after forgoing CPR rather than cessation of neurologic function despite any possible intervention. The waiting time after cardiac asystole to organ procurement varies among NHBD protocols, with some support for a uniform interval of 5 minutes. However, there are rare case reports of spontaneous return of cardiac function after more than 5 minutes of asystole, and uncertainty remains whether the neurologic criteria for death are satisfied after 5 minutes of asystole. As a result, some argue for extending the time period between asystole and organ procurement to 10 minutes [17].

Some clinicians are concerned about an apparent conflict of interest if parents are approached about organ donation following a decision to withdraw LSMT. Also, any organ preservation procedures started before death may create a conflict of interest between the ongoing treatment of the dying patient and preserving the viability of transplantable organs. Will parents assume that withdrawing LSMT was to obtain the child's organs? To avoid this interpretation, some argue that any discussion about NHBD organ procurement should be in response to a family-initiated question about organ donation. Also, the location and process of withdrawing LSMT should be considered carefully. Some withdraw LSMT in the operating room after the child has been prepared for organ procurement. There may be considerable pressure exerted on clinicians managing the child to hasten death so that organ procurement can take place within the predetermined time limit.

Research with Critically Ill Children in the Pediatric Intensive Care Unit

The regulations in the United States for the protection of human research subjects rest on two foundations: (1) voluntary and informed consent and (2) the independent review of the research risks. An ethical and responsible researcher is often added as the third foundation needed for the protection of human research subjects. The essential difference between research and standard clinical practice is researchers' commitment to generating knowledge while being responsible for the patients who are the human subjects of the research. For any research to be performed, the risks should be minimized and reasonable with respect to any anticipated benefits to the subjects and/or the importance of the resulting knowledge. Because children generally cannot give voluntary and informed consent to their own research participation, there are further restrictions on the research risks to which a parent may expose a child. The federal regulations allow children to participate in minimal risk research based on an analogy to parental authority to make decisions about risk exposure in everyday life. The regulations also allow children with a disease or condition to be exposed to slightly more than minimal risk in nontherapeutic research if the child's experience is similar to everyday life with that condition and the anticipated knowledge is of vital importance for understanding or benefiting that condition [15].

The term *therapeutic research* is misleading in that not all interventions or procedures included in a research study may offer the prospect of direct benefit to the subject. There are likely to be nontherapeutic aspects of the research, such as an extra blood test or chest radiograph. The nontherapeutic parts of the research need to be no more than a "minor increase over minimal risk" and cannot be justified by the anticipated benefit of other parts of the overall research study. The risks of interventions that offer direct benefit can be more than minimal. However, the risks must be justified by the anticipated benefit, and the balance of anticipated benefit to the risk should be at least as favorable as that presented by available alternatives. Readers are referred to the recent report of the Institute of Medicine for a more complete discussion of the ethical and regulatory issues in pediatric research [15].

A general ethical principle is that individuals who are capable of voluntary and informed consent be approached first about research participation. Also, children should be included in research only if scientifically necessary. An unintended result is that the majority of marketed medications are not labeled for use in children, especially in the setting of intensive care. Clinicians are left with a difficult choice of using medications *off label* and risking increased toxicity or decreased efficacy or not using a medication and potentially denying a child an important therapeutic advance. Over the past decade, the United States has granted 6-month patent extensions for the performance of requested pediatric studies, resulting in new pediatric labeling for many important drugs. However, pediatric clinicians continue to use medications in an *off label* and thus innovative way.

Innovative therapy can be defined as a new and/or unproven intervention done primarily for the benefit of the patient, with no intent to gather new information. As with the *off label* use of medications, innovative therapies may be more hazardous than research partly because they are not subject to peer review and toxicity has not been systematically assessed. Although innovative medical and surgical interventions are not subject to research regulations, some argue that clinicians have a moral obligation to submit innovative therapies to formal evaluation. Others express concern that the institutional system for review of research protocols lacks the timeliness and expertise needed to evaluate innovative treatments. Research in pediatric critical care is further hampered by the lack of existing infrastructure to conduct multicenter studies. For any given condition, the numbers of children cared for in a single institution are generally insufficient for an adequately powered clinical trial.

A special problem in the intensive care setting is the difficulty of studying interventions for life-threatening conditions, such as neuroprotection after successful cardiopulmonary resuscitation, where the experimental intervention needs to be administered either during or shortly after the initial event. Under these circumstances, it may be difficult if not impossible to obtain meaningful voluntary and informed consent from a parent. Before 1996, such research was conducted using *deferred consent* by which parents were asked for consent after the intervention had been performed. Recognizing that this approach was effectively a waiver of prospective consent, regulations were established that would allow for an exception from the requirement to obtain informed consent under certain conditions. For research that offers the prospect of direct benefit, the requirement to obtain prospective informed consent could be waived provided that (1) the human subjects are in a life-threatening situation; (2) available treatments are unproved or unsatisfactory; and (3) obtaining informed consent is not feasible. The feasibility of informed consent depends on the subject's condition, the difficulty of identifying potential subjects ahead of time, and the need to administer the experimental intervention within a relatively short time period. The regulations require a process of community consultation and public disclosure, after which an institutional review board (with federal oversight) could approve the research. Although somewhat cumbersome and little used in pediatrics to date, this process allows for community involvement in the ethics and design of research so that the development of new interventions for life-threatening conditions facing critically ill children can move forward despite the difficulty of obtaining meaningful informed consent [22].

References

1. American Academy of Pediatrics, Committee on Bioethics. Ethics and the care of critically ill infants and children. Pediatrics 1996;98(1):149–152.
2. Nelson LJ, Nelson RM. Ethics and the provision of burdensome, harmful or futile therapy to children. Crit Care Med 1992;20(3):427–433.
3. Helft PR, Siegler M, Lantos J. The rise and fall of the futility movement. N Engl J Med 2000;343:293.
4. Contro NA, Larson J, Scofield S, et al. Hospital staff and family perspectives regarding quality of pediatric palliative care. Pediatrics 2004;114: 1248–1252.
5. Freyer DR. Care of the dying adolescent: special considerations. Pediatrics 2004;113:381–388.
6. Nelson RM, Brodwin P. Professional power and the cultural meanings of biotechnology. In: Murray TH, Mehlman MJ, eds. Encyclopedia of Ethical, Legal, and Policy Issues in Biotechnology. New York: John Wiley & Sons; 2000:888–896.
7. Luce JM, Alpers A. End-of-life care: what do the American courts say? Crit Care Med 2001;29(2 Suppl):N40–N45.
8. Dyck AJ. An alternative to the ethic of euthanasia. In: Reiser S, Dyck A, Curran W, eds. Ethics in Medicine: Historical Perspectives and Contemporary Concerns. Cambridge, MA: MIT Press; 1977:529–535.
9. Nelson LJ, Rushton CH, Cranford RE, Nelson RM, Glover JJ, Truog RD. Forgoing medically provided nutrition and hydration in pediatric patients. J Law Med Ethics 1995;23(1):33–46.
10. American Academy of Pediatrics, Committee on Bioethics and Committee on Hospital Care. Palliative care for children. Pediatrics 2000; 106(2 Pt 1):351–357.
11. American College of Critical Care Medicine and Society of Critical Care Medicine. Guidelines for ICU admission, discharge and triage. Crit Care Med 1999;27(3):633–638.
12. American Academy of Pediatrics, Committee on Bioethics. Informed consent, parental permission, and assent in pediatric practice. Pediatrics 1995;95(2):314–317.
13. American Academy of Pediatrics, Committee on Bioethics. Religious objections to medical care. Pediatrics 1997;99(2):279–281.
14. American Academy of Pediatrics, Committee on Child Abuse and Neglect and Committee on Bioethics. Foregoing life-sustaining medical treatment in abused children. Pediatrics 2000;106(5):1151–1153.
15. Institute of Medicine, Committee on Clinical Research Involving Children, and Field MJ and Behrman RE, eds. Ethical Conduct of Clinical Research Involving Children. Washington, DC: The National Academies Press; 2004.
16. American Academy of Pediatrics, Committee on Bioethics. Institutional ethics committees. Pediatrics 2001;107(1):205–209.
17. Bell MD. Non-heart beating organ donation: old procurement strategy—new ethical problems. J Med Ethics 2003;29:176–181.
18. Capron AM. Brain death—well settled yet still unresolved. N Engl J Med 2001;344:1244–1246.
19. Lazar NM, Shemie S, Webster GC, Dickens BM. Bioethics for clinicians: 24. Brain death. CMAJ 2001;164:833–836.
20. American Academy of Pediatrics, Committee on Hospital Care and Section on Surgery. Pediatric organ donation and transplantation: policy statement: organizational principles to guide and define the child health care system and/or improve the health of all children. Pediatrics 2002;109(5):982–984.
21. Koogler T, Costarino AT Jr. The potential benefits of the pediatric nonheartbeating organ donor. Pediatrics 1998;101(6):1049–1052.
22. Morris MC, Nadkarni VM, Ward FR, Nelson RM. Exception From Informed Consent for Pediatric Resuscitation Research: Community Consultation for a Trial of Brain Cooling After In-Hospital Cardiac Arrest. Pediatrics 2004;114(3):776–781.

4

The Patient's Family in the Pediatric Intensive Care Unit

Sol J. Goldstein and I. David Todres

I feel terrible. I've had awful thoughts about him. I just want to get out of here. Out of the unit. Out of the hospital.

Mother in the pediatric intensive care unit

Introduction

The physical space of the pediatric intensive care unit (PICU) is usually filled with a symphony of sounds and noises that signify alarm situations. Tension reigns high amidst the hustle and bustle of activity as the staff cares for seriously and acutely ill children. Everyone associated with the unit lives and contends with this world of tension and learns to cope with the overabundance of stimuli. The young patients are dealing with their illnesses and their physicians as passive recipients of the treatment by the medical profession. In this chapter, we examine what happens to the families of the young patients; how the child's illness affects them during the child's stay on the unit; how this may affect them in the future; and the impact on the family dynamics between all of them as a result of the child's stay on the PICU. We first explore what these families experience and follow up with suggestions as to how to help them deal with this. We then take advantage of this opportunity to deal with the "family" of health care workers in the PICU and, most important, to explore how to deal with the families who are both peripheral yet a central part of the PICU, namely, our own partners and children.

The Parents

Parents see themselves as the people who will protect their children, keep them from harm, and keep them safe from those who would hurt them. The greater the danger to the child, the less inhibited are the parents in their approach to defending them. Witness the mother who will attack the bear that holds her child in its arms!

When parents bring their child to the PICU, they surrender that child to the care of the personnel of that unit. Physical treatment of the child will often involve the child being pierced, cut, and manipulated in such a way that would be unacceptable to anyone else dealing with this child. On the unit, however, all too frequently this is entirely necessary to save the life of the child. The child is benefited psychologically by the presence nearby of the parents, who are there as a source of comfort and as a tie and bond to the natural family constellation [1]. This means, however, that all too frequently the parents are witness to the child being subjected to procedures that are uncomfortable and distressing to him. Anyone else who would do such things to their child would be severely challenged. Here, however, the parents must stand by and cooperate with the health care providers and hope that this will eventually bring their child back to health, and as protectors they would be able to take over once again as the parents. The parents are then forced into the position of being passive participants, able to help their child only through cooperating with the staff whose treatment is, in reality, visualized psychologically as an assault upon the child. As one parent pointed out, *These people are being abusive of my child. They are doing to him something which he does not want to have done, which is not his choice, which is hurting him. They are holding him down and not giving in to his protests. Is this not abuse?*

The parent whose child is in the PICU must, therefore, transcend the usual strengths required by a parent in order to deal with his or her children to reach a new level. In doing so, this would allow that parent to deal with those caring for the child in a spirit of acceptance and cooperation. The parents must resist the impulse to avenge the hurt being done to the child and to cooperate with the medical staff. They must trust this will help their child and that the child will grow to forgive them for not having protected them from the medical helpers.

D.S. Wheeler et al. (eds.), *Science and Practice of Pediatric Critical Care Medicine*,
DOI 10.1007/978-1-84800-921-9_4, © Springer-Verlag London Limited 2009

Regression on the Part of the Parent

To deal with what is happening, the parent must retreat from the role of being the major decision maker and protector of the child. Parents need to give the leadership role over to the medical staff that are caring for and making decisions about their child. In addition, they give themselves over to hope and expectations and, not infrequently, to prayer and pleading of a higher being for the child's health. High anxiety comes with the unknown factors involved with the child in the PICU. Onto all of this superimpose the presence or absence of blame on oneself and others, depending on the reason for the child being in the PICU. Now it is relatively easy to account for a temporary regression that may display itself to the PICU staff as excessive demanding, questioning their future activities, suspiciousness, hostility, and even untoward aggressiveness toward those caring for the child [2]. If not dealt with promptly and sensitively, this may lead further to complaints filed about the medical care and the personnel involved or, worse still, verbal or physical attacks upon the staff. One of the authors (S.G.) recalls such an incident where a child died as a result of complications following cardiac surgery:

I was sitting in their hotel room with the family who had come from South America. Although they had been initially almost speechless, after a few hours they were talking to me about the fact that they had been assured at home that if they brought their child to this particular hospital, their child would be cured of its disability. They would not have to worry about the cardiac surgery. We spoke about the frustration of this and examined where they might be feeling blame. Suddenly, father rose from his chair, approached the window of the hotel room, pounded on it, and yelled "Its God's fault, its God's fault. God let us down." Someone needed to be blamed, it needed to be verbalized, and hopefully the blame was best expressed against a being away from the unit.

The Issue of Blame

We live in a society where blame is an integral part of our belief system. If something has gone wrong, somebody, somewhere, is responsible. They are to be punished for, admonished for, or berated for what they have done to cause bad things to happen or for what they have not done in order to prevent bad things from happening. It seems that it is simpler to deal with overwhelming feelings when a source of blame is placed on a person or a thing. In this way, one does not have to face the impossible task of dealing with overwhelming feelings of helplessness in the face of an emotional onslaught. When one is incapable of doing anything to change one's position, some comfort may, nevertheless, be gained from blaming others for the predicament in which they find themselves. This is a mechanism that is used by both adults and children in dealing with overwhelming emotional onslaught. When working with the family it is important to acknowledge to the members that this is a feeling that may be present. How to deal with these feelings is approached later in this chapter.

Unacceptable Feelings

Parents will often refer to their time on the unit as being like a nightmare. This may, in fact, be a good analogy. A nightmare is a situation in which one is horrified by being in a terrifying predicament and desperately looking for a way to get out. One way of extricating themselves from this nightmare is for the child to die. This is an unacceptable thought to most parents, yet the thought nevertheless does occur to them, even fleetingly. They are usually horrified by this, feel very guilty, and will do anything to keep their partner and others from knowing this thought. Yet, it is an entirely normal thought. In fact, this is a way of escaping the horrible nightmarish situation.

Bargaining

Many examples of bargaining exist, including parents who offer to give up smoking, to be more faithful in their marriage, to begin to attend church or synagogue regularly, to begin to operate more ethically in their business, to do more charity work, in return for their child's recovery. When one is desperate and searching for any way to ensure the health of the child on the unit, parents will offer almost anything in return. This is a form of what we call *magical thinking*—an offering of psychological sacrifices in order to achieve what one hopes for. Parents will often think, however, if others find out what they were doing they will consider them to be *weird* or *crazy*.

Self-Deprivation

Frequently we have found that parents, while sitting in the child's room or in the parents' lounge of the PICU, feel that they are not allowed to enjoy any pleasure in life. These feelings vary and may exhibit themselves in various ways. For example, they may not allow themselves to go out for a good meal during the day or evening, to get a good night's sleep, to go back home to be with the rest of the family for an evening, or to go to a movie during the hours when the child on the unit is asleep or unavailable to them. The parents feel as if any pleasure is something that is not allowed because it would be contrary to the experience that their child is going through. Often, they would not even allow themselves to think of anything lighthearted or humorous. They feel that anything that has given them comfort in the past is not to be allowed. The message, in essence, is, *How can we enjoy anything at all while our child's life is at risk—while our child is suffering and we cannot help?*

The Siblings

The authors are unaware of any family that has within it more than one child where there is an absence of sibling rivalry. It is entirely normal for siblings to be competitive with one another and vie for the attention of their parents. When one child enters the spotlight within the family, the others are usually quite envious and often quite resentful of their brother's or sister's presence. Others in the family try to get more attention from their parents and gain their own share of the spotlight or favorite person. Frequently, these children even entertain unconscious or near-conscious thoughts about eliminating that sibling and taking the spotlight for themselves. When the sibling is ill and in the PICU, they are often fraught with guilt for having had such thoughts and feeling any resentment toward the child now having so much of the parental attention.

Now, not only is the child receiving all the parental attention but he or she is also using the very energy from mother and father who need to devote themselves to doing whatever they can to deal with the serious illness of the child. They might ask themselves, how could they as siblings demand anything of their father and mother when their needs are so trivial in comparison to those of their sibling? How bad can they be that they entertain such negative thoughts about both their suffering parents and their suffering sibling? The siblings feel that they should be able to put their own needs aside and not resent all the attention given to the sick sibling.

In a related story we recall dealing with a father who was struggling with the birth of a severely deformed infant. One morning he stated very clearly that he had come to an unequivocal decision, along with his wife, to place the infant for adoption by an agency. They felt they could no longer handle the situation with the infant. They came to this decision after an incident when their other child had come to the father crying because she had fallen, skinned her knee, and wanted some comfort. The father had turned in a fit of anger towards her and yelled at her because she was being *such a suck* when her sister was in the hospital unable to breathe and having difficulty in simply staying alive. He related the look of horror on his little 3-year-old daughter's face. At that moment, he felt strongly that he would not speak to her again in that way and that this situation was no longer tolerable. He felt that he could not take away her childhood and development because of the misfortune of the severely limited newborn.

This attitude occurs over and over again within the families of the children in the PICU. The gap between the mundane, everyday chores at home and the life and death situation in the PICU becomes difficult to bridge. While the ill child is in the PICU, everyday life does go on, and the rest of the children still have their day-to-day needs. For example, they may complain about their homework assignment, or falling and bumping their knee, or not being able to watch a favorite television program. This response is entirely normal on the part of the children. They may feel badly for the sick sibling but still require their own needs to be met.

The children may have desires to visit with their sibling in the PICU, or they may choose not to. They may express these desires, or they may choose to keep them to themselves. This may depend on the freedom to interchange and debate these situations with one another and with their parents. The siblings will often have questions and issues to discuss with their parents, yet they are worried that they will overburden the already exhausted and challenged parents.

How to Handle All of the Above

There is much about the PICU and what the family is exposed to and involved with that is beyond our control. However, one has to look at what can be done. Health care providers working with these families must maximize everything positive and possible. It is important for families to be involved in these processes and activities. Ultimately, the parents' involvement is of help to the child and the staff. Table 4.1 highlights the details that follow.

It is important to provide an environment for the family that will minimize their stress. Families have often stated that facilities that allow them to be comfortably close to their child with appropriate privacy are extremely helpful. The introduction of a harpist on our unit has been found to help relieve the stress of patients, families, and staff!

It is an unfortunate reality that, in the PICU, the parents are deprived of their ability to participate as active parents. They have to stand by and observe the medical staff do their work. However, we as the medical staff should make certain that as much as possible the parents should be appropriately involved in the caretaking

TABLE 4.1. Suggestions for physicians dealing with families.

1. Arrange for a quiet room to sit with the family, unhurried and away from the demands of the unit.
2. Talk to them in simple terms about what is happening to their child, what you are attempting to do, and the chances for and against the child's recovery.
3. Ask them for their questions and their input, respecting cultural and religious perspectives and recognizing the need for interpreter service.
4. Empathize with the frustrations, fears, temptations, and anxieties with which they struggle.
5. Do not judge them on their thoughts. Instead, acknowledge and validate their feelings.
6. Try to meet with them regularly and more frequently, even for short periods, to keep them updated on their child's condition.
7. Designate a specific team member to deal with the family when the stay in the PICU is prolonged. Families have difficulty relating to multiple physicians.
8. Encourage the family's continued involvement with the other members of the family.
9. Always remember to bear with them and tolerate their silence as well as their own ways of expressing their emotions.
10. When the parent has been directly responsible for what has happened to the child, take whatever action is required to provide for the immediate and future safety of that child as well as the other children in the family. Do so, however, without being judgmental of the people involved.

of the child. We also must recognize, however, that while they are on the unit the parents are still under the supervision of the medical staff. The parents need to realize that the children who are at home and not on the unit as a patient need the comfort of the parents. When the parents become involved in looking after the needs of their other children, they will feel that much the better for this, since they are now functioning in their regular capacity. The children themselves will not feel so deprived by the parents and, therefore, resentful of the child on the unit as their parents begin to fulfill their needs. They all need to speak to one another, to discuss both positive and negative feelings about the illness of the sibling. The parents must recall that the children need to be parented and not judged for the feelings that they entertain about the child on the unit. One will find, usually, that even with the absence of discussion about the initial resentment, the children will begin to talk about that sibling—relating stories between all of them. The parents and children might be best served through bringing up how the afflicted child's illness has disrupted their family and its normal functioning. They could verbalize their understanding of how resentful and conflicted the children at home might be feeling. They may even get themselves to apologize to the other children for not having been as available or good humored as they usually are.

For all concerned, this is salutary. Questions about what will happen to this child in the PICU and specific concerns about the sick child need to be addressed. Hopefully, the parents will be able to share with the children any positive aspects of the case or to be able to talk to them about how worried they are, too. This may be helped by assistance from one of the trained personnel from the PICU (e.g., social workers, child life specialists, or chaplains). We have found social workers committed to the unit to be invaluable in helping to identify families' concerns and providing suggestions for coping. At times chaplains assigned to the unit can be an important resource for the families' spiritual distress. Families should be given the option of having a chaplain made available to them.

It is important that parents are apprised of what tests their child will have to undergo, when to expect the test, and when the results will be available. Delays in communicating this information to families lead to a great deal of distress. Also, informing families of their child's progress while in the operating room for many hours will help to relieve anxiety on their part.

It is equally important that the personnel from the PICU make the parents aware of some of the conflicts that have been mentioned above. This includes conflicted feelings of resentment toward the medical staff for what they are doing; while thankful for the efforts being put forth toward helping their child, parents may be blaming of one another, medical staff, or the deity [2]. All of these feelings need to be discussed in the context of being normal feelings so that those who experience them are not labeled *weird* or *crazy*. Similarly, the personnel dealing with these parents can bring up the topics of bargaining, self-deprivation, blame, and guilt at wishing this nightmare to end. This should be the accepted and usual way in which families deal with these crises. The parents should be told that they cannot do anything more than they are doing for themselves and for the child. It should be emphasized that leading a family life that approaches the norm as much as possible will help the parents and the children at home. The team has to impart to them that they are all working toward the same purpose—to help the child toward recovery and for the family to alleviate stress. There will be times, however, that they have to be guided to look at the reality of the situation at the cost of giving up on false hopes. On the other hand, one should not dispel all hope. Those of us who work with the parents must recognize that they are coming from different life experiences, varied ethnic and religious backgrounds, and disparate belief systems. These need to be respected because people deal with their lives in many different ways during times of crisis [3,4]. What is, however, common to all of them is their function as parents, and this must be encouraged at all times for the betterment of both the parents and the children.

One must remember that during the times of crisis of a child in the PICU, the family is going through all types of bargaining and will frequently turn to religion and to their clergy for help. We must recognize these people and their individual beliefs, listen to them, and try to work with them in an effort to have them understand what the staff is attempting to accomplish and allow their input with their religious view of illness, death, and dying, as long as the health of the child is not compromised. Enlist the help of the hospital chaplains.

One of the authors recalls clearly an incident wherein a child from a culture and country quite different from ours was on the unit and doing very poorly. The child, in fact, was dying despite the best efforts of the team. The staff was quite perturbed when the child's father showed up on the unit with a little box containing a mixture of ashes that he had obtained from someone's fireplace and the blood of a rooster that he had slaughtered within the past hour. They were refusing to allow him to spread this on the floor at the foot of the child's bed. In fact, they were horrified at what they considered a voodoo practice. These doubts continued until a senior staff member, a native of New Zealand, asked the question, *Can it be less help to them than we and our treatments are being at this time? Would it harm anyone to allow this?* We all learned a very valuable lesson.

The authors have found that sometimes what seems obvious to health care providers is not obvious to the parents. We must make these things understandable to them, in an accepting manner, while discussing some of these difficult thoughts in a matter-of-fact way, without judgment [5]. It is helpful to open a discussion between parents and staff, parents and children, or parents and children

and staff in a manner that can be most helpful to everyone. A comment like *you will find yourself at times to feel very resentful of those of us who are around and working with your child and who appear to be quite happy or free of stress despite the fact that you are feeling so sad and stressed* or *there are times when you will feel like striking out in anger and frustration for some of the procedures that we have done on your child, but we are doing them in order to help the child and not because we wish to hurt him or her.* Another frequently helpful comment is, *This is a nightmarish situation for all of you. We do hope that everyone here will be able to get through this to help your child.* The person dealing with the family has to make it clear to the parent that nothing that they have done has produced this illness. The exception to this is of course a case where parents have been clearly abusive or neglectful of children. You may even bring up the fact that *succeeding at something or enjoying something does not take away from your child's chances at getting better. Allowing yourself to go to a movie, enjoy a good meal, or have a good night's sleep will not deprive your child of chances of getting better.*

What does one do when one or both of the parents is partially or wholly to blame for what has happened to the child? This situation might occur if the child's illness is a byproduct or direct result of a genetically determined aberration or anomaly in which the parent is a carrier of the same defective gene or if the child's affliction is a consequence of the parent's having been involved in or caused an accident that resulted in the child's injury. The accident could have been caused by ignorance, carelessness, or even negligence on the part of the parent. The person dealing with the family is working with parents in distress. If one or both parents are involved in harmful activities that endanger the child or others in the family, then we as professionals must do whatever is required to protect the children from such caretakers. This would involve the reporting of harmful acts by the family to the appropriate authorities so the children will be protected.

As helping staff and qualified health care professionals, we need to remember that we are not judges or police personnel. We must deal with our own feelings within ourselves and discuss them with colleagues, especially mental health professionals assigned to the unit. To help parents of a child in distress, we must recognize that our negative feelings aroused by their behavior will not help the child or the family. The therapeutic dealings with abusive and destructive parents may be the most difficult task of the staff of the unit. As staff members we must deal with and separate ourselves from these abuses.

When the child's predicament is cause by an actual accident we must recognize how very difficult this is for the parents. We must devote our energies to relieve them of their guilt by clarifying for them the fact that they did not wish to hurt their child. One has to repeat for them the fact that what they did to their child happened by chance and was not something that they purposely set out to do. One may even say that having had angry feelings with this child in the past, or having felt exasperated in dealing with the child in the past, has nothing to do with what actually happened in the accident.

In essence the role of the supportive worker with the parents is to first bring them away from self-blame, self-deprivation, and the blaming of others. It is important to openly discuss matters that parents unconsciously perhaps feel uncomfortable bringing into the open. Parents need to know that they are not alone in having thought this way. Let them know that they are not being judged by the staff for thinking this way and they should not be judging themselves. If they are experiencing thoughts and feelings that they consider evil or crazy or weird, let them know that these are not uncommon for people who are going through what they are experiencing. What they are experiencing is akin to a nightmare, and they have no choice other than to go through it with the staff's support. As parents, they need to support one another, because the return to health will be accomplished through concentrating on parenting their children.

Does this require special expertise? It is our contention that every health care professional should lend an empathic and nonjudgmental ear and allow families to speak as much as they need. It is important to show tolerance and allow them to come to their own resolutions rather than bombarding them with advice. A person experienced in the ways of the PICU and its effects on the family can be of great assistance by allowing parents to hope without giving false hope. It is not the profession so much as the sensitivity of the deliverer of the message that is of most importance.

Presence of Families at Resuscitation and Performance of Complex Procedures

Until fairly recently, there existed a "blanket policy" of excluding families of critically ill children from viewing resuscitation and complex procedures performed on their children. This practice was based on the premise that these procedures would cause family distress, and their presence might affect the staff performance of these procedures. A number of recent studies have challenged this approach, demonstrating that family presence not only did not generally produce undue psychological distress but was seen by families as a positive benefit to them and to the patient [6,7]. Some authors of studies of adult patients and families have challenged this. McClenathan et al. [8] surveyed professionals regarding family-witnessed resuscitation and showed that the majority of critical care professionals do not support the current recommendations of emergency cardiovascular care and cardiopulmonary resuscitation guidelines of 2000. In a survey study by Helmer et al. [9], members of the Emergency Nurse Association and American Association for Surgery of Trauma were much more in favor of family presence at resuscitation following trauma. It appears that the special bond between parent and child makes this an important and necessary consideration for pediatric patients [9]. Acceptance of family presence is higher among nurses than physicians and increases among physicians of rising seniority [10]. There is evidence that the bereavement process is eased if a family member witnesses the resuscitation. Our practice has been to offer the parents the choice with the understanding that if they prefer not to, that is an acceptable choice that would be supported. It is essential that the family presence is guided by a staff member who ensures that it is continuously supported to meet their needs. When medical and nursing staffs have had previous experience with the presence of family during resuscitation, they are more accepting of this practice [11].

Dealing with the Difficult Family

The family that is identified as being difficult is usually the one that (1) challenges our decisions; (2) interferes with the treatment process by not complying with the rules of the unit, such as the limitation of number of visitors or of the time of the visits to the unit; (3) threatens law suits or complaints to professional bodies; (4) complains to other parents of children of the unit; (5) refuses to speak or be spoken to by anyone other than the director of the unit; (6) constantly consults with others who may not know or understand the workings of the unit or the manifestations of the child's disease and its sequela—for example, other parents, outside physicians, clergy, or relatives; (7) is outwardly and openly abusive of those dealing with their child; and (8) wishes to perform rituals or to carry out religious activities that are quite foreign to those working on the unit. When dealing with such people we, once again, have to avoid being judgmental but deal with family members as distressed people who are attempting to take some control over what is happening to the child on the unit—to fulfilling the parenting role. They are uncomfortable in a passive role, are distressed by what is going on, and are attempting to deal with the situation. We have to recognize that admonishing, arguing, and being defensive in our dealings with such family members and their advisors is of little use and could actually be injurious to all concerned.

Difficult families are usually best handled by assigning one staff member, usually a mental health professional, to deal with them on a regular basis and to act as a mediator with other staff members. The head of the treatment team should be readily available to this staff member and to the family. The person dealing with this family should meet in a private room away from the scene of all the action. The staff member's role is to listen to the complaints of the family with an open mind in an attempt to understand their complaints from their point of view. The staff person should be cognizant that the family is reacting with panic, is highly anxious, and is tense. It must be made clear, however, that under no circumstances are they to abuse any of the people who are caring for their child. One way of explaining this to the anxious family is to point out that you yourself would do anything to ensure the happiness and contentment of the person taking care of you or your child should either of you require someone's help. More gets accomplished through kindness and understanding than it does through berating, admonishing or belittling. It is imperative that you set this tone in dealing with the difficult family.

Listen closely to the complaints of the *difficult family*. Sometimes their requests and complaints do contain valid and good criticisms. From these complaints have often come many positive changes to our entire system. Do you recall the days when parents were not even allowed to visit in the hospitals with their children because the children "cried and carried on" when they left? Now we recognize and welcome the parents staying with their children whenever this is possible because it benefits all.

When you speak with threatening families, try to tell them that you do hear and appreciate their concerns and fears and will do what can be done within reason. Point out, however, that you are limited to what is possible and beyond that nothing can be done. Tell them that you cannot and will not try to stop them from lodging their complaints but you wonder whether this will help anything, including whether this would help them feel better or help their child get better.

When family issues center around breaking hospital rules about visitation—the number of people visiting the child or the length of time being spent with the child—examine why the rules are there and whether they can be bent. A discussion should be held with the staff to consider whether visits that interfere with staff routines are simply inconvenient or are really affecting the treatment of children on the unit. Staff may consider being flexible about visitation rules when visits are not inconveniencing the child or the other children in the PICU and are not interfering with patients' treatments.

We must recall that the morale of the staff of the unit is of utmost importance. If a family cannot be dealt with by the staff, a transfer to another hospital or a meeting with the ombudsman of the hospital should be offered to the family. It should be pointed out that we do not wish to hold them or their child in the unit against their wishes. If it is their desire to leave, the staff needs to explain that this will not be opposed even though the staff might advise against it. It is the "difficult" families that make the discussions at the regular sessions with the mental health professional lively, animated, and often most helpful.

Imparting Bad News

All health care providers recognize that breaking bad news to families of children in the PICU is something we cannot avoid [12]. The first rule is to make certain that we do not delay, equivocate, or hesitate in doing so. Each piece of bad news must be shared before parents suddenly become overwhelmed with too much bad news at once. It is a natural tendency to avoid telling bad news and often to avoid the family all together. The staff needs to deal with the bad news as one would with the immunization process: start with smaller doses to allow for the build up of the handling of the bad news. It is important to meet with the parents in a secluded place away from the bedside, unless the situation dictates that there is no choice. Sit down with the parents and whoever is involved in their support system such as other family members, friends, and clergy. Communication should be straightforward and honest, offering hope if there is any, while being as succinct and clear as possible. If the family asks, offer alternatives if possible. If they request plans and direction, then offer the help of those on your team who can help with this. When communicating bad news to families, allow them to talk, cry, and express their frustrations. Your communication tone should be empathic rather than defensive, while expressing the knowledge that you and the team have, are, and will continue to do their best.

Appropriate team members need to be available for families. Impress upon them that they will be involved in all decisions. The staff member should encourage families to recognize that this does not mean that they can make clinical and therapeutic decisions that would appear not to be in the best interests of the child.

Remember that frequently families requiring your support want and need silence—a silence that should not be broken because of your discomfort. Showing empathy, support, understanding, and patience is the best practice. The discomfort and pain of the family is yours to help them deal with, not your own to express to them. Be available to them and let them know of this.

End-of-Life Care

At times the PICU team will have to deal with the family in an end-of-life situation [13,14]. The family's functioning at this time will depend much on their values, previous experiences of a loss, how they coped with it, and their religious and spiritual beliefs. At this time, too, intense emotions erupt, including anger, denial, guilt,

and distrust. The family needs to trust the PICU team. Open honesty, respect, and compassion need to be shown to the dying patient and family because these are important determinants of family satisfaction [15]. It is helpful to work together with the family with a focus on the child's quality of life and relief of pain and other symptoms. In this regard, the palliative care team can be especially helpful, and their resources should be integrated into the care of the child and the family. Giving the family confusing messages of hope and despair adds to the family's burden. The PICU team needs to respect the family's religious and cultural beliefs as to how the child should die [16]. It is important that a bereavement follow-up meeting is arranged for the family to help them come to terms with the loss of their child. Usually this takes place 8–12 weeks after the death of the child [17].

Working with the family of the dying child demands heroic effort and compassion. What positive effect it can have for the family in their grief is well illustrated in the following letter received by the nurses in our PICU [18]:

In the almost three weeks that we were in the pediatric ICU (PICU), we witnessed at least two if not three deaths besides our son's. We know that death is a part of your job and therefore must be dealt with as each sees fit. As I envision it, it must be put in a spot where you are able to handle it. For many it means not letting yourself get too attached to the patient. For many it must mean not letting yourselves feel, much like we reacted, when the others died. But even knowing this, after our son died, I have to admit that I found myself wondering if "you" (the staff) thought about him—and us.

I thought you probably did but realized that the next child was needing you and that your lives no longer involved us. You HAD to move on, whether you thought about us or not. . . .

It seems funny that we'd be so happy to see people we barely knew but your visit and the effort it took to come, signifies a great deal. It meant that you DID care about our baby. Our gratitude for this cannot be overstated, and the solace we derived from your caring was—and is—immense. And since grief and these ceremonies are for the living, it meant that you cared about us, too. Please know that we genuinely appreciate the gesture. At the heart of our pleasure at seeing you, I've come to realize, is that here were two people who actually knew our son as the dear little individual he was. Friends of many years and many in our families did not share, for obvious reasons, in his preciously short life—as did you. It made your visit all the more poignant. A special thanks for that. Please do not feel that your encouragement helped to give us false hope. Hope is what got us through those three weeks. Despair could wait.

Leaving the Intensive Care Unit

Finally, we must recognize that the work of the helping professionals is not finished once the people leave the unit [19]. Follow-up sessions with the family may be indicated in order to help them reintegrate the child into the home so that the child is accepted by the siblings. The child needs to be accepted and not punished for having been the center of the family attention for so long. Neither should the child be set up as the *angelic child* who was so close to death that they can now do no wrong. Parents might become overly protective and overly indulgent at the expense of their other children. The follow-up sessions also allow us to gauge how the family is returning to equanimity after such a traumatic experience. The sessions help to mitigate relentless suffering, dreaming about, reliving, and rethinking the ordeal in the PICU [20].

The Staff of the Pediatric Intensive Care Unit as a Family

Each and every staff member of the PICU is to all intents and purposes a member of one family. All members of this family—professional, technical, clerical, and maintenance staff—need to be recognized for their unique and varied contributions toward the healthy functioning of the unit as a whole. The presence on the intensive care unit of a middle-aged cleaning lady who spoke with a heavy ethnic accent was appreciated by patients' families, who frequently made reference to her encouragement and her empathic comments about how difficult it was for certain families on given days.

The staff needs to be helped to recognize the value of their support of, and respect for, each other as they work to care for critically ill children and their families while dealing with the *politics* of the institution. The team leader must be able to oversee all of this and to help facilitate the smooth working of the unit where the contributions of individual members of the team are valued.

In general the staff need to learn the rules of working together under extremely stressful circumstances and making proper use of the Cs—Constructive Confrontation, Clarification, and Collaboration—or the benefit of all concerned. The presence of a mental health specialist is helpful to understand the particular dynamics involved in the PICU and operative in the families of the patients. Such a specialist could be a valued consultant to various team members and especially to the leader.

The entire staff must recognize that successful treatment of patients includes dealing with their families, which requires both the cooperation and interaction of a multitude of people. Each person needs to recognize that his or her role is a crucial one while respecting that it is interdependent with the roles of each and every other member of the PICU team. This will lead to a sensitive and sensible interplay between everyone concerned and ultimately to the benefit of the family culture so important to the PICU.

The leader must impart to his or her team the need to balance one's adult executive functions in working on the unit each day with equally important play activities that are childlike. These play activities have constantly changing rules, a lack of direct purpose, and a goal of solely achieving psychological pleasure. Again, the mental health expert can be of utmost use in assisting the staff in distinguishing between childlike play and the less beneficial, purposeful, organized, and rule-governed games of adults. In addition, we recommend regular communication sessions for team members where problems can be dealt with through direct, goal-oriented communication and airing of differences to reach solutions.

The Other Families of the Intensive Care Unit

It is our experience that there are other important families involved in the PICU—the families of each staff member. One of the dangers that PICU staff face is minimizing the hurts of the children in our own families. A PICU staff person may spend the day carrying out procedures on children on life support, inserting arterial lines, maintaining blood gases, and resuscitating children. After such a day it would not be farfetched to predict the response of one of the parents on returning home, who could even be forgiven for becoming easily exasperated by a 4-year-old demanding to be played with or crying because the request for chocolate milk has not been fulfilled at a moment's notice. How often do we have to keep ourselves back from saying to our children, "Don't be such a baby. You hardly bumped your head and you are crying so hard. Do you know what it is like to really be hurt?" Our children's hurts and needs, no matter how trivial they seem to be in comparison to the needs of the children on the PICU, are real and urgent. In our role as parents it is important for us to be able to deal with and fulfill them. We need to remember that our 3-year-old daughter's hurt feelings are the most important hurt feelings that we have to deal with when she approaches us; just as our 4-year-old budding basketball star's jammed thumb is as important to us as any aberration of blood gases on the unit may be.

Once, an intensive care physician spoke about feeling terrible, that he could not share his work with his children because he felt that *this might gross them out*. It is our feeling that, on the contrary, while we should not be sharing intimate details with what goes on there, there is nothing wrong with letting our children know that the people who work the PICU are no less the heroes than are the firemen and policemen in our society. The PICU staffs are dealing with life and death situations that are the aberrant exceptions to the lives of most of the people in our society. They live their work lives while constantly confronting the exceptions to the rule that everything will go on well in life.

We cannot help but quote the 3-year-old daughter of one of the authors (S.G.) who said one evening at the dinner table, *You are so much nicer a daddy on the days you are at the hospital because you don't yell at us for spilling the milk all over*. She seemed, even at that tender age, to have grasped the point of all of this, namely, that being aware of the terrifying problems of patients on the unit makes spilled milk a small and laughable problem.

References

1. American Academy of Pediatrics, Committee of Hospital Care, Institute for Family-Centered Care. Family-centered care and the pediatrician's role. Policy statement. Pediatrics 2003;112:691–696.
2. Groves JE, Beresin EV. Difficult patients, difficult families. New Horizons 1998;6:331–343.
3. Kleinman A, Eisenberg L, Good B. Culture, illness and care: clinical lessons from anthropologic and cross-cultural research. Ann Intern Med 1978;88:251–258.
4. Betancourt JR. Cultural competence—marginal or mainstream movement? N Engl J Med 2004;351:953–955.
5. Todres ID, Earle M, Jellinek MS. Enhancing communication: the physician and family in the pediatric intensive care unit. Pediatr Clin North Am 1994;41:1395–1404.
6. Clark AP, Aldridge MD, Guzzetta CE, Nyquist-Heise P, et al. Family presence during cardiopulmonary resuscitation. Crit Care Nurs Clin North Am 2005;17:23–32.
7. Boudreaux ED, Francis JL, Loyacano T. Family presence during invasive procedures and resuscitations in the emergency department: a critical review and suggestions for future research. Ann Emerg Med 2002;40:193–205.
8. McClenathan BM, Torrington KG, Uyehara CFT. Family member presence during cardiopulmonary resuscitation; a survey of US and international critical care professionals. Chest 2002;122:2204–2211.
9. Helmer SD, Smith RS, Dort JM, Shapiro WM, Katan BS. Family presence during trauma resuscitation: a survey of AAST and ENA members. J Trauma 2000;48:1015–1024.

10. Mitchell MH, Lynch MB. Should relatives be allowed in the resuscitation room? J Accid Emerg Med 1997;14:366–369.

11. Sacchetti A, Carraccio C, Leva E, Harris RH, Lichenstein R. Acceptance of family member presence during pediatric resuscitation in the emergency department: effects of personal experience. Pediatr Emerg Care 2000;16:85–87.

12. Fallowfield L, Jenkins V. Communicating sad, bad, and difficult news in medicine. Lancet 2004;363:312–319.

13. Van der Feen JR, Jellinek MS. Consultations to end-of-life treatment decisions in children. In: Steinberg ED, Youngner SJ, eds. End-of-Life Decisions: A Psychosocial Perspective. Washington, DC: American Psychiatric Press; 1998.

14. Sahler OJZ, Frager G, Levetown M, Cohn FG, Lipson MA. Medical education about end-of-life care in the pediatric setting: principles, challenges, and opportunities. Pediatrics 2000;105:575–584.

15. Kirk P, Kirk I, Kristjanson LJ. What do patients receiving palliative care for cancer and their families want to be told? A Canadian and Australian qualitative study. BMJ 2004;328:1343–1347.

16. Barakate LP, Sills R, LaBagnara S. Management of fatal illness and death in children or their parents. Pediatr Rev 1995;16:419–423.

17. Cook P, White DK, Ross-Russell RI. Bereavement support following sudden and unexpected death: guidelines for care. Arch Dis Child 2002;87:36–39.

18. Todres ID, Armstrong A, Lally P, Cassem EH. Negotiating end of life issues. New Horizons 1998;6:374–382.

19. Wharton RH, Schalich WO. From recovery through rehabilitation: you can get there from here. New Horizons 1998;6:363–373.

20. Jellinek MS, Catlin EA, Todres ID, Cassem EH. Facing tragic decisions with parents in the NICU: clinical perspectives. Pediatrics 1992;89:119–122.

5
Scoring Systems in Critical Care

Thomas J. Cholis III and Murray M. Pollack

Introduction

Scoring systems have become commonplace. Clinical scores, such as the Apgar score and Glasgow Coma Scale (GCS) score, are used daily to influence health care decisions for individual patients. The Pediatric Risk of Mortality (PRISM) and other physiology-based scores (e.g., the Acute Physiology and Chronic Health [APACHE] score) have become the standards in critical care medicine in determining the degree of the severity of illness within a unit. These scoring systems examine common variables and predict the patient's mortality risk. By providing objective severity of illness information, these scores allow comparisons of therapies, units, and hospitals by contrasting expected outcomes to observed outcomes. In addition, hospitals can use objective severity of illness data to assess quality by comparing their care facility to similar facilities or historical controls. In the current climate of health care cost-consciousness, the implications of comparing various institutions with the utilization of health care [1] can have an important effect on the reimbursement and evaluation of intensive care units.

Development

An important aspect of creating a scoring system is ensuring that the system fills a specific need within the clinical realm. Perhaps most important to a successful scoring system is the seemingly simple process of choosing an outcome. The outcome predicted by the scoring system must be clearly defined and separated from the predictive variables. Death or survival is a clear, separate, and easy outcome to determine. Other examples, such as discharge to home or extubation for a defined period of time, are also clearly defined clinical outcomes. Conversely, functional status and quality of life are not clearly defined and therefore are subject to physician bias and interpretation. A scoring system using a subjective outcome has a higher likelihood of not being successfully validated.

Developing a scoring system depends on choosing clear, easily defined predictor variables that are clearly defined and adhering to methodologic standards. The predictor (independent) variables should be selected a priori and should be objective, exhaustive, well defined, and mutually exclusive. Predictor variables should not overlap. For example, using the heart rate and the Apgar scores as separate variables or outcomes from one another would *double count* heart rate because it is a component of the Apgar score [2]. The predictor variables should also be well defined and easily applied outside the initiating institution. This requirement increases the chances that the scoring system will be externally valid. Choosing predictor variables can involve a wide range of data information, including the following: physiologic status, physiologic reserve, diagnoses, and therapeutic response [3].

The scoring systems most commonly used in the intensive care unit (e.g., APACHE, PRISM) use physiologic data points as their most important predictor variables. This naturally appeals to critical care physicians as the monitoring and maintaining of physiological stability is intrinsic to the care of the critically ill patient. Physiologic reserve is a similarly commonly used variable, usually reported as chronic disease state and age. The extremes of age are often used to estimate physiologic reserve. For example, a history of prematurity is often used for evaluating physiologic reserve as low birth weight predicts increased mortality risk. Furthermore, diagnoses appeal to clinicians as they apply to the understanding of a disease process. For example, the diagnosis of respiratory syncytial virus (RSV) in a previously healthy 2 year old has a very different implication than an RSV diagnosis in a former premature infant with cyanotic heart disease. Certain scoring systems have attempted to use diagnostic coding [4] as an initial variable along with the associated pathophysiology of the disease associated with a mortality outcome.

Subjectively derived scoring systems rely on experts to select variables that are important. Potential advantages are that such scoring systems are quicker and less expensive to derive. However, the determination by experts of the clinical scores subjects the scores to the experts' bias. Therefore, these scores may perform less well than objectively derived scores. The initial APACHE system [5] is an excellent example of how a subjective scoring system should be initiated. By choosing specific, easily defined variables, determining the weight, importance, and interaction among these variables, and identifying a clearly derived outcome, the authors of the initial APACHE system maximized the validity of their subjective

D.S. Wheeler et al. (eds.), *Science and Practice of Pediatric Critical Care Medicine*,
DOI 10.1007/978-1-84800-921-9_5, © Springer-Verlag London Limited 2009

scoring system. The experts selected 34 potential measurements and then weighted the separate variables to reflect their contribution to the outcome. For example, they subjectively estimated that a pH <7.15 had an equivalent mortality risk as a mean arterial pressure of less than 50.

The objective method for scoring system development generally requires a large database to determine statistically important predictors. For example, the PRISM [6] score objectively assessed the variables in the Physiologic Stability Index (PSI), a pediatric subjectively determined severity of illness score. Thus, the contribution of the individual variable to the outcome (survival/death) was determined statistically, not by clinical experts. The time, cost, and expertise required to collect a large, reliable database are disadvantages to this methodology. Another disadvantage is that the subject population, if not sufficiently encompassing, will present a population bias. The importance of a deviation from normal of a physiologic variable would be different in a unit that has a very unique practice pattern compared with the *routine* treatment practice. For example, the Clinical Risk Index for Babies [7] was developed in 1993 but incorporated data from the pre-surfactant era when neither surfactant nor antenatal corticosteroid use was widely available. Clearly these two therapies had a large effect on outcome, and reassessment of the score became necessary [8]. This study was then further updated [9] and statistically analyzed to improve its calibration.

Multivariable analyses are the standard for developing objective scoring systems. Various types of statistical analyses can address specific outcomes within the scoring system. Dichotomous variables (e.g., survival or death) or continuous variables (length of stay) [10] can be statistically accommodated. An important aspect of logistic regression analysis is that there are a sufficient number of outcomes for the number of predictor variables. A traditional rule suggests that there should be at least 10 of the least common outcomes [11,12] for each predictor variable included in the prediction model to avoid errors.

Judging the usefulness and applicability of clinical scores is important. The data needed for the predictive variables within the system should be easily obtained and readily available. The more routinely collected variables (e.g., vital signs) increase applicability of the scoring system compared with variables that depend on uncommon tests. Inter-rater and intra-rater reliability provide important information when assessing a scoring system. A weakness of subjective assessments (e.g., physicians assessing pain on a 1 through 10 score) is the large inter-rater variability. Objective variables (e.g., vital signs) improve inter-rater reliability.

Content and construct validity are also important. Content validity is *what makes sense* to experts. Subjectively derived scores generally have good content validity because they appeal to the common sense of clinicians. Scoring systems with high content validity more easily become ensconced in the medical field. The Apgar score had subjectively chosen variables at the time of its creation. Clearly, the appeal of an easy and readily assessable score with high content validity can help achieve great success as a scoring system. Construct validity, on the other hand, is the statistical performance that a score does what it is intended to do. External validity refers to the applicability of the score to a separate patient population than the initial study. Internal validity is separating out specific subsections of the patient population from which the score was derived. For example, applying a score to a specific subsection such as congenital heart disease patients should mirror the same scoring system performance as the entire patient popula-

tion. Typically if a system has poor internal validity, it is unlikely to have good external validity.

Three statistical methods used to assess performance are the chi-squared goodness-of-fit test, the z-score, and receiver operating character (ROC) curve analysis [13,14]. The goodness-of-fit test evaluates a score's calibration by comparing the predicted versus observed outcomes over the range of illness. The z-score compares the observed to the predicted numbers of outcomes over all illness strata and expresses the ratio in terms of a normalized curve. The ROC curve analyzes the index's performance over the range of cutoff points. These cutoff points are determined by the sensitivity (true positives, correct prediction outcome) and specificity (true negative, correct alternate prediction). The area underneath the curve is a measure of the score's overall performance and is the best measure of discrimination. The most accurate scoring system has a single point that correctly assesses outcome, creating an ROC area of 1.0. A scoring system equivalent to chance has an index of 0.5. The closer the area index is to 1, the better the discrimination of the scoring system.

Finally, Laupacis et al. [11] recommend that scoring systems maintain a *sensibility* standard. A key component is the expected use of the scoring system. For example, scoring systems focused on clinical variables in the trauma bay require different variables and ease of calculation than a mortality-risk model. The GCS score requires quick, easily obtainable variables in contrast to the physiologic variables of PRISM. Because mortality-risk scores compare and contrast severity of illness and individual hospitals, they require a higher standard of statistical accuracy and reliability.

Clinical Score Uses

Scoring systems are developed for a diverse range of clinical and statistical situations. Each application requires different predictor variables and statistical calculation for the intended purpose. As an example, the Apgar and PRISM scores have very different intentions. A quick clinical score to rapidly assess newborns has different statistical necessities than one to assess and contrast intensive care unit performances.

An important use of scoring systems is external benchmarking [1], which compares institutional performance to an external standard of institutions. Benchmarking for pediatric intensive care units (PICUs) is the comparison of individual PICUs to other PICUs. The performance measure most commonly used in PICU benchmarking is the standardized mortality rate, where the observed mortality rate is divided by the expected mortality rate based on the clinical scoring system. A single unit's performance can be compared and contrasted with those of other facilities in the benchmarking group as well as the historical units used to develop and calibrate the severity score. If the standardized outcome is lower or higher than expected, an explanation for the difference should be sought. Before the use of the APACHE and the PRISM scores, only ICU crude mortality rates could be compared, which inadequately accounted for the varying degrees of illness in different ICUs. For example, adult ICU mortality rates ranged from 6.0% to 43.0% in the early 1980s, demonstrating the need for correction by severity of illness.

Scoring systems have helped set national as well as local health care policies. For example, the Leapfrog group recently recommended pediatric intensivist presence in PICUs based on research comparing intensivist versus nonintensivist PICU models using

PRISM scores to control for severity of illness. Internal benchmarking is the comparison of performances within the same institution. Internal benchmarking allows institutions to assess their changes over time by comparing outcomes while ensuring that changes in patient case mix has not accounted for the performance measure change. Generic benchmarking is the term used to describe the comparison between the standard or previous method of care to a new method or technology.

Scoring systems have multiple other uses. They are very common in the medical literature. Most modern clinical research reports use a physiology-based score to control for severity of illness in the patient populations. This allows the researchers, reviewers, and readers to account for differences between the study groups. Clinical scores such as the Croup score [15] have been used as endpoints in therapeutic trials. Care maps and pathways for physicians and staff taking care of patients also use clinical scoring systems to assess in making therapeutic decisions. For example, the GCS score [16] is used to rapidly assess neurologic status and provides information relevant to the need for tracheal intubation or observation in trauma patients (e.g., GCS <8). Physicians have considered using scoring systems for prognostication [17] as well. Object risk assessment could help physicians to make a treatment plan, counsel family members, and settle interdisciplinary disagreements.

Scoring Systems Examples

One of the earliest modern scoring systems was the Apgar system, whereby newborn infants were assessed by their physiologic status. Although in her initial publication of the scoring system Dr. Apgar recommended the score not be applied to individual patients [2], it is frequently used to make clinical assessments and supplement clinical judgment. The GCS score was presented in 1974, and, although it initially was published without statistical validation, it became standard of care worldwide to assess neurologic status and to predict outcome. These scores both had extraordinarily high content validity, greatly aiding their inclusion into clinical practice.

Disease-Specific Scoring Systems

Disease-specific scoring systems have a high clinical appeal to physicians and health care providers. Scoring systems based on the pathophysiology of a specific disease emphasize the nuances and progression of current comprehension of the disease. Meningococcemia, a disease with a high pediatric mortality rate and a well-recognized clinical symptomatology, lends itself perfectly for these types of scoring systems. Numerous scoring systems have been developed to predict mortality in pediatric patients with meningococcemia. These scoring systems contain known variables within the disease process, including temperature and the presence of certain physical examination findings, such as ecchymosis and nuchal rigidity [18]. However, when trialed against the more generic forms of scoring systems [19], these systems have not proven to be as effective.

The Therapeutic Intervention Scoring System

Proposed in 1974, the Therapeutic Intervention Scoring System (TISS) [20] was the first quantitative scoring method to measure severity of illness, albeit indirectly. The TISS score had 76 thera-

peutic and monitoring interventions from 1 to 4 based on degree of complexity and invasiveness. The TISS points increase as the severity of illness increases. For example, pulmonary artery catheter placement is usually performed for only the sickest of patients, so it receives a higher TISS score than, say, nasogastric tube placement. However, the TISS score has institutional bias associated with it because it depends on therapeutic and monitoring philosophies, which vary among institutions. The TISS score remains an excellent tool for tracking therapeutic interventions and indirectly reflects cost of care.

The Acute Physiology and Chronic Health Score

The APACHE [5] system was published in 1981 as a scoring method that was devised subjectively as a prediction system for severity of illness and probability of mortality. The original APACHE was prospectively trialed with 582 patients in both a university hospital and a community hospital. The sensitivity and specificity were 97% and 49%, respectively. Positive and negative predictive values were 90% and 79%, respectively. The APACHE scoring system was further refined in 1985 and 1991 (APACHE II and III, respectively) to improve the scoring system. The second APACHE system dropped the number of variables from 34 to 12 and was externally and internally validated among 12 hospitals. The third version was prospectively analyzed [21] from 40 hospitals (17,440 patients), which predicted within 3% (ROC = 0.90).

The Pediatric Risk of Mortality Score

The PRISM score was objectively derived from the Physiologic Stability Index to reduce the number of variables and objectively assess their contribution to mortality risk using a multivariate logistic regression model. The initial PRISM score had 14 variables, with 23 ranges of these variables. Because objective scoring systems frequently require updating, PRISM III was developed and tested in 32 PICUs with over 11,000 patients [22]. The PRISM III initially had two prediction algorithms associated with the PRISM score for the first 12 and the first 24 hours of care, although current recommendations are to use only the prediction models based on the first 12 hours of care. It is the standard mortality risk assessment score used today. The PRISM III score is intermittently recalibrated and information concerning its performance is available on the pediatric intensive care unit evaluations (PICUEs) Web site [23].

The Pediatric Index of Mortality

The Pediatric Index of Mortality (PIM) was developed in eight Australian and British PICUs with only 5,695 patients. This model used eight variables [24] collected from the time of initial contact by the ICU team through the first hour of admission. This model was developed because of the idea that poorly managed patients would have worse physiology and therefore have a higher severity of illness and a higher PRISM score, rewarding poor management. There is no evidence to suggest that this proposition is correct. There are also some conceptual problems with the PIM score. First, single-measurement admission values are often subject to random variation or even *gaming* by the users, thus biasing the results [25]. Second, the time period for the data sampling is actually a variable time period starting when the ICU team contacts the patients (e.g., on transport or in the emergency department), creating the potential for large institutional biases. Third, the adult experience with the Mortality Prediction Model (MPM), the admission score upon which PIM is modeled, and physiology-based scores such as APACHE and the Simplified Acute Physiology Score (SAPS) have consistently shown better performance with the physiology-based scores.

Conclusion

The use and number of clinical scoring systems has grown substantially in the past 20 years. Intensivists use scoring systems in research, literature, and clinical practice to assess clinical patient status, mortality risk, prognostication, and quality of care. The comprehension of the methods to develop the scoring systems, including the selection of variables and statistical evidence associated with the systems, is an important aspect of a critical care physician's training and knowledge base.

References

1. Galvin R, Milstein A. Large employers' new strategies in health care. N Engl J Med 2002;347:939–942.
2. Apgar V. A proposal for a new method of evaluation of the newborn infant. Anesth Analg 1953;32:260–267.
3. Pollack MM. Prediction of outcome. In: Fuhrman BP, Zimmerman JE, eds. Pediatric Critical Care, 2nd ed. New York: Mosby; 1998:152–161.
4. Willson, D, Horn SD, Smout R, Gassaway J, Torres A. Severity assessment in children hospitalized with bronchiolitis using the pediatric component of the Comprehensive Severity Index. Pediatr Crit Care Med 2000;1:127–132.
5. Knaus WA, Zimmerman JE, Wagner DP, Lawrence DE. APACHE—acute physiology and chronic health evaluation: a physiology based classification system. Crit Care Med 1981;9:591–597.
6. Pollack MMP, Ruttimann UE, Getson PR. Accurate prediction of the outcome of pediatric intensive care. N Engl J Med 1987;316:134–139.
7. The International Neonatal Network. The CRIB (Clinical Risk Index for Babies) score: a tool for assessing initial neonatal risk and comparing performance of neonatal intensive care units. Lancet 1993;342:193–198.
8. Pollack M, Kock M, Bartel D, et al. A comparison of neonatal mortality risk prediction models in very low birth weight infants. Pediatrics 2000;105:1051–1057.
9. Parry G, Tucker J, Tarnow-Mordi W. CRIB II: an update for the clinical risk index for babies score. Lancet 2003;361:1789–1791.
10. Hand DJ. Statistical methods in diagnosis. Stat Methods Med Res 1992;1:49–67.
11. Laupacis A, Sekar N, Stiell IG. Clinical prediction rules. A review and suggested modifications of methodological standards. JAMA 1997;277:488–494.
12. Harrell FE Jr, Lee KL, Mark DB. Multivariable prognostic models: Issues in developing models, evaluating assumptions and adequacy, and measuring and reducing errors. Stat Med 1996;15:361–387.
13. Flora JD. A method for comparing survival of burn patients to a standard curve. J Trauma 1978;18:701–705.
14. Lemeshow S, Hosmer DW. A review of goodness-of-fit statistics for use in the development of logistic regression models. Am J Epidemiol 1982;115:92–106.
15. Auseoj M, Saenz A, et al. The effectiveness of glucocorticoids treating croup: meta-analysis. BM. 1999;319:595–600.
16. Teasdale G, Jennett B: Assessment of coma and impaired consciousness. A practical scale. Lancet 1974;2:81–84.
17. Pollack MM. Appendix: prognostication scores. In: Field MJ, Behrman R, eds. When Children Die: Improving Palliative and End-of-Life Care for Children and Their Families. Washington, DC: Institute of Medicine of the National Academies; Chapter 2, also see www.nap.edu/catalog/1039.html.
18. Alistair PJT, Sills JA, Hart CA. Validation of the Glasgow Meningococcal Septicemia Prognostic Score: a 10-year retrospective survey. Crit Care Med 1991;19:26–30.
19. Leteurtre S, Leclerc F, Martinot A, et al. Can generic scores (Pediatric Risk of Mortality and Pediatric Index of Mortality) replace specific scores in predicting the outcome of presumed meningococcal septic shock in children? Crit Care Med 2001;29:1239–1246.
20. Keene AR, Cullen DJ. Therapeutic intervention scoring system: update 1983. Crit Care Med 1983;11:1–3.
21. Knaus WA, Wagner DP, Draper EA, et al. The APACHE III prognostic system: risk prediction of hospital mortality for critically ill hospitalized adults. Chest 1991;100:1619–1636.
22. Pollack MM, Patel K, Ruttimann U. PRISM III: an updated pediatric risk of mortality score. Crit Care Med 1996;24:743–752.
23. Pediatric Intensive Care Unit Evaluations. www.picues.org.
24. Shann F, Pearson G, Slater A, et al. Paediatric Index of Mortality (PIM): a mortality prediction model for children in intensive care. Intensive Care Med 1997;23:201–107.
25. Pollack MM, Patel KM, Ruttimann U, et al. Frequency of variable measurement in 16 pediatric intensive care units: influence on accuracy and potential for bias in severity of illness assessment. Crit Care Med 1996;24:74–77.

6

Outcomes and Quality: Definitions, Assessment, and Analysis

Susan L. Bratton and James P. Marcin

Growing Need to Measure and Assess Outcomes and Quality in Pediatric Critical Care

Background

Despite tremendous growth in medical knowledge and technology, translation of advances into clinical practice has been imperfect. Recent reports by the Institute of Medicine (IOM) [1–3], the Institute for Health Care Improvement [4], and the Agency for Healthcare Research and Quality (AHRQ) [5,6] have highlighted medical errors and frequent gaps in health care delivery and safety. Mandates from payers [7,8], state and federal regulators [9,10], accrediting bodies [11,12], as well as the public are increasing pressure on the health system to consistently document care quality and test methods for improvement. These same forces are marshaling financial pressure for health systems to make this information available to the public as well as to the purchasers of health care. Public accounting of outcomes and quality measures in health care may help to increase quality, lower costs, and help to restore public trust in the health system [1,13].

Quality efforts depend on identifying and tracking outcomes and other measures. High-acuity, error-prone departments, such as intensive care, require focused quality efforts. Intensive care units (ICUs) provide care for complex patients who frequently have multiorgan system dysfunction and a variety of co-morbidities. Care involves integration of clinical, physiologic, and laboratory data and often requires a high number of interventions per patient. All of these factors add to the complexity of their care as well as to the risk adjustment needed to determine standardized outcome measures for performance evaluation. Organizations such as the Leapfrog Group [14], the IOM [2], and the AHRQ have emphasized structural changes in ICU physician staffing (including pediatric ICUs [PICUs]) as one of three primary interventions to improve hospital-based medical care. The Leapfrog Group estimates that ICU mortality would decrease 30% in the United States if all patients were managed or co-managed by critical care medicine physicians [14].

Delivery of intensive care medicine is complicated, serving patients with diverse disease processes that require collaborative teams to produce better clinical outcomes and improve patient and family satisfaction at lower costs. This requires better co-ordinated care and enhanced communications with all hospital areas and departments. However, most efforts to define quality measures have been targeted to hospital-based care of adult patients [14–16]. Even national recommendations regarding case volume of high-risk procedures are limited to adult disease states such as coronary artery bypass grafting, percutaneous coronary interventions, abdominal aortic aneurysm repair, pancreatic resections and esophageal resections, with surgery for congenital heart disease as the sole targeted high-risk pediatric procedure [14,15]. Nevertheless, the outcomes and quality assessment movement will soon impact children's hospitals and pediatric critical care [17–19].

Definition of Quality

The IOM has defined *health care quality* as "the degree to which health services for individuals and populations increase the likelihood of desired health outcomes and are consistent with current professional knowledge" [20]. To assess health care quality, many measures are needed to quantitatively determine outcomes and quality. However, a notable constraint to quality improvement, particularly among pediatric health care, is the lack of structured research and explicit measures defining health outcomes.

Classification of Quality Problems

Health care quality problems are classified into three categories: underuse, overuse, and misuse. *Underuse* is the failure to provide a health service when it would provide a favorable outcome for the patient. Missed childhood vaccinations are an example of underuse. A pediatric acute care example of underuse is failure to provide patients with asthma an action plan to guide them to modify their asthma therapy during an exacerbation. *Overuse* occurs when a health service is provided under circumstances in which its potential harm exceeds possible benefit. An outpatient example would

D.S. Wheeler et al. (eds.), *Science and Practice of Pediatric Critical Care Medicine*,
DOI 10.1007/978-1-84800-921-9_6, © Springer-Verlag London Limited 2009

be prescription of antibiotics for cold symptoms, and an inpatient example is hospital admission for an otherwise healthy child with uncomplicated pneumonia before a trial of oral antibiotics. *Misuse* occurs when the patient receives an appropriate service but in a manner that leads to a preventable complication. *Misuse* and *errors* are not synonymous because not all errors result in adverse events or injury. An example of misuse is the treatment of streptococcal pharyngitis with amoxicillin leading to a rash in a child with a known penicillin allergy. Inpatient examples of misuse abound, including preventable adverse drug events and preventable surgical complications. In summary, the health system must strive to consistently deliver effective care to those who can benefit from it, to always reframe from providing inappropriate services, and to eliminate preventable complications [21].

Other important outcome and quality terms include *near miss*, which is any incident that could potentially lead to patient harm. An *adverse event* is any untoward medical occurrence. *Adverse drug reactions* are all noxious and unintended responses to a medication administered at usual doses. A *serious adverse event* is any event that results in death, is life threatening, requires inpatient hospitalization, prolongs existing hospitalization, or results in persistent or significant disability. A *preventable death* occurs when the patient received poor care that likely resulted in the patient's death. *System factors* are any elements or factors that influence how health care is delivered in a health care setting. System factors can be categorized as patient, task, provider, team, ICU **environment**, and institutional environment factors.

Framework for Outcomes and Quality Changes

The framework to address outcomes and quality improvement is important. The goal of measurement is to characterize and learn how to improve the system and care delivery. Strategic planning is critical and requires input from staff with direct patient care responsibilities. Ideas should be generated to improve the current system of care delivery. Caregivers must work cooperatively, and support from many groups may be needed. Once an outcome or quality issue has been identified, the measurement system must fit the improvement system [20]. The improvement team must have a measurement system that tests for changes and then be able to implement those efforts that result in improvements. Thus the ability to measure and follow outcomes is critical to improving the system.

Defining a Measure

Outcome and quality measures can be used for different purposes, including external reporting to regulatory agencies or for internal assessment and improvement efforts. *Benchmarking* refers to when outcomes and quality measures are compared among similar institutions for the purposes of comparing or ranking. To develop an outcome or measure of quality, one needs to prioritize the area for assessment. This area should be important and affect satisfaction with care, morbidity, mortality, or cost of care.

Outcomes and quality measures need to be clear, easily defined, and relevant, fulfilling a specified need. The measurement of the outcomes should also be time specific and adhere to well-defined methodologic standards [22]. Types of measurements include rates, continuous time measurements, and time to event ratios. For instance, one can evaluate late medication administra-

tion as an overall late medication rate, an overall average time of administration, or an absolute number of late medications administered.

The data collected, including the outcomes, quality measures, and contributing or circumstantial data, should have sufficient specifications that they can reliably be collected. Reliability, or the reproducibility of data collection, is improved by detailed data specification, well-developed collection instruments, and adequate training of data collectors [22]. The process should be pilot tested to ensure that the data collection system functions well and to determine if the collected information is believed to be important. The process then requires close examination to define the unit of analysis and the measure of performance. Finally, pilot data are needed to determine baseline performance [23]. Graphical representation of the data is frequently more compelling to care delivery teams than are tabular data, and both time-series charts and flow charts are helpful to show change in performance over time and the effects of quality initiatives [24].

Outcomes to Measure

One of the first models to evaluate health care quality was developed by Donabedian [25]. He proposed measuring three elements of health care: structure, process, and outcomes. Structure of care refers to hospital, provider, or patient characteristics (e.g., does the hospital have magnetic resonance imaging capability?). Process of care refers to the technical or interpersonal delivery of medical care (e.g., does the medical team provide state-of-the-art therapies or use clinical guidelines or pathways?). Outcomes of care refer to clinical endpoints (e.g., mortality rates or satisfaction of care). Lohr defined outcomes as the 5 Ds: death, disease, disability, discomfort, and dissatisfaction [26]. For an outcome to be a valid measure, it must be closely related to processes of care that can be modified to affect the outcome. For example, measuring the rate of inhaled corticosteroid use among patients with asthma is a valid process measure because the use of corticosteroids has been shown to reduce need for urgent asthma care [22].

Standard Intensive Care Unit Outcomes

Some states such as California require that pediatric ICUs collect standardized mortality data [27]. The most commonly used mortality scoring systems are the Pediatric Risk of Mortality (PRISM III) [28,29] and the Pediatric Index of Mortality (PIM2) [30]. The PRISM III includes demographic data as well as physiologic and laboratory data collected during the first 12 to 24 hours of ICU admission. The PIM2 data are collected at the time of admission to an ICU, and the time required to collect scoring data is less than required for PRISM III. Both systems perform well for large groups of PICU patients [31]. However, because death in the PICU is relatively uncommon, organ dysfunction has also been used as a measure of illness severity and a clinical outcome for therapeutic trials [32–34]. The Paediatric Logistic Organ Dysfunction (PELOD) score is a valid tool for measuring the severity of multiple organ dysfunction syndrome in the PICU [35–37]. Other examples of standard ICU benchmarking data include rates of catheter-associated bloodstream infections [38–44] and ventilator-acquired pneumonia [44].

Other Opportunities for Measurement

Other outcomes and quality measures frequently evaluated include extubation failure [45,46], unplanned extubation [47], catheter-associated thrombosis, skin breakdown, and medication errors [48–59]. Decisions regarding areas to measure and target for improvement should be driven by error event data that highlight either common or high-risk errors. The AHRQ has developed quality indicators that can be assessed using administrative data [60]. These indicators were developed after a comprehensive literature review, analysis of ICD-9-CM codes, review by a clinician panel, implementation of risk adjustment, and empirical analyses.

There are three modules measuring various aspects of quality. *Prevention quality indicators* identify hospital admissions that evidence suggests could have been avoided, at least in part, through high-quality outpatient care. *Inpatient quality indicators* reflect quality of care inside hospitals, including inpatient mortality for medical conditions and surgical procedures. These inpatient quality indicators include mortality for medical conditions and surgical procedures as well as utilization of procedures for which there are questions of overuse, underuse, or misuse. *Patient safety indicators* also reflect quality of care inside hospitals but focus on potentially avoidable complications and iatrogenic events. The indicators also target volume of procedures for which there is evidence that a higher volume of procedures may be associated with lower mortality.

In a recent paper, Sedman et al. [18] applied the patient safety indicators algorithms to the comparative database of the National Association of Children's Hospitals and Related Institutions from 1999 to 2002. They established mean rates in children's hospitals for each of the safety indicator events. Although some of the safety indicators appeared to be appropriate when applied to the pediatric population (e.g., foreign body left in during procedure, iatrogenic pneumothorax, infection caused by medical care, decubiti, and venous thrombosis), others were likely not valid measures of safety in pediatric patients (e.g., failure to rescue and mortality in low-risk Diagnostic Related Groups [DRGs]) [18]. The AHRQ has plans to develop pediatric-specific quality indicators in the near future.

The Plan-Do-Study-Act Cycle

Langley et al. [61] described a method to generate improvements in complicated systems. Three fundamental questions must first be answered: What change is to be accomplished? How will one determine if the change is an improvement? What changes can be made that will result in an improvement? The framework for changing the system is the Plan-Do-Study-Act (PDSA) cycle (Figure 6.1). The PDSA cycle is shorthand for testing a change in the real work setting by planning it, trying it, observing the results, and acting on what is learned. After testing a change on a small scale, learning from each test, and refining the change through several PDSA cycles, the team can implement the change on a broader scale to include the entire ICU or other ICUs within the organization [62]. Several examples of PDSA cycles in PICU care have recently been published [47,63–66]. One study involved decreasing unplanned extubation in a PICU. The planned interventions included identification of high-risk patients (toddlers), institution of a ventilator weaning protocol, institution of a sedation protocol, addition of

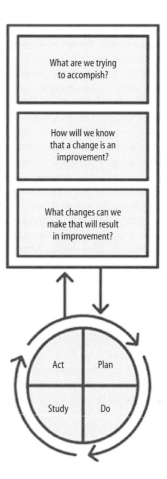

FIGURE 6.1. Plan-Do-Study-Act cycle. (Adopted from Berwick [62]. Copyright 1996 with permission from the BMJ Publishing Group.)

policies regarding number of personnel needed for turning and procedures such as chest radiographs, and continued staff education regarding patients and times of risk for unplanned extubation. The authors reported a steady decline in the number of unplanned extubations over the 5 years of study [47].

Targeting Outcome Measures

The IOM has set forth a vision for improved health care in the 21st century. The key elements for improvement are that health care should be *safe*—avoiding injury from care intended to help them; *effective*—providing services based on scientific knowledge; *patient centered*—providing care that is respectful and responsive to individual patient values; *timely*—reducing wait times for both those who receive and those who give care; *efficient*—avoiding waste; and, finally, *equitable*—providing care that does not vary because of personal characteristics [1]. These goals can be used to help focus outcome and quality measures for the ICU, the hospital, and the health system caring for pediatric patients. Each of these elements with some applications in critical care will be discussed.

Safe Care

Safety has traditionally been monitored by ICU morbidity and mortality meetings where complications and deaths are discussed.

Although such meetings are useful, they rarely addressed near-miss errors and traditionally do not evaluate errors that do not cause harm. The IOM and Leapfrog Group have strongly advocated increased use of technology to decrease errors [1,2,14]. The most frequently discussed issue is computerized order entry. Estimates predict that, with such systems, medication errors would decrease by over half [14]. However, because of cost constraints, less than 10% of hospitals in the United States have implemented such technology. Pediatric hospitals require specialized computer software given the large range of patient sizes, which further complicate implementation.

A new and exciting technology for increasing safety for infusion delivery is "smart pumps," which incorporate sophisticated computer technologies for storing drug information (i.e., drug library), making calculations, and checking entered information against dosing parameters [57,59]. These features offer a ready safety net for nurses to check the medication order. A recent study reported on a hospital program that implemented the use of smart pumps for 32 standard concentration medications, thereby significantly decreasing the number of medication errors captured in the hospital's incident reporting system compared with the year prior to the intervention [59]. Use of technology as a safety net in the pressure-filled area of critical care is an important method to decrease human errors.

Monitoring Systems

The AHRQ's Physiologic Stability Index (PSI) is a tool to help health system leaders identify potential adverse events occurring during hospitalization [67,68]. The AHRQ is providing the software as a service to hospitals to help identify and problem solve unsafe events [69]. An initial pediatric study using the PSI on the 2000 Healthcare Cost and Utilization Project dataset estimated that patient safety events incurred >1 billion dollars in excess charges for U.S. children in 2000. Young patients and those insured by Medicaid had a significantly greater risk of an adverse safety event, and almost all PSIs were associated with significant and substantial increases in length of stay, charges, and in-hospital deaths [70].

Effective Care

The IOM has defined effective care as "providing services based on scientific knowledge to all who can benefit and refraining from providing services to those not likely to benefit (avoiding underuse and overuse, respectively)" [1].

Standardized Mortality

The most recognized method for assessing the effectiveness of ICU care has been the standardized mortality ratio, which is the ratio of actual mortality divided by the predicted mortality based on mortality scores. Scores less than 1 reflect lower mortality than predicted by the patient's severity of illness, whereas scores greater than 1 reflect higher than predicted mortality (see Chapter 5). Currently the two most commonly used general PICU scoring systems are the Pediatric Risk of Mortality (PRISM III) [28,29] and the Pediatric Index of Mortality (PIM2) [30,31]. Recently, Jenkins and Gauvreau [71] reported a Risk Adjustment for Congenital Heart Surgery Score (RACHS -1) that used expert consensus and empirical data for risk of mortality after congenital heart surgery. This scoring system is new, but it may prove helpful when comparing

outcomes of surgery across centers to identify differences in performance [72,73].

Collaborative Data Sharing

The National Association of Children's Hospitals and Associated Institutions (NACHRI) [74] and the Virtual PICU [75] have jointly developed the Virtual PICU Performance System (VPS), which is a clinical database of children's hospitals that allows standardized data sharing and benchmarking among PICUs. All participating ICUs collect information on quality control, patient and hospital measures, diagnoses, interventions, discharge, organ donation, and PIM2 scores. The VPS can be used to track and trend individual and aggregate clinical patient data, facilitate patient flow, document patient care, or collect data for multisite research studies. It can also be used to compare patient mix, performance, and outcomes with peer ICUs.

Another large organization that allows comparison among peer institutions is the Child Health Corporation of America (CHCA) [19]. The CHCA members contribute to the Pediatric Health Information Dictionary (PHIS), which can be used for both clinical and financial comparative data. The PHIS includes diagnostic and demographic data as well as extensive charge information. Although the PHIS contains a flag for ICU admission, the database does not contain physiologic data. Severity of illness assessment includes a case mix index [76] and the All-Patient Refined (APR) DRG severity of illness scores [77]. The CHCA also has a collaborative called the Child Health Accountability Initiative to develop pediatric outcome and quality measures. Current efforts are directed to patient safety, pediatric medication error reduction, treatment of bronchiolitis, and pain management [78]. The PHIS data have been used to demonstrate the effects of evidence-based bronchiolitis clinical care guidelines across time and institutions [79].

The Kids' Inpatient Database (KID) is one in a family of databases and software tools developed as part of the Healthcare Cost and Utilization Project (HCUP) sponsored by the AHRQ. The KID for 2000 included 1.9 million hospital discharges from 27 state inpatient databases on patients 20 years of age or less. The KID can be used to study uncommon conditions, such as congenital anomalies; the economic burden associated with specific procedures or conditions; and the pediatric conditions most often associated with particular outcomes such as death in the hospital. However, KID does not include a marker for care in a PICU or severity of illness assessment [80].

Case Volume

Generally, a relationship between high case volume and improved health care outcomes has been described [14,72,81]. Presently, the AHRQ only includes congenital heart surgery as a quality indicator for hospital-level public reporting of high-risk pediatric procedures [14]. However, leaders in child health quality have targeted common pediatric surgical conditions such as appendicitis and tonsillectomy for analysis particularly related to safety [82]. Studies suggest that children admitted to PICUs [83] and those with uncommon problems such as intussusception have fewer complications and better outcomes when diagnosed and treated at larger volume pediatric centers [84]. Application of complex technologies such as extracorporeal life support has also been shown to be more successful in high-volume centers [85–87], and pediatric critical care providers need to help establish guidelines for conditions or technologies that are best delivered at regionalized centers [88,89].

Guidelines

Guideline use has not been extensively enumerated for pediatric critical care practice. Variation in ICU practice has been shown in management of common diseases such as asthma [90], presenting opportunities to standardize and improve care. Recent exceptions are the guidelines for treatment of pediatric patients with asthma [91], diabetic ketoacidosis [92], septic shock [93], and severe traumatic brain injury [94]. Currently studies have not evaluated whether implementation of these guidelines has been widespread or has improved outcomes. National efforts regarding implementation for the treatment recommendations of adults with septic shock [95] have been highlighted with a goal to decrease mortality by 25% [96].

Patient-Centered Care

Provision of "care that is respectful of and responsive to individual patient preferences, needs and values and ensuring that patient values guide all clinical decisions" [1] is a goal outlined by the IOM. Involvement of the patients and their families in medical decisions will vary by patient, with some intimately involved with decisions desiring detailed information, and other families will be more comfortable with providers making recommendations while keeping the family abreast of the child's condition. Although communication with families still remains an art [97,98], hospitals are becoming more friendly to families, and many ICUs have unrestricted or minimally restrictive family visiting rules. Many providers welcome parents during rounds when medical decisions are discussed. Currently, assessment of family-centered care relies on survey instruments. Some that have been used include the Picker Pediatric Inpatient Survey and the Multi-Dimensional Assessment of Parental Satisfaction [82], which are pediatric specific. Heyland et al. [99] reported on a survey used for families of adult ICU patients.

Timely Care

Timeliness can be characterized in two important ways. One measure involves timely and effective communication and wait times. More important in ICU care is the availability of resources to prevent harmful delay in care. Presence of critical care medicine physicians to direct care in the ICU has been shown to decrease mortality [14], and pediatric patients have greater survival when they receive care in a PICU [100,101]. Critically ill and injured children may not live close to a PICU. Most PICUs are in urban areas, and acutely ill patients may have to be stabilized in a community hospital before transfer. Proximity to a PICU has been shown to decrease mortality caused by trauma [102]. However, innovative use of technology in the form of telemedicine has been shown to effectively triage less complicated rural pediatric patients to receive care in their community hospital with a pediatric critical care consultation or if more severely ill to be transferred to a referral PICU [103]. Telemedicine has also been used for diagnosis of children with congenital heart disease [104] and for immediate support to remote locations during pediatric resuscitations [105].

Timeliness in transfer of information is critical in complex care situations. Multiple personnel and processes must interact, and communication is key. Studies of PICU patients have shown increased mortality at night, suggesting areas for improvement [106]. When all care providers are able to participate in care and exchange opinions regarding a patient's condition, timely interventions can be made [107,108]. Improved electronic transfer of information can help ensure seamless communication and eliminate illegible hard copies of records, which are currently a barrier to information flow.

Efficient Care

Waste avoidance is a logical concept; however, the quality of care should not be jeopardized. The staffing of most PICUs in the United States shows similar nurse- and physician-to-patient ratios with the exception of the smallest units (one to six beds) [89]. However, nursing shortages may well adversely impact pediatric care in the future. Increasing ICU beds increases the fixed costs of the ICU, and units that have excess beds typically have a greater number of patients admitted for monitoring (low acuity) rather than for receiving ICU-specific therapies such as mechanical ventilation or administration of vasoactive medications (high acuity). Such benchmarking allows ICUs to determine their proportion of low-acuity patients and a measure of ICU efficiency [109–111].

Patients who are more gravely ill stay longer, so clinical scoring systems are needed to calculate predicted length of stay (LOS). The standardized LOS is the ratio of the actual LOS and the predicted LOS. Technology utilization per day (e.g., mechanical ventilation) and standardized LOS can be compared for ICU efficiency benchmarking. Pediatric Intensive Care Unit Evaluations [112], NACHRI [76], the VPICU-VPS [75], and CHCA [19] offer such comparisons to their members.

Equitable Care

Finally, the quality of care should not vary by personal characteristics or geograph location. However, examples of worse health outcomes for poor and minority children abound [70,113–118]. Worse critical care outcomes may be due to lesser access to primary care [119,120], lower parental recognition of disease signs or symptoms leading to delay in diagnosis [115,121], greater risk for injuries [122], or to processes of ICU care such as hospital location [102] and discrimination [123,124]. Critical care medicine providers and the health care system must work to make health care equitable for all children in our care.

Conclusion

Outcomes in critical care are expanding to include not only risk-adjusted mortality but many other outcomes and processes. Providers must work within the system to improve data capture and quality assessments. Collaborative use of data and more universal definitions of important outcomes and health measures will allow ICUs to better gauge their status and target areas for improvement. Innovative use of technology can be implemented to limit risk from human error. A change in culture is evolving with a new focus on quality and outcomes and a growing need to track and compare them and demonstrate improvements.

References

1. Institute of Medicine, Committee on Quality of Health Care in America. Crossing the Quality Chasm: A New Health System for the 21st Century. Washington, DC: National Academy Press; 2001.

2. Institute of Medicine, Committee on Quality of Health Care in America. To Err is Human: Building a Safer Health System. Washington, DC: National Academy Press; 2000.

3. Institute of Medicine, Committee on Identifying Priority Areas for Quality Improvement. Priority Areas for National Action: Transforming Health Care Quality. Washington, DC: National Academies Press; 2003.

4. Institute for Healthcare Improvement. Critical Care. Available at: http://www.ihi.org/IHI/Topics/CriticalCare. Accessed November 2004.

5. Clancy CM, Scully T. A call to excellence. Health Aff (Millwood) 2003;22:113–115.

6. United States Agency for Healthcare Research and Quality. National Healthcare Disparities Report. Rockville, MD: U.S. Dept. of Health and Human Services, Agency for Healthcare Research and Quality; 2003.

7. Anthem Blue Cross and Blue Shield Join with Nine Hospitals and the American College of Cardiology to Reward Quality. Available at: http://www.anthem.com/jsp/antiphona/bcbs/int_primary.jsp?content_id=PW_035971. Accessed February 18, 2003.

8. Niagara Health Quality Coalition. Alliance for Healthcare Quality: Indicators of Inpatient Care in New York Hospital. Available at: http://www.myhealthfinder.com/newyork/doc/interpret.php. Accessed November 2004.

9. Center for Medicare and Medicaid Services. The Premier Hospital Quality Incentive Demonstration: Rewarding Superior Quality Care. http://www.cms.hhs.gov/quality/hospital/PremierFactSheet.pdf. Accessed November 2004.

10. Texas Health Care Information Council. Indicators of Inpatient Care in Texas Hospitals, 2002. Available at: http://www.thcic.state.tx.us/IQIReport2002/IQIReport2002.htm. Accessed November 2004.

11. Joint Commission of Accreditation of Healthcare Organizations: Performance Measurement in Health Care. Available at: http://www.jacho.org/pms/index.htm. Accessed November 2004.

12. National Association of Children's Hospitals and Related Institutions. Benchmarking and Data. Available at: http://www.childrenshospitals.net/Template.cfm?Section=Benchmarking_and_Data&Template=/TaggedPageDisplay.cfm&TPLID=53&ContentID=5973. Accessed November 2004.

13. Kaiser Family Foundation. National Survey on Consumers' Experiences with Patient Safety and Quality Information. Menlo Park: Kaiser Family Foundation; 2004.

14. The Leapfrog Group. The Leapfrog Safety Practices 2003: The Potential Benefits of Universal Adoption. Available at: http://www.leapfroggroup.org/media/file/Leapfrog-Birkmeyer.pdf. Access date: November 2004.

15. Agency for Healthcare Research and Quality. AHRQ Guide to Inpatient Quality Indicators. Available at: http://qualityindicators.ahrq.gov/downloads/iqi/iqi_guide_rev3.pdf. Accessed November 2004.

16. McGlynn EA, Asch SM, Adams J, et al. The quality of health care delivered to adults in the United States. N Engl J Med 2003; 348:2635–2645.

17. National Association of Children's Hospitals and Related Institutions. Benchmarking and Data: 2004 PICU Focus Group. Available at: http://www.childrenshospitals.net/Template.cfm?Section=Benchmarking_and_Data&Template=/. Accessed: November 2004.

18. Sedman A, Harris JM, Schulz K, et al. The relevance of the agency for health care research and quality patient safety indicators for children's hospitals. Pediatrics 2005;115:135–145.

19. Child Health Corporation of America. Performance Improvement CHCA Patient Safety for Children Initiative. Available at: http://www.chca.com/servpediat.html. Accessed November 2004.

20. Lohr KN, Schroeder SA. A strategy for quality assurance in Medicare. N Engl J Med 1990;322:707–712.

21. Chassin MR, Galvin RW. The urgent need to improve health care quality. Institute of Medicine national roundtable on health care quality. JAMA 1998;280:1000–1005.

22. Laupacis A, Sekar N, Stiell IG. Clinical prediction rules. A review and suggested modifications of methodological standards. JAMA 1997; 277:488–494.

23. Pronovost PJ, Nolan T, Zeger S, Miller M, Rubin H. How can clinicians measure safety and quality in acute care? Lancet 2004;363:1061–1067.

24. A Resource from the Institute of Healthcare Improvement. Available at: http://www.ihi.org/IHI/Topics/Improvement/ImprovementMethods/Tools/Run+chart.htm. Accessed November 2004.

25. Donabedian A. Evaluating the quality of medical care. Milbank Mem Fund Q 1966;44(Suppl):166–206.

26. Lohr KN. Outcome measurement: concepts and questions. Inquiry 1988;25:37–50.

27. California Children's Services Department of Health Services. California Children's Service (CCS) Manual of Procedures, CCS Standards for Pediatric Intensive Care Units. Sacramento: State of California; 1999.

28. Pollack MM, Patel KM, Ruttimann UE. The Pediatric Risk of Mortality III—Acute Physiology Score (PRISM III-APS): a method of assessing physiologic instability for pediatric intensive care unit patients. J Pediatr 1997;131:575–581.

29. Pollack MM, Patel KM, Ruttimann UE. PRISM III: an updated Pediatric Risk of Mortality score. Crit Care Med 1996;24:743–752.

30. Slater A, Shann F, Pearson G. PIM2: a revised version of the Pediatric Index of Mortality. Intensive Care Med 2003;29:278–285.

31. Slater A, Shann F. The suitability of the Pediatric Index of Mortality (PIM), PIM2, the Pediatric Risk of Mortality (PRISM), and PRISM III for monitoring the quality of pediatric intensive care in Australia and New Zealand. Pediatr Crit Care Med 2004;5:447–454.

32. Vincent JL, de Mendonca A, Cantraine F, et al. Use of the SOFA score to assess the incidence of organ dysfunction/failure in intensive care units: results of a multicenter, prospective study. Working group on "sepsis-related problems" of the European Society of Intensive Care Medicine. Crit Care Med 1998;26:1793–1800.

33. Le Gall JR, Klar J, Lemeshow S, et al. The Logistic Organ Dysfunction system. A new way to assess organ dysfunction in the intensive care unit. ICU Scoring Group. JAMA 1996;276:802–810.

34. Marshall JC, Cook DJ, Christou NV, et al. Multiple organ dysfunction score: a reliable descriptor of a complex clinical outcome. Crit Care Med 1995;23:1638–1652.

35. Leclerc F, Leteurtre S, Duhamel A, et al. Cumulative influence of organ dysfunctions and septic state on mortality of critically ill children. Am J Respir Crit Care Med, published ahead of print on October 29, 2004 as doi:10.1164/rccm.200405–630OC.

36. Leteurtre S, Martinot A, Duhamel A, et al. Validation of the paediatric logistic organ dysfunction (PELOD) score: prospective, observational, multicentre study. Lancet 2003;362:192–197.

37. Leteurtre S, Martinot A, Duhamel A, et al. Development of a pediatric multiple organ dysfunction score: use of two strategies. Med Decis Making 1999;19:399–410.

38. Stover BH, Shulman ST, Bratcher DF, et al. Nosocomial infection rates in US children's hospitals' neonatal and pediatric intensive care units. Am J Infect Control 2001;29:152–157.

39. O'Grady NP, Alexander M, Dellinger EP, et al. Guidelines for the prevention of intravascular catheter-related infections. The Hospital Infection Control Practices Advisory Committee, Centers for Disease Control and Prevention, U.S. Pediatrics 2002;110:e51.

40. Berenholtz SM, Pronovost PJ, Lipsett PA, et al. Eliminating catheter-related bloodstream infections in the intensive care unit. Crit Care Med 2004;32:2014–2020.

41. Richards MJ, Edwards JR, Culver DH, Gaynes RP. Nosocomial infections in pediatric intensive care units in the United States.

National Nosocomial Infections Surveillance System. Pediatrics 1999;103:e39.

42. Yogaraj JS, Elward AM, Fraser VJ. Rate, risk factors, and outcomes of nosocomial primary bloodstream infection in pediatric intensive care unit patients. Pediatrics 2002;110:481–485.

43. Odetola FO, Moler FW, Dechert RE, VanDerElzen K, Chenoweth C. Nosocomial catheter-related bloodstream infections in a pediatric intensive care unit: risk and rates associated with various intravascular technologies. Pediatr Crit Care Med 2003;4:432–436.

44. Elward AM, Warren DK, Fraser VJ. Ventilator-associated pneumonia in pediatric intensive care unit patients: risk factors and outcomes. Pediatrics 2002;109:758–764.

45. Kurachek SC, Newth CJ, Quasney MW, et al. Extubation failure in pediatric intensive care: a multiple-center study of risk factors and outcomes. Crit Care Med 2003;31:2657–2664.

46. Randolph AG, Wypij D, Venkataraman ST, et al. Effect of mechanical ventilator weaning protocols on respiratory outcomes in infants and children: a randomized controlled trial. JAMA 2002;288:2561–2568.

47. Sadowski R, Dechert RE, Bandy KP, et al. Continuous quality improvement: reducing unplanned extubations in a pediatric intensive care unit. Pediatrics 2004;114:628–632.

48. Kaushal R, Bates DW, Landrigan C, et al. Medication errors and adverse drug events in pediatric inpatients. JAMA 2001;285:2114–2120.

49. Fernandez CV, Gillis-Ring J. Strategies for the prevention of medical error in pediatrics. J Pediatr 2003;143:155–162.

50. Stucky ER. Prevention of medication errors in the pediatric inpatient setting. Pediatrics 2003;112:431–436.

51. Mullett CJ, Evans RS, Christenson JC, Dean JM. Development and impact of a computerized pediatric antiinfective decision support program. Pediatrics 2001;108:e75.

52. Kaushal R, Barker KN, Bates DW. How can information technology improve patient safety and reduce medication errors in children's health care? Arch Pediatr Adolesc Med 2001;155:1002–1007.

53. Cullen DJ, Sweitzer BJ, Bates DW, et al. Preventable adverse drug events in hospitalized patients: a comparative study of intensive care and general care units. Crit Care Med 1997;25:1289–1297.

54. Parshuram CS, Ng GY, Ho TK, et al. Discrepancies between ordered and delivered concentrations of opiate infusions in critical care. Crit Care Med 2003;31:2483–2487.

55. Pinheiro J, A. M, Lesar T. Systematic steps to diminish multi-fold medication errors in neonates. J Pediatr Pharmacol Ther 2003;8:266–273.

56. Mitchell A, Sommo P, Mocerine T, Lesar T. A standardized approach to pediatric parenteral medication delivery. Hosp Pharm 2004;39:433–459.

57. Malashock C, Shulls S, Gould D. Effect of smart infusion pumps on medication errors related to infusion device programming. Hosp Pharm 2004;39:460–469.

58. Cimino MA, Kirschbaum MS, Brodsky L, Shaha SH Assessing medication prescribing errors in pediatric intensive care units. Pediatr Crit Care Med 2004;5:124–132.

59. Parker HB, Grant MJ, Cash J, O'Connell M, Larsen GY. Standard drug concentrations and smart pump technology reduce continuous medication infusion errors in pediatric patients. Pediatrics 2004;5:510.

60. AHRQ. Inpatient Quality Indicators Overview. Available at: http://www.qualityindicators.ahrq.gov/iqi_overview.htm. Accessed November 2004.

61. Langley GJ, Nolan KM, Nolan TW. The Foundation for Improvement. Silver Springs, MD: API Publishing; 1992.

62. Berwick DM. A primer on leading the improvement of systems. BMJ 1996;312:619–622.

63. Slonim AD, LaFleur BJ, Ahmed W, Joseph JG. Hospital-reported medical errors in children. Pediatrics 2003;111:617–621.

64. Osmon S, Harris CB, Dunagan WC, et al. Reporting of medical errors: an intensive care unit experience. Crit Care Med 2004;32:727–733.

65. Intensive Care Unit Safety Reporting System. Available at: http://www.icusrs.org. Accessed November 2004.

66. Kilbride HW, Powers R, Wirtschafter DD, et al. Evaluation and development of potentially better practices to prevent neonatal nosocomial bacteremia. Pediatrics 2003;111:e504–e518.

67. Zhan C, Miller MR. Administrative data based patient safety research: a critical review. Qual Saf Health Care 2003;12(Suppl 2):ii58–ii63.

68. Zhan C, Miller MR. Excess length of stay, charges, and mortality attributable to medical injuries during hospitalization. JAMA 2003;290:1868–1874.

69. AHRQ Quality Indicators. Patient Safety Indicators Overview. Available at: http://www.qualityindicators.ahrq.gov/psi_overview.htm. Accessed November 2004.

70. Miller MR, Zhan C. Pediatric patient safety in hospitals: a national picture in 2000. Pediatrics 2004;113:1741–1746.

71. Jenkins KJ, Gauvreau K. Center-specific differences in mortality: preliminary analyses using the Risk Adjustment in Congenital Heart Surgery (RACHS-1) method. J Thorac Cardiovasc Surg 2002;124:97–104.

72. Jenkins KJ, Newburger JW, Lock JE, et al. In-hospital mortality for surgical repair of congenital heart defects: preliminary observations of variation by hospital caseload. Pediatrics 1995;95:323–330.

73. Kuhlthau K, Ferris TG, Iezzoni LI. Risk adjustment for pediatric quality indicators. Pediatrics 2004;113:210–216.

74. National Association of Children's Hospitals and Related Institutions. Benchmarking and Case Mix Index. Available at: http://www.childrenshospitals.net/Template.cfm?Section=Case_Mix&Template=/TaggedPage/TaggedPageDisplay.cfm&TPLID=79&ContentID=7064. Accessed November 2004.

75. National Association of Children's Hospitals and Related Institutions. Benchmarking and Data: Software and Tools: VPICU. Available at: http://www.childrenshospitals.net/Template.cfm?Section=Sotware_Tools&CONTENTID=7423&TEMPLATE=/ContentManagement/ContentDisplay.cfm. Accessed November 2004.

76. National Association of Children's Hospital and Related Institutions. Description of Methodologic and Hospital Specific Factors Affecting the Calculation of Children's Hospital DRG Case Mix Index. Available at: http://www.childrenshospitals.net/Template.cfm?Section=Search&Template=/Search/SearchDisplay.cfm. Accessed October 2004.

77. National Association of Children's Hospitals and Related Institutions. Summary of Current Status of All Patient Refined Diagnosis Related Groups. Available at: http://www.childrenshospitals.net/Content/ContentGroups/Benchmarking_and_Data1/Classification_Research/APR-DRGs1/Summary_of_Current_Status_APR-DRGs.htm. Accessed November 2004.

78. Dougherty D, Simpson LA. Measuring the quality of children's health care: a prerequisite to action. Pediatrics 2004;113:185–198.

79. Todd J, Bertoch D, Dolan S. Use of a large national database for comparative evaluation of the effect of a bronchiolitis/viral pneumonia clinical care guideline on patient outcome and resource utilization. Arch Pediatr Adolesc Med 2002;156:1086–1090.

80. Overview of the Kids' Inpatient Database (KID). Available at: http://www.hcup-us.ahrq.gov/Data. Accessed November 2004.

81. Halm EA, Lee C, Chassin MR. Is volume related to outcome in health care? A systematic review and methodologic critique of the literature. Ann Intern Med 2002;137:511–520.

82. Beal AC, Co JP, Dougherty D, et al. Quality measures for children's health care. Pediatrics 2004;113:199–209.

83. Marcin JP, Song J, Leigh JP. The impact of pediatric intensive care unit volume on mortality: A hierarchical instrumental variable analysis. Pediatr Crit Care Med 2005 (in press).

84. Bratton SL, Haberkern CM, Waldhausen JH, Sawin RS, Allison JW. Intussusception: hospital size and risk of surgery. Pediatrics 2001;107:299–303.

85. Kolovos NS, Bratton SL, Moler FW, et al. Outcome of pediatric patients treated with extracorporeal life support after cardiac surgery. Ann Thorac Surg 2003;76:1435–1442.

86. Haefner SM, Bratton SL, Annich GM, Bartlett RH, Custer JR. Complications of intermittent prone positioning in pediatric patients receiving extracorporeal membrane oxygenation for respiratory failure.
Chest 2003;123:1589–1594.

87. Bartlett RH, Roloff DW, Custer JR, Younger JG, Hirschl RB. Extracorporeal life support: the University of Michigan experience. JAMA
2000;283:904–908.

88. Rosenberg DI, Moss MM. Guidelines and levels of care for pediatric
intensive care units. Pediatrics 2004;114:1114–1125.

89. Odetola F, Clark SJ, Freed GL, Bratton SL, Davis MD. A national survey
of pediatric critical care resources in the United States. Pediatrics.
2005 (in press).

90. Roberts JS, Bratton SL, Brogan TV. Acute severe asthma: differences
in therapies and outcomes among pediatric intensive care units. Crit
Care Med 2002;30:581–585.

91. Global Initiative for Asthma. National Institutes of Health. Pocket
guide for asthma management and prevention in children. Available
at: www.ginasthma.con/ped.pdf. Accessed November 2004.

92. Dunger DB, Sperling MA, Acerini CL, et al. ESPE/LWPES consensus
statement on diabetic ketoacidosis in children and adolescents. Arch
Dis Child 2004;89:188–194.

93. Carcillo JA, Fields AI. Clinical practice parameters for hemodynamic
support of pediatric and neonatal patients in septic shock. Crit Care
Med 2002;30:1365–1378.

94. Adelson PD, Bratton SL, Carney NA, et al. Guidelines for the acute
medical management of severe traumatic brain injury in children and
adolescents. Crit Care Med 2003;31:S417–S490.

95. Hollenberg SM, Ahrens TS, Annane D, et al. Practice parameters for
hemodynamic support of sepsis in adult patients: 2004 update. Crit
Care Med 2004;32:1928–1948.

96. Institute for Healthcare Improvement. Critical Care: Sepsis. Available
at: http://www.ihi.org/IHI/Topics/CriticalCare/sepsis. Accessed
November 2004.

97. Burns JP, Mello MM, Studdert DM, et al. Results of a clinical trial
on care improvement for the critically ill. Crit Care Med 2003;31:2107–
2117.

98. Hardart GE, Truog RD. Attitudes and preferences of intensivists
regarding the role of family interests in medical decision making for
incompetent patients. Crit Care Med 2003;31:1895–1900.

99. Heyland DK, Rocker GM, Dodek PM, et al. Family satisfaction with
care in the intensive care unit: results of a multiple center study. Crit
Care Med 2002;30:1413–1418.

100. Pollack MM, Katz RW, Ruttimann UE, Getson PR. Improving the
outcome and efficiency of intensive care: the impact of an intensivist.
Crit Care Med 1988;16:11–17.

101. Pollack MM, Alexander SR, Clarke N, et al. Improved outcomes from
tertiary center pediatric intensive care: a statewide comparison of
tertiary and nontertiary care facilities. Crit Care Med 1991;19:
150–159.

102. Odetola FO, Miller W, Davis MM, Bratton SL. The relationship
between the location of pediatric intensive care unit facilities and
child mortality from trauma: a county-level ecologic study. J Pediatr
(in press).

103. Marcin JP, Nesbitt TS, Kallas HJ, et al. Use of telemedicine to provide
pediatric critical care inpatient consultations to underserved rural
Northern California. J Pediatr 2004;144:375–380.

104. Sable CA, Cummings SD, Pearson GD, et al. Impact of telemedicine on
the practice of pediatric cardiology in community hospitals. Pediatrics 2002;109:e3.

105. Kon AA, Marcin JP. Using telemedicine to improve communication
during pediatric resuscitations. J Telemed Telecare 2005 (in press).

106. Arias Y, Taylor DS, Marcin JP. Association between evening admissions and higher mortality rates in the pediatric intensive care unit.
Pediatrics 2004;113:e530–e534.

107. Baggs JG, Schmitt MH, Mushlin AI, et al. Association between nurse–
physician collaboration and patient outcomes in three intensive care
units. Crit Care Med 1999;27:1991–1998.

108. MacIntyre NR. Evidence-based ventilator weaning and discontinua-
tion. Respir Care 2004;49:830–836.

109. Pollack MM, Getson PR, Ruttimann UE, et al. Efficiency of intensive
care. A comparative analysis of eight pediatric intensive care units.
JAMA 1987;258:1481–1486.

110. Ruttimann UE, Pollack MM. Variability in duration of stay in pediatric intensive care units: a multiinstitutional study. J Pediatr 1996;128:
35–44.

111. Ruttimann UE, Patel KM, Pollack MM. Length of stay and efficiency
in pediatric intensive care units. J Pediatr 1998;133:79–85.

112. Pediatric Intensive Care Unit Evaluations: Assessing Quality and Efficiency: Scientific Background and Research. Available at: http://www.
childrensnationalmedicalcenter.com/picues/scientific_quality.aspx
Accessed November 2004.

113. Naclerio AL, Gardner JW, Pollack MM. Socioeconomic factors
and emergency pediatric ICU admissions. Ann N Y Acad Sci 1999;896:379–
382.

114. Keenan HT, Foster CM, Bratton SL. Social factors associated with
prolonged hospitalization among diabetic children. Pediatrics 2002;
109:40–44.

115. Bratton SL, Roberts JS, Watson RS, Cabana MD. Acute severe asthma:
outcome and Medicaid insurance. Pediatr Crit Care Med 2002;3:
234–238.

116. Kuehl KS, Baffa JM, Chase GA. Insurance and education determine
survival in infantile coarctation of the aorta. J Health Care Poor
Underserved 2000;11:400–411.

117. DeMone JA, Gonzalez PC, Gauvreau K, Piercey GE, Jenkins KJ. Risk
of death for Medicaid recipients undergoing congenital heart surgery.
Pediatr Cardiol 2003;24:97–102.

118. Tilford JM, Simpson PM, Yeh TS, et al. Variation in therapy and
outcome for pediatric head trauma patients. Crit Care Med
2001;29:1056–1061.

119. Ponsky TA, Huang ZJ, Kittle K, et al. Hospital- and patient-level characteristics and the risk of appendiceal rupture and negative appen-
dectomy in children. JAMA 2004;292:1977–1982.

120. Brown R, Bratton SL, Cabana MD, Kaciroti N, Clark NM. Physician
asthma education program improves outcomes for children of low-
income families. Chest 2004;126:369–374.

121. Kuehl KS, Loffredo CA, Ferencz C. Failure to diagnose congenital
heart disease in infancy. Pediatrics 1999;103:743–747.

122. Marcin JP, Schembri MS, He J, Romano PS. A population-based analysis of socioeconomic status and insurance status and their relationship with pediatric trauma hospitalization and mortality rates. Am J
Public Health 2003;93:461–466.

123. Haas JS, Goldman L. Acutely injured patients with trauma in Massachusetts: differences in care and mortality, by insurance status. Am J
Public Health 1994;84:1605–1608.

124. Erickson LC, Wise PH, Cook EF, Beiser A, Newburger JW. The impact
of managed care insurance on use of lower-mortality hospitals by
children undergoing cardiac surgery in California. Pediatrics 2000;
105:1271–1278.

7

Pediatric Intensive Care Unit Administration

Lorry R. Frankel

Introduction

As discussed in Chapter 1, pediatric critical care medicine is a relatively new specialty. The pediatric intensive care unit (PICU) developed as a geographically distinct special care unit within the hospital dedicated solely to the care of critically ill or injured infants and children. However, whereas other units have continued to evolve and further subspecialize—witness the development of the modern medical ICU, surgical ICU, cardiothoracic ICU, neurosurgical ICU, burn unit, and so forth—the PICU has, for the most part, remained multidisciplinary in concept, perhaps stemming from the relatively limited number of available PICU beds. For example, a 1990 survey identified a total of 301 PICUs in the United States. Nearly half of these units had between 4 and 6 beds, while only 6% had more than 18 beds. Interestingly, only 79.6% of these PICUs had a full-time medical director, and a pediatric intensivist was available in only 73.2% [1].

Since 1995, there has been an increase in the total number of PICU beds in the United States, with the largest growth in the number of PICUs with 15 or more beds [2]. The number of PICU beds appears to be increasing at a faster rate than that of the pediatric population, although the reasons for this discrepancy are not known [2,3]. Europe too has witnessed a growth in the number of PICU beds, although considerable differences in the structure, organization, and staffing of these PICUs are apparent [4]. The impact of this growth, both in the United States and abroad, remains to be evaluated. Several studies have documented significantly improved outcomes when children receive care in the PICU versus the adult intensive care unit [5–10]. Unfortunately, despite the growth in the number of PICU beds, many critically ill children still do not have access to quality pediatric intensive care. The continued need for distribution of relatively scarce resources has led to the concept of regionalization of pediatric intensive care,

further driving the need for multidisciplinary PICUs that provide care for both medical and surgical patients.

The Specialized Pediatric Cardiac Intensive Care Unit

The development of pediatric cardiac surgical programs has had a profound effect on the specialty of pediatric intensive care. With the field of congenital heart surgery rapidly expanding, many cardiothoracic surgeons and hospital administrators have expressed a desire to develop specialized pediatric cardiac intensive care units (PCICUs) dedicated solely to the care of critically ill neonates, infants, and children with congenital heart disease. One commonly cited advantage of a dedicated PCICU is that it concentrates medical and nursing expertise in one area of the hospital [11,12]. However, even in the absence of a separate, geographically distinct PCICU, the majority of programs prefer to cohort all their postoperative cardiothoracic surgery patients in one area of the PICU. These patients are then managed by a select group of physicians and nurses both interested and skilled in cardiac intensive care. Few, if any, studies have assessed the impact of this kind of administrative structure on outcome, and, even if the separation of the medical and nursing staffs into this structure provides better outcomes, the economic cost may be exorbitantly high. Thus a careful analysis for the development of a separate PCICU should be done before embarking on the development of a separate and distinct ICU, which may be seen only to fragment care despite the goal of promoting better outcomes.

Clearly, the need for specialized pediatric cardiac intensivists is controversial, and there are strong advocates to vehemently argue either point. Whether the critical care needs of infants and children with congenital heart disease are better served by individuals with dual board certification in pediatric critical care medicine and pediatric cardiology is a matter of debate and is beyond the scope of this chapter. Some experts would argue that additional training in pediatric cardiac intensive care lasting between 9 to 12 months beyond pediatric cardiology fellowship training is sufficient, and guidelines for this training period have been proposed by a joint task force sponsored by the American College of Cardiology, American Heart Association, and American Board of Pediatrics [13]. The debate on this subject is likely to continue for many years, although

D.S. Wheeler et al. (eds.), *Science and Practice of Pediatric Critical Care Medicine*,
DOI 10.1007/978-1-84800-921-9_7, © Springer-Verlag London Limited 2009

the fact remains that the field of pediatric cardiac intensive care is growing at a tremendous pace. As this *sub-subspecialty* of pediatric critical care medicine evolves, it will be most interesting to see how outcomes will be affected.

National Standards for Pediatric Intensive Care Unit Organization and Administration

In 1993, The American Academy of Pediatrics and the Pediatric Section of the Society of Critical Care Medicine published specific guidelines and levels of pediatric intensive care [14]. These guidelines were revised and published in the journals *Pediatrics* and *Critical Care Medicine* in 2004 [15,16]. Both the 1993 and 2004 guidelines established minimum acceptable standards and levels of care for PICUs based on the concept of categorization into Level I and Level II PICUs. The primary differences between Level I and Level II PICUs involve the types of physicians staffing the PICU (in terms of subspecialty support) and available hospital resources. For example, both a Level I and Level II PICU should be staffed by properly trained pediatric intensivists. However, although the availability of surgical subspecialties such as pediatric general surgery, neurosurgery, and cardiovascular surgery is essential to a Level I PICU, it is not mandated for a Level II PICU [15,16]. In addition, although 24-hour access to magnetic resonance imaging (MRI) services is essential for Level I classification, it is not required for Level II classification [15,16].

Level I PICU services should be available to the most critically ill and injured children, although, given the shortage of pediatric intensivists and other geographic limitations, Level II services may be a reasonable alternative. For example, a critically ill child may be resuscitated and stabilized at a Level II PICU before transfer to a Level I PICU, if clinically necessary. For this reason, cooperative agreements and communication between Level I and Level II PICUs should be established [15,16]. Issues pertaining to categorization and regionalization of emergency medical services and pediatric intensive care are further discussed later in this textbook.

Organization of the Pediatric Intensive Care Unit Team

The clinical expertise required to safely and effectively manage critically ill infants and children housed in a multidisciplinary PICU encompasses many different disciplines. Because most PICUs serve as regional referral facilities and care for both surgical and medical patients, a collaborative working relationship must exist for all health care providers working in the PICU setting to allow the safe and efficient management of these very complex patients. The PICU must be organized in such a manner that the multidisciplinary approach to the care of these children is done with evidence-based approaches and technical expertise that permits for state- of-the-art delivery of clinical care. To accomplish these goals, an administrative structure must be developed that embraces this level of cooperation and collegiality.

Pediatric intensive care units are specially designed and equipped facilities that require specialized nurses, respiratory therapists, pharmacists, social workers, and physicians trained in pediatric critical care medicine. Both Level I and Level II PICUs are truly multidisciplinary in nature and must therefore have a management structure that is representative of the personnel who work in the PICU [15,16]. The medical director of the PICU must be initially board certified in pediatrics, anesthesiology, or pediatric surgery with additional qualifications in pediatric critical care medicine (American Board of Pediatrics), pediatrics and critical care medicine (American Board of Anesthesiology), and surgical critical care medicine (American Board of Surgery), respectively. If the medical director is not a pediatrician, a pediatric intensivist (as defined above) should be appointed as a co-director of the PICU [15,16]. The medical director works closely with the nursing leadership and the other physicians (including consultants) to promote integration of critical care services.

An associate medical director from another field may also be helpful and should also be so credentialed by the American Board of Pediatrics, the American Board of Anesthesiology (critical care medicine), or American Board of Surgery (surgical critical care medicine). The associate medical director can assist in various administrative tasks required to run a busy PICU. For example, assistance from an anesthesiologist may be helpful in developing clinical pathways for sedation and pain management and protocols needed to facilitate the transfer of patients from the operating room to the PICU. A pediatric surgeon with interests in trauma care is instrumental in developing the appropriate protocols required for the care of the injured child.

Studies clearly document that having a full-time pediatric intensivist dedicated to the PICU improves patient care and outcome [7,9,10,17]. However, the shortage of properly trained pediatric intensivists necessitates that the attending physician may delegate the care of patients to a physician at least at a postgraduate level of year 2 (PGY2) or to an advanced practice nurse or physician's assistant [15,16]. Nonphysician providers, or physician extenders, must receive proper credentialing and training, and these individuals provide care under the direction of the attending physician. In addition, Level I designation requires the in-house presence of a PGY3 or above (in addition to the PGY2 or physician extender). Level I designation further requires that the attending physician be available within 30 minutes to assist with patient care, when necessary [15,16].

In addition to the appropriately trained and credentialed medical personnel in the PICU, a nursing administrative staff must be appointed and dedicated to the care of the critically ill infant and child. A nurse manager with substantial pediatric experience is essential for both Level I and Level II designation. A master's degree in either pediatric nursing or administration is desirable, but not required. The nurse manager should also have a background in critical care nursing (preferably pediatrics) and must have the managerial skills to hire, train, and retain nursing staff, as this is the back bone of the PICU setting. An advanced practice nurse— either a clinical nurse specialist or nurse practitioner—should be available to provide clinical leadership and education in the nursing care of critically ill and injured children. The clinical nurse specialist must have a master's degree in nursing, pediatric critical care nurse specialist certification, and clinical expertise in pediatric critical care [15,16]. Critically ill or injured children should be cared for by pediatric critical care nurses who have completed a clinical and didactic orientation and training period before assuming full responsibility for patient care. At a minimum, training and certification in Pediatric Advanced Life Support (PALS) or its equivalent should be required. The PICU nurse manager and clinical nurse specialist should work closely to develop and implement a program for nursing orientation and yearly competency review in these areas.

Allied health care and ancillary support professionals who also participate in the care of the critically ill child must have a partnership with the administrative leadership in the PICU. Respiratory therapy, social services, and pharmacy should have liaisons that are able to articulate and develop plans for PICU management that assist in the care delivered by the various practitioners in the intensive care setting. Thus, a strong administrative group in the PICU consists of leaders from medicine, nursing, respiratory therapy, social services, and pharmacy. The major responsibilities of the administrative leadership in the PICU include but are not limited to (1) developing policies and procedures for the PICU; (2) improving quality assurance; (3) enhancing continuing education; (4) training PICU personnel; (5) developing outreach programs to educate the community; (6) reviewing budgets for both personnel and capital equipment; and (7) developing goals to improve care and to develop a better team approach to care for these complicated patients.

Developing Policies and Procedures

The development of policies and procedures is a necessity for the day-to-day functioning of the PICU. By working together, the PICU administrative team can develop, review, and revise patient care protocols. These protocols can then be used to assist in the standardization of care plans that reflect the multidisciplinary approach to care of the critically ill child. Such efforts may result in the development of admission and discharge criteria; chain of command; care of vascular access catheters; administration of sedation; code policies; roles of the PICU attendings, fellows, residents, hospitalists, and nurse practitioners; order writing; and so forth. When available, national guidelines and standards should be utilized [18–20].

Improving Quality Assurance

Quality assurance (QA) programs are designed to continually look at care delivered to patients and to find ways to improve on them so that patients receive safe and efficient care. Examples of QA programs include policies directed toward reduction of nosocomial infection rates (i.e., bloodstream infections, ventilator associated pneumonias, urinary tract infections), inadvertent extubations, medication administration errors, readmission to the PICU within 24 to 48 hours following transfer out of the PICU, length of PICU stays, adverse neurologic outcomes, and the unanticipated PICU admissions from various areas within the hospital, as well as development of rapid response teams, implementation of mock code programs, and a careful and structured review of all mortalities and significant morbidities (e.g., intravenous infiltrations that require plastic surgical consultation). A good QA program encourages an honest and open approach to patient care data and information. This encourages maximum participation from all of the personnel who work in the PICU [21–23]. Quality assurance is discussed in greater detail in subsequent chapters in this textbook.

Enhancing Continuing Education and Training New Personnel

The PICU administrative team should also develop and implement a plan for educating and training new personnel, as well as ensuring the continuing education of experienced personnel. Obviously, a significant amount of teaching occurs at the bedside. This is critically important to educate the bedside personnel who are caring for the patient. However, additional educational activities are needed to allow PICU personnel to have learning opportunities away from the bedside. Such activities may include a skills lab in which the staff have the opportunity to work with newer infusion pumps, monitors, or other equipment commonly used in the PICU. Also, didactic sessions or seminars may be helpful to bring everyone up to date with new topics or best practices such as ventilator management, agents commonly used for sedation, management for shock, or case reviews. Case reviews may be most helpful for review situations where the outcome could have been improved. These may include sentinel events, root cause analyses, or code reviews.

Training and education of PICU personnel in the nuances of critical care management are critical in the retention and promotion of the nursing and ancillary staff. This requires the allocation of clinical nurse specialists and nurse educators who assist in both bedside teaching and in developing ongoing educational programs for the staff. Continuing education is extremely important in maintaining job satisfaction among the staff and developing a stronger PICU team. A unique approach to satisfying the educational needs is to have a monthly staff seminar on a pertinent topic or a quarterly educational conference that emphasizes a topic germane to the PICU. Such a topic might be the approach to the pediatric trauma victim with a series of lectures from both the PICU medical staff and the relevant surgeons (i.e., trauma surgery, orthopedic surgery, and neurosurgery). These educational conferences help to establish the team dynamics needed to make the PICU function in a cohesive and cooperative manner. Other training modalities may include simulation-based training whereby the staff uses simulators to improve both clinical and technical skills in an environment that emphasizes close observation and feedback. Finally, the most important part of this is a collaborative approach to the educational component that reinforces the team work needed to care for the critically ill infant and child.

Developing Outreach Programs to the Community

In addition to providing in-house educational opportunities, the PICU should have a regional responsibility to educate the referring physicians and referral hospitals in the evaluation, stabilization, and emergency preparedness to care for complex patients. These educational activities may include periodic case reviews and discussions, a formalized lecture series, and morbidity and mortality conferences designed for physicians, nurses, and others. Not only do these outreach efforts educate the local communities, it is further hoped that pediatric care is improved and that relationships with these smaller facilities is improved.

Reviewing Budgets for Personnel and Capital Equipment

It is imperative for the PICU administrative team to collaborate on the budget for the PICU in order to understand the financial aspects of critical care management for both capital equipment and personnel. A periodic review by the nurse manager and the medical director of the budget and performance against budget are key to understanding how the unit must contribute to the hospital's bottom line. This permits a better understanding of resource utilization, costs, and reimbursement so that the PICU team can practice in a financially responsible environment. By having a clearer understanding of the financial aspects of critical care one can develop capital equipment requests designed to replace equipment in the PICU as well as purchase new items designed to improve patient care. Obviously, capital requests must be reviewed in a timely fashion, and thus it is the responsibility of the hospital administration to make certain that both the medical directors and the nurse managers have enough notification to research the various equipment requests. In addition, because the PICU is an environment where much collaboration occurs in the care of very high risk and complicated patients and often the need arises to provide more medical supervision to the PICU, a careful examination of the physician coverage needs for the unit must be part of the budgetary process as well. Having qualified personnel providing critical care is of great importance. This ensures the availability of expertly skilled personnel needed to care for the critically ill patient. By including this in the hospital budget, one would be able to add necessary individuals required for the care of these patients. These individuals may be additional physicians (pediatric intensivists, hospitalists, house officers, and so forth) or physician extenders (physician assistants or nurse practitioners). Thus a reasonable understanding of the revenues generated by the PICU and the costs needed to run the PICU will enable one to understand the profit margins generated and how to reinvest these into the PICU for future growth or divert some to the other vital components of the hospital.

Developing Goals to Improve Care

As more and more institutions are moving toward performance directed or outcomes based standards of care, PICUs must develop goals and methods to achieve these standards. Goal setting requires input from both management and staff. In addition, the goals should parallel the parent organization and be modified to reflect what is absolutely reasonable in the PICU. Such examples may include, but are certainly not limited to, improving patient and parental satisfaction using tools such as standardized questionnaires and comparing these results with like institutions, reducing nosocomial infection rates by a predetermined rate, improving communication in the PICU by developing goal sheets, developing a primary health care group to care for patients who have required prolonged PICU stays (usually more than 1 week), improving educational programs for the staff, and creating a work environment that respects all the staff and encourages their input into patient care.

Administration and Management

The creation of a critical care committee is helpful to formulate policies, review incident reports, develop QA programs, and formulate educational agendas for the PICU. In addition, this committee can review the adverse events that have occurred and thereby develop educational opportunities that surround these untoward events. The critical care committee must meet on a regular basis, and it is helpful to have a set agenda. The committee should hear reports from the other contributors to the PICU, such as pharmacy, respiratory therapy, social services, laboratory, radiology, and pathology. This multidisciplinary approach supports the overall collaborative nature of pediatric intensive care. This committee should also report on a regular basis to the hospital's medical board.

Because of the many bioethical issues associated with many of the patients with life-threatening conditions, the PICU will potentially have a close working relationship with the hospital's ethics committee. This committee serves as a review board when ethical conflicts arise regarding patient care. These conflicts may be between physicians, physicians and other health care team members, or the health care team and the family. Often it is best to try and resolve such conflicts via a care conference or a series of care conferences where the family meets with various members of the medical and health care teams to better understand their child's illness and the ethical quandary in which the health care team finds itself. Many times these ethical conflicts resolve themselves with honest communication between the family members and the health care providers.

Children who are *chronically* critically ill (generally defined by a PICU length of stay of more than 1 week) pose unique challenges to the PICU team as well. The use of weekly interdisciplinary rounds becomes a necessity for these patients for a number of reasons. Some are very complex and require multiple subspecialist input for the comprehensive care required. This input may come from other medical services, social services, regional referral centers, convalescent facilities, case managers, and so forth. The opportunity to discuss on a weekly basis these complex patients enables all of the team members to get on the same page and thus provide a more comprehensive approach to the care of the child. This may also help the family with discharge planning, especially if special equipment is needed or a referral to another facility is needed before the child can go home.

Conclusion

Thus one can see that the PICU environment can be a very complex organization with many different services caring for the patients in an intensive care setting. Therefore, it is required to have an administrative structure in place that enable the team to care for the patient, emphasizing a multidisciplinary approach to safe and effective patient care. It is imperative that the PICU is seen as an area within the hospital where the child receives the best possible care by a comforting and skilled staff who are able to address many of the patient's as well as the family's concerns and thereby promote optimal outcomes.

References

1. Pollack MM, Cuerdon TC, Getson PR. Pediatric intensive care units: results of a national survey. Crit Care Med 1993;21:607–614.
2. Randolph AG, Gonzales CA, Cortellini L, Yeh TS. Growth of pediatric intensive care units in the United States from 1995 to 2001. J Pediatr 2004;144:792–798.
3. Odetola FO, Clark SJ, Freed GL, Bratton SL, Davis MM. A national survey of pediatric critical care resources in the United States. Pediatrics 2005;115:e382–e386.
4. Nipshagen MD, Polderman KH, DeVictor D, Gemke RJ. Pediatric intensive care: result of a European survey. Intensive Care Med 2002;28:1797–1803.
5. Ramenofsky ML, Luterman A, Quindlen E, Riddick L, Curreri PW. Maximum survival in pediatric trauma: the ideal system. J Trauma 1984;24:818–823.
6. Haller JA, Shorter N, Miller D, Colombani P, Hall J, Buck J. Organization and function of a regional pediatric trauma center: does a system of management improve outcome? J Trauma 1983; 23:691–691.

7. Pollack MM, Katz RW, Ruttiman UE, Getson PR. Improving the outcome and efficiency of intensive care: the impact of an intensivist. Crit Care Med 1988;16:11–17.

8. Haller JA, Beaver B. A model: systems management of life threatening injuries in children for the state of Maryland, USA. Intensive Care Med 1989;15(Suppl 1):S53–S56.

9. Pollack MM, Alexander SR, Clarke N, Ruttimann UE, Tesselaar HM, Bachulis AC. Improved outcomes from tertiary center pediatric intensive care: a statewide comparison of tertiary and nontertiary care facilities. Crit Care Med 1991;19:150–159.

10. Pollack MM, Cuerdon TT, Patel KM, Ruttimann UE, Getson PR, Levetown M. Impact of quality-of-care factors on pediatric intensive care unit mortality. JAMA 1994;272:941–946.

11. Chang AC. Pediatric cardiac intensive care: current state of the art and beyond the millennium. Curr Opin Pediatr 2000;12:238–246.

12. Chang AC. How to start and sustain a successful pediatric cardiac intensive care program: a combined clinical and administrative strategy. Pediatr Crit Care Med 2002;3:107–111.

13. Allen HD, Bricker JT, Freed MD, et al. AC/AHA/AAP recommendations for training in pediatric cardiology. Pediatrics 2005;116:1574–1596.

14. Committee on Hospital Care of the American Academy of Pediatrics and Pediatric Section of the Society of Critical Care Medicine. Guidelines and levels of care for pediatric intensive care units. Pediatrics 1993;92:166–175.

15. Rosenberg DI, Moss MM. American Academy of Pediatrics Section on Critical Care/American Academy of Pediatrics Committee on Hospital Care. Guidelines and levels of care for pediatric intensive care units. Pediatrics 2004;114:1114–1125.

16. Rosenberg DI, Moss MM. American College of Critical Care Medicine of the Society of Critical Care Medicine: guidelines and levels of care for pediatric intensive care units. Crit Care Med 2004; 32:2117–2127.

17. Pollack MM, Patel KM, Ruttiman E. Pediatric critical care training programs have a positive effect on pediatric intensive care mortality. Crit Care Med 1997;25:1637–1642.

18. American Academy of Pediatrics. Committee on Hospital Care and Section of Critical Care. Society of Critical Care Medicine. Pediatric Section Admission Criteria Task Force. Guidelines for developing admission and discharge policies for the pediatric intensive care unit. Pediatrics 1999;103:840–842.

19. Pediatric Section Task Force on Admission and Discharge Criteria, Society of Critical Care Medicine in conjunction with the American College of Critical Care Medicine and the Committee on Hospital Care of the American Academy of Pediatrics. Guidelines for developing admission and discharge policies for the pediatric intensive care unit. Crit Care Med 1999;27:843–845.

20. Jaimovich DG. Committee on Hospital Care and Section on Critical Care. Admission and discharge guidelines for the pediatric patient requiring intermediate care. Crit Care Med 2004;32:1215–1218.

21. Rafkin HS, Hoyt JW. Objective data and quality assurance programs. Current and future trends. Crit Care Clin 1994;10:157–177.

22. Garland A. Improving the ICU: part 1. Chest 2005;127:2151–2164.

23. Garland A. Improving the ICU: part 2. Chest 2005;127:2165–2179.

8

Nursing Care in the Pediatric Intensive Care Unit

Franco A. Carnevale

Role of the Pediatric Critical Care Nurse

The increasing complexity of pediatric critical care has required a corresponding evolution in the sophistication of pediatric critical care nursing (PCCN). The role of the nurse in this setting is multifaceted [1]. First, the nurse serves as a form of *total systems monitor*—continually examining all the physiologic monitors and treatment devices, along with the child's body. This requires the acquisition of *peripheral vision*. A skilful nurse learns to adjust settings on critical care equipment so it can serve as an extension of her own sensory system. The nurse has to perform routine *maintenance* activities (e.g., medication preparation, blood procurement) while remaining attentive to the child's physiologic status—continually *tuned in* to the immediate recognition of any disruption in the child's condition.

Second, in the event of any irregularity, the nurse must instantly judge the significance of the event and initiate an appropriate response. Such irregularities are frequently attributable to equipment artifacts or to *normal* patient functions such as movement or coughing that may trigger a variety of electronic alarms. The nurse has to immediately determine the importance of such events by *scanning* the child's body and surrounding equipment and discern whether this implies a threat to the patient or not. If a significant problem is detected, then the nurse has to implement the required intervention (e.g., manual ventilation, airway suctioning). In cases of uncertainty or serious problems, the nurse will need to notify the physician. However, this notification needs to be done with discretion given the competing demands on the physician's time.

Third, the nurse has a primary responsibility for ensuring patient safety [1], although this is not exclusively a nursing responsibility. She needs to prevent adverse events through the use of appropriate security measures (e.g., bedside rails, restraints, medication preparation procedures, infusion pump settings).

Fourth, the nurse is also responsible for maintaining a bedside environment that fosters the psychosocial adaptation of the child and family [2]. She has to be attentive to the patient's psychological condition by addressing expressed needs while continually anticipating additional needs, inferred from a strong understanding of children's coping with critical illness. This involves the use of basic comforting skills, play therapies (in collaboration with child life specialists), as well as selected psychotherapeutic interventions (e.g., empathic listening, cognitive reframing), in collaboration with members of the mental health disciplines. She is also required to attend the needs of the child's family, recognizing the extraordinary distress that can result from the illness and the benefit that the child will derive from the family's successful adaptation to the situation.

Fifth, the nurse also functions as an *integrator* of patient information. The nurse is in continual contact with a vast body of bedside and laboratory patient information. Consequently, the nursing record serves as an integrated record of patient data that provides (1) a vital reference source for other health care professionals, (2) a log for subsequent shifts that need to compare data against prior events, and (3) a permanent record for retrospective reviews (e.g., morbidity and mortality analyses or quality improvement audits). The nurse also serves as a *live* patient data source. Given the rapid pace with which events unfold in the pediatric intensive care unit (PICU), the nurse is required to keep abreast of all that is going on with her assigned patient, to help ensure integrated coordinated patient care.

Turning to a *pilot in a cockpit* metaphor, PCCN typically involves highly routine surveillance functions, vigilantly attending to a multitude of cues to ensure an early recognition of *turbulence* or *system failure*. Such events must be immediately recognized and the corrective interventions should be expediently and effectively implemented while ensuring the comfort and safety of the *passengers*. Pediatric critical care nursing practiced in this manner will help ensure optimal outcomes in terms of patient survival and morbidity, as well as child and family adaptation to the stresses of the experience. This nursing requires an education, administration, and innovation and research infrastructure that will foster and support the expert nursing practice outlined. The remainder of this chapter discusses these infrastructural elements.

The female gender has been used solely for convenience purposes for all references to "nurses." No gender bias is implied.

D.S. Wheeler et al. (eds.), *Science and Practice of Pediatric Critical Care Medicine*,
DOI 10.1007/978-1-84800-921-9_8, © Springer-Verlag London Limited 2009

Education

Orientation of New Staff

Typically, entry-level nursing education programs provide some basic exposure to general pediatric nursing, but little direct experience in critical care (neither adult nor pediatric) is offered. Academic programs in critical care nursing or PCCN are generally restricted to graduate advanced practice programs for clinical nurse specialists or nurse practitioners.

Newly hired PICU nurses will typically have little or no prior PCCN training. Such training is usually acquired *on the job*. Given the critical condition of the PICU patient population and the need to provide no margin for *learning curve* errors, employers have a responsibility for developing closely supervised education programs that will expediently enable the new PICU nurse to acquire baseline knowledge and skills to manage less critical patients. Ultimately there is a gradual advancement in the complexity of assigned patients as expertise evolves.

New recruits, who usually have no prior PICU experience, arrive with (1) related experience such as neonatal critical care, (2) general pediatric experience, (3) adult critical care experience, (4) neither pediatric nor adult critical care experience (e.g., general adult medicine), or (5) no experience at all (i.e., a new graduate). Although the direct hiring of the latter candidates is a hotly contested point, they can successfully adapt to a PICU setting, given adequate educational, mentoring, and administrative support.

In light of these commonly diverse backgrounds, every PICU needs to maintain an orientation program for new staff that can be readily tailored to the variable needs of new staff [3]. An orientation program should consist of (1) 1 to 2 weeks of introductory reviews and (2) a 3- to 4-week clinical preceptorship directly supervised by a senior PICU nurse (4 to 8 weeks for a new graduate). The introductory reviews should include (1) assigned readings, drawing selected chapters from seminal PCCN textbooks [4,5]; (2) lectures that review basic critical care theory (e.g., evaluation of vital functions, hemodynamic evaluation, blood gas interpretation, neurologic evaluation, critical care pharmacology); (3) demonstration and practice of common procedures (e.g., airway suctioning, manual ventilation, blood procurement from arterial catheter); (4) discussion of the role of the PICU nurse; (5) overview of pertinent psychosocial issues; (6) introduction to key members of the PICU team; and (7) review of key PICU policies and procedures and other textual resources available to nurses. Such reviews can be conducted with a cohort group of new recruits.

The Clinical Preceptorship

The clinical preceptorship should enable new staff to directly care for PICU patients [3]. This implies a co-assignment with a senior nurse committed to serve as a clinical preceptor. Ideally, the new nurse will work with one sole preceptor throughout the preceptorship, to ensure pedagogical continuity. The preceptor–preceptee dyad should be initially counted as one sole nurse, in terms of workload assignment, to ensure that the preceptor can provide the required level of support and supervision. Patient acuity and the level of preceptee autonomy should be gradually increased at a pace where the learner is capable of safely caring for a stable patient without continuous and direct supervision by the final two to three assigned shifts of the preceptorship.

Sometimes, the learner's background and capabilities enable a rapid progression, whereas for others this process may need to be slowed to a point where the preceptorship needs to be extended. In these latter cases, performance limitations need to be explicitly stated for the learner and an additional training plan will need to be developed. The preceptorship is formally terminated when the learner has fulfilled all of the required skill and knowledge objectives or, on occasion, if it is judged that the learner will not be able to continue her employment in the PICU. Candidates successfully completing their preceptorship may benefit from a subsequent (formal or informal) mentorship wherein they can derive ongoing clinical and professional guidance from either their original preceptors or other appropriate senior staff.

Clinical preceptors supporting such a program should be provided with the educational and administrative support that is necessary to successfully fulfill this critical role. In addition to advanced expertise in PCCN, preceptorship also requires a body of knowledge and skills that are not readily acquired through clinical care. This includes an understanding of (1) adult learning principles, (2) bedside instructional techniques, (3) clinical performance appraisal, and (4) dynamics of the preceptee–preceptor relationship. This can be acquired through a combination of classroom activities and direct coaching from an experienced nursing educator. Preceptors require administrative support wherein they can readily negotiate preceptee patient assignments (*workload* as well as *type* of patient) according to the preceptee's learning needs, discuss any performance problems that arise, and review any general issues that may help improve the unit's preceptorship program.

Senior Staff Development

This discussion has focused exclusively on the learning needs of newly hired staff. However, orientation and preceptorship programs only provide for a basic level of PCCN training. Additional educational programs are also required to ensure the ongoing development of PICU nursing staff [3]. Most importantly, nurses need ready access to advanced experts in PCCN (e.g., exemplary senior nurses, clinical nurse specialists, nurse practitioners) as well as pediatric critical care physicians and other experts (e.g., respiratory technologists) who can provide bedside coaching for the management of emerging issues in everyday practice.

Structured classroom-type programs should also be developed. These can be topic specific: (1) Pediatric Advanced Life Support course; (2) an intermediate level workshop examining selected PCCN functions (e.g., stabilization of a postoperative cardiac surgery patient, continuous renal-replacement therapy); (3) review session on analgesia and sedation; or (4) trauma management workshop.

Some senior staff development programs are also required. For example, the Montreal Children's Hospital PICU has a 10-day PCCN course for senior nursing staff (which has been running for over 20 years) that provides an advanced review of critical care topics. This includes a thorough review of recent practices, ongoing debates, and emerging trends through lectures, case reviews, assigned readings, homework exercises, and student presentations (Table 8.1). Such programs help prepare senior staff to manage the most complex PICU patients while serving as clinical leaders and mentors for junior staff.

TABLE 8.1. Senior staff development course for pediatric intensive care unit nursing: principal topics.

Mechanics of ventilation
Control of breathing
Gas exchange and transport
Myocardial mechanics
Cardiac electrophysiology
Hemodynamic physiology
Critical care pharmacology
Fluids, electrolytes, and nutrition
Cerebral injury
Seizures
Sepsis
Immune function
Coagulopathies
Shock
Trauma
Hepatic dysfunction
Renal dysfunction
Analgesia and sedation
Extracorporeal membrane oxygenation and ventricular assist devices
Ethics

Administration

Structure

It is important that the PICU nursing manager understands the complexity of the nursing service required in a PICU [6]. The manager commonly determines (1) the appropriate number of staff required for a given mix of patients, (2) support services that are made available to nurses, (3) access to educational programs and resources, and (4) the number and type of new staff that will be recruited. Thus, the manager can profoundly enable or disable the functioning of a PICU nursing team. Such a manager should ideally have a strong background in PCCN as well as nursing management. The PICU should be co-managed by the medical director and nursing manager, each holding primary responsibility for his or her respective discipline while jointly managing areas of common concern (e.g., quality improvement). This structure facilitates reciprocal problem solving and support, which have been associated with improved patient outcomes [7].

Staffing

The most prominent administrative problem raised in PCCN relates to nursing staffing levels. What nurse/-patient ratios are required to provide necessary care? This problem is related to increasing concerns about cost containment and nursing shortages in the face of rising demands for PICU services. Nurse/patient ratios have obvious implications for nursing staff satisfaction and morale but have also been linked to patient outcomes. Evidence emerging out of other settings indicates that low nursing staffing levels are directly related to increased patient morbidity [8,9]. This problem has been scarcely examined within the PICU setting, although a recent study has reported that patients are more likely to experience unplanned extubations if they are assigned to a nurse caring for two patients rather than one [10].

The American Academy of Pediatrics Section on Critical Care and the American Academy of Pediatrics Committee on Hospital Care have jointly published *Guidelines and levels of care for pediatric intensive care units* [11]. This article indicates that nurse/patient ratios should vary according to patient needs, ranging from 2 to 1 to 1 to 3. However, no further detail is provided on how specific staffing determinations should be made. A recent international consultation revealed that there do not exist any widely accepted PICU nursing staffing standards, with a corresponding diversity of viewpoints on how this problem ought to be managed [12,13].

Ball has examined the utility of nursing workload measures as a means for addressing this problem in critical care in general [14]. She questions the validity of such tools for these purposes, arguing that nursing staffing requirements should be based on patient needs and on the nursing care that would meaningfully address these rather than a count of tasks performed. Furthermore, no accepted tool exists for the measurement of PCCN workload. Although validated PICU acuity measures are available, these do not directly correlate with nursing workload. It appears that the best available means for determining workload is the judgment of nursing managers. This further justifies the necessity that such managers possess a strong grasp of PCCN.

Innovation and Research

Although PICU nurses share numerous concerns and interests with physicians and other health care professionals, a number of topics have gained particular importance in PCCN. These are related to problems that more immediately concern nurses, although not exclusively. In fact, the PCCN literature has taken the lead in examining topics that are highly relevant to other critical care practitioners as well.

This literature is accessible through excellent PCCN textbooks [4,5] and a number of highly respected critical care nursing journals (as well as non-nursing journals). *Pediatric Intensive Care Nursing* is an international journal exclusively devoted to PCCN. The PICU nurses needing to consult colleagues about additional clinical problems can do so through the international PCCN Internet discussion group *PICU-Nurse-International* (http://health.groups.yahoo.com/group/PICU-Nurse-International/).

The PCCN literature examines physiologic, psychosocial, and ethical problems, as well as some of the educational and administrative issues discussed earlier [15]. A selection of topics reviewed in this literature include the evaluation and management of analgesia and sedation [16–19], prone positioning [20], pressure ulcers [21], airway suctioning practices [22], environmental noise [23], and PICU ethical dilemmas [24,25]. Pediatric critical care nursing researchers have demonstrated a particular interest in psychosocial problems. This research has examined parental needs and stressors [26–29], sibling experiences [29], the experience of the critically ill child [29–31], the experience of the entire family as a whole [29,32], and family presence during resuscitation [33].

A major finding of this psychosocial research is that *families are not visitors* [2,29]. Family members are attempting to fulfill their respective family functions in the PICU (e.g., parenting)—they are not visiting. The extent to which the experiences of individual family members can be favorably supported, these members will derive benefits that can also benefit the critically ill child. Family presence and participation in the patient's care can foster both the patient's and the family's well being. Therefore, the PICU should ensure that families have access to essential physical comforts, as well as supportive psychosocial services. In light of the long-term psychological consequences that critical illness may entail for the child and family, these families could also benefit from integrated long-term follow-up services. Finally, the PICU setting is one of the primary sites of child deaths in pediatrics. The PICU staff should thus be sensitive to caring for the special needs of dying children and their families [34].

Conclusion

Pediatric critical care nursing is a major component of excellent pediatric critical care. The provision of this specialized nursing entails significant training and administrative support while continually drawing on ongoing PCCN clinical innovations and research to adapt nursing care to new understandings of the needs of critically ill children and their families. The strength of a PICU's service is inescapably tied to the quality and rigor of care that the nursing team can provide, in collaboration with the entire pediatric critical care team.

References

1. Benner P, Hooper-Kyriakidis P, Stannard D. Clinical Wisdom and Interventions in Critical Care: A Thinking-in-Action Approach. Philadelphia: WB Saunders; 1999.
2. Carnevale FA. The injured family. In: Moloney-Harmon PA, Czerwinski SJ, eds. Nursing Care of the Pediatric Trauma Patient. St. Louis: WB Saunders; 2003:107–117.
3. Czerwinski S, Martin ED. Facilitation of learning. In: Curley MAQ, Moloney-Harmon P, eds. Critical Care Nursing of Infants and Children, 2nd ed. Philadelphia: WB Saunders; 2001:85–106.
4. Curley MAQ, Moloney-Harmon P, eds. Critical Care Nursing of Infants and Children, 2nd ed. Philadelphia: WB Saunders; 2001.
5. Hazinski MF. Manual of Pediatric Critical Care. St. Louis: Mosby; 1999.
6. Fagan MJ. Leadership in pediatric critical care. In: Curley MAQ, Moloney-Harmon P, eds. Critical Care Nursing of Infants and Children, 2nd ed. Philadelphia: WB Saunders; 2001:71–83.
7. Knaus WA, Draper EA, Wagner DP, et al. An evaluation of outcome from intensive care in major medical centres. Ann Intern Med 1986; 104:410–418.
8. Cho SH, Ketefian S, Barkauskas VH, et al. The effects of nurse staffing on adverse events, morbidity, mortality, and medical costs. Nurs Res 2003;52:71–79.
9. Aiken LH, Clarke SP, Sloane DM, Sochalski J, Silber JH. Hospital nurse staffing and patient mortality, nurse burnout, and job dissatisfaction. JAMA 2002;288(16):1987–1993.
10. Marcin JP, Rutan E, Rapetti PM, Brown JP, Rahnamayi R, Pretzlaff RK. Nurse staffing and unplanned extubation in the pediatric intensive care unit. Pediatr Crit Care Med 2005;6(3):254–257.
11. Rosenberg DI, Moss MM, American Academy of Pediatrics Section on Critical Care, and American Academy of Pediatrics Committee on Hospital Care. Guidelines and levels of care for pediatric intensive care units. Pediatrics 2004;114(4):1114–1125.
12. Carnevale FA. PICU Nurse–Patient Ratios—in search of the "right" numbers. Pediatr Intensive Care Nurs 2001;2(1):7–9.
13. Clarke T, Mackinnon E, England K, Burr G, Fowler S, Fairservice L. A review of intensive care nurse staffing practices overseas: what lessons for Australia? Intensive Crit Care Nurs 2000;16(4):228–242.
14. Ball C: Patient:nurse ratios in critical care—time for some radical thinking. Intensive Crit Care Nurs 2001;17(3):125–127.
15. Carnevale FA. Key issues in critical care nursing. In: Fink M, Abraham E, Vincent JL, Kochanek P, eds. Textbook of Critical Care, 5th ed. Philadelphia: Elsevier; 2005:2217–2223.
16. Franck LS, Naughton I, Winter I. Opioid and benzodiazepine withdrawal symptoms in paediatric intensive care patients. Intensive Crit Care Nurs 2004;20(6):344–351.
17. Johnston CC, Stevens B, Craig KD, et al. Developmental changes in pain expression in premature, full-term, two- and four-month-old infants. Pain 1993;52:201–208.
18. Puntillo KA: Dimensions of procedural pain and its analgesic management in critically ill surgical patients. Am J Crit Care 1994;3:116–122.
19. Alexander E, Carnevale FA, Razack S. Evaluation of a sedation protocol for intubated critically ill children. Intensive Crit Care Nurs 2002; 18:292–301.
20. Curley MA, Thompson JE, Arnold JH. The effects of early and repeated prone positioning in pediatric patients with acute lung injury. Chest 2000;118:156–163.
21. Curley MA, Quigley SM, Lin M. Pressure ulcers in pediatric intensive care: incidence and associated factors. Pediatr Crit Care Med 2003;3: 284–290.
22. Ackerman MH, Ecklund MM, Abu-Jumah M. A review of normal saline instillation: implications for practice. Dimens Crit Care Nurs 1996; 15(1):31–38.
23. Milette IH, Carnevale FA: I'm trying to heal. . . . Noise levels in a pediatric intensive care unit. Dynamics 2003;14(4):14–21.
24. Carnevale FA. Ethical care of the critically ill child: a conception of a "thick" bioethics. Nursing Ethics (in press).
25. Kirschbaum MS. Life support decisions for children: what do parents value? ANS Adv Nurs Sci 1996;19(1):51–71.
26. Fisher MD. Identified needs of parents in a pediatric intensive care unit. Crit Care Nurse 1994;14(3):82–90.
27. Kirschbaum MS. Needs of parents of critically ill children. Dimens Crit Care Nurs 1990;9:344–352.
28. Miles MS, Carter MC, Elberly TW, et al. Toward an understanding of parent stress in the pediatric intensive care unit: overview of the program of research. Mater Child Nurs J. 1989;18:181–186.
29. Carnevale FA. "Striving to recapture our previous life"—the experience of families of critically ill children. Off J Can Assoc Crit Care Nurs 1999;9(4):16–22.
30. Rennick JE, Johnston CC, Dougherty G, et al. Children's psychological responses after critical illness and exposure to invasive technology. J Dev Behav Pediatr 2002;23:133–144.
31. Carnevale FA. The experience of critically ill children: narratives of unmaking. Intensive Crit Care Nurs. 1997;13:49–52.
32. Youngblut JM, Lauzon S. Family functioning following pediatric intensive care unit hospitalization. Issues Compr Pediatr Nurs 1995;18:11–25.
33. Latour JM. Perspectives on parental presence during resuscitation: a literature review. Pediatr Intensive Care Nurs 2002;3(1):5–8.
34. Widger KA, Wilkins K. What are the key components of quality perinatal and pediatric end-of-life care? A literature review. J Palliat Care 2004;20(2):105–112.

9

The Physician–Scientist in the Pediatric Intensive Care Unit

Thomas P. Shanley

A fool is a man who never tried an experiment in his life.

Erasmus Darwin (1792)

Introduction

The advancement of clinical practices in medical subspecialties has nearly always relied on successful experimentation. Biomedical research has substantially impacted human health and, as a result, nearly every aspect of living over the past century. Technological and scientific advances during the past decade have resulted in a fundamental change in the way that basic disease processes are viewed. These tremendous advances have led to the eradication of diseases, have cured previously fatal illnesses and anomalies, and have substantially increased the average life span. However, some aspects of medicine, in particular critical care medicine, have failed to fully enjoy this impressive success. For example, mortality from sepsis has only modestly been impacted over the past two decades, and only recently has a substantial impact on mortality from acute lung injury/acute respiratory distress syndrome been significantly appreciated.

To continue to impact on the diseases that plague children in the pediatric intensive care unit (PICU) setting, we must impart the skills necessary for performing the required clinical and basic science research to practicing intensivists. It is well-trained physician–scientists who will provide insight into the molecular pathogeneses of diseases, design novel therapeutic agents and strategies, test their clinical effectiveness and safety, and measure overall outcomes and cost-effectiveness of novel approaches. As a result, advancement of our field relies on the successful training of physician–scientists in pediatric critical care medicine.

A "Call to Arms"

Recent occurrences have laid the groundwork for immense research opportunities in pediatric critical care medicine. Just after the start of the new millennium, the journals *Science* and *Nature* respectively announced the completion of the Human Genome Project by Celera and the National Institutes of Health (NIH) [1,2]. The realization of this vision, once considered by many as the ultimate pinnacle of science, came to fruition largely as a result of the great advances in molecular biology over the past decades. The completion of this crucial task has identified an estimated 30,000 genes in the human genome. However, with alternative splicing variants, single nucleotide polymorphisms, and post-transcriptional modifications, it is estimated that these genes encode for some 300,000 separate proteins in humans. The need for advanced informatics tools to be applied to this new science of *genomics* necessary to integrate and correlate huge numbers of data have driven the age of *bioinformatics*.

Simultaneously, there has been a recent recognition that children should be incorporated into clinical trials. Under the auspices of the Food and Drug Administration Modernization Act of 1997, incentives are in place that encourage drug companies to perform studies in children. At the NIH, leadership has been put in place that represents the voice of pediatric intensivists not only at the National Institute of Child Health Development (NICHD) but also at other branches of the NIH, such as the National Heart, Lung, and Blood Institute (NHLBI) and General Medical Science (NIGMS). Networks, such as the Pediatric Acute Lung Injury and Sepsis Investigators (PALISI) group and virtual PICU (vPICU), are evolving with the goal of uniting academic divisions of pediatric critical care in order to devise strategies by which clinical trials can be designed through sharing of resources, revenue, and patient data. At the same time, a general consensus exists that there is a critical shortage of pediatrician–scientists [3,4].

Finally, as the understanding of the pathogeneses of diseases reaches the cellular and molecular levels, the gap between medicine and molecular biology will disappear. It is imperative that all physicians caring for critically ill children in this new era have a thorough understanding of the applicability of molecular biology to clinical medicine. The challenge for the physician–scientist in the year 2006 and beyond will be to bring these new findings from the bench to the bedside. Thus, in this exciting time, the potential for enormous research growth exists. It is imperative that the pediatric

D.S. Wheeler et al. (eds.), *Science and Practice of Pediatric Critical Care Medicine*,
DOI 10.1007/978-1-84800-921-9_9, © Springer-Verlag London Limited 2009

TABLE 9.1. Key questions for the pediatric critical care community.

1. Are pediatric intensivists contributing to the further understanding of critical illness?
2. Are pediatric intensivists contributing to the intellectual advancement of medicine and the rich intellectual and academic milieu in the universities in which they find themselves?
3. Are intensivists obtaining extramural funding for university-wide interactive and collaborative research efforts?
4. Are intensivists training future generation physician–scientists adequately?

critical care community can affirmatively answer several key questions (Table 9.1). At this important juncture of our existence as a subspecialty, we must answer each question affirmatively for the sake of our dedicated profession and those children we care for.

Newly Revised Requirements for Subspecialty Training

One of the most important of these tasks is to determine how best to train future physician–scientists. In 1978, the Task Force on the Future of Pediatric Education (FOPE) was charged with carefully examining the manner by which pediatric specialists and, subsequently, subspecialists were trained. More recently, a funded, 3-year initiative called FOPE II was assigned the task of re-evaluating the 1978 report and providing new directions for change as pediatrics entered the 21st century [5,6]. In March 2002, the American Board of Pediatrics (ABP) distributed a report from the Task Force of the Future of Pediatric Education II (FOPE II). This group was assigned the specific task of re-examining the manner by which subspecialty residents (i.e., fellows) were being trained in the United States. Under the auspices of FOPE II, the ABP assigned a Subspecialties Committee to review the current fellowship training requirements and determine if they are sufficient to meet the needs of both the public and the pediatric medical community. As a result of these discussions, a revised set of requirements has been established calling for fellowship training programs to incorporate into their curriculum mastery of each of six general competencies identified by the Accreditation Council for Graduate Medical Education (ACGME): medical knowledge, patient care, professionalism, interpersonal and communication skills, practice-based learning and improvement, and systems-based practice; and an additional requirement to engage fellows in specific areas of scholarly activity that will facilitate the acquisition of those skills (see http://www.abp.org/) necessary for becoming an effective subspecialist and advancing pediatric *research*. In order to accomplish this, what the requirements practically called for was that all fellows engage in *projects of substantive scholarly exploration and analysis that require critical thinking* in any number of areas, including basic, clinical, or translational research; health service research; quality improvement; bioethics; education; or public policy. The requirement to have a *Scholarship Oversight Committee* charged with overseeing the progress and completion of the scholarly activity is intended to ensure acquisition of these necessary skills.

In their report, the Subspecialties Committee acknowledged that the 1996 statement from the Federation of Pediatric Organizations (FOPO) that "the principal goal of fellowship training should be the development of future academic pediatricians" remains a relevant one. However, the subcommittee recognized the various career pathways available for academic pediatric subspecialists and thus

thought it inappropriate to restrict fellow trainees only to a physician–scientist pathway. As a result, the committee stated that the requirement for "evidence of a meaningful accomplishment in research" previously mandated by the ABP failed to achieve its intended goal and thus discontinued it, replacing it with a broader goal of providing skills associated with *academic scholarship*. It was implied that programs should enjoy greater flexibility in designing curriculum by providing expert training in such diverse fields as medical education, history, law, ethics, public policy, health administration, and finances, in addition to those *traditional* areas of basic science and clinical research. As a result of these discussions, the Subspecialties Committee stated the following recommendations:

1. Existing pathways should be structured to allow greater flexibility in training curricula to prepare subspecialty pediatricians for multiple career choices. There should be some modification of existing pathways to allow greater flexibility in the duration and content of clinical training.
2. A new training pathway entitled "Accelerated Research Pathway" should be established. This pathway is intended to assist in the development of highly skilled clinical and laboratory investigators.
3. The requirement for "evidence of a meaningful accomplishment in research" should be discontinued and replaced with a curriculum to provide a broad foundation for scholarly activities.
4. The Subboards should develop additional content specifications for the subspecialty examinations based on the required competencies and assist in the development of assessment instruments to evaluate required competencies as defined by the ACGME [7].

Thus, it is within the context of these proposed guidelines that both mentors and trainees must design the optimal curriculum for the individual embarking on his or her early research training career.

What the New Proposals Suggest

One of the principal recommended guidelines in the 1996 FOPO statement agreed upon by the Subspecialties Committee is that "each fellow should have a mutually agreed upon research mentor who is capable of fostering the trainee's career development and that a research advisory committee should be established to guide and assist the trainee further." Among all other factors, identification of a mentor may have the greatest impact on the eventual success of a trainee's research training. It is therefore imperative that both fellows, who are judging the merits of individual training programs, as well as junior faculty candidates, who are assessing the support to be enjoyed in a new position, develop a sense of the ease or difficulty by which this may be achieved. There are certain factors that can assist this process before one embarks on an unproductive journey.

First, inquire about the recent history of research training and career development among the past fellows and current junior faculty. Do graduates of the fellowship program publish? Have they obtained academic positions upon graduation from the program? Are the current fellows enthusiastic about the mentoring they are receiving for their scholarly pursuit? Are the junior faculty supported? Have they obtained intramural and/or extramural funding? How many of the faculty are committed to extraclinical scholarly pursuits? Determining the answers to these questions is crucial in evaluating the likelihood of the program/division to support the scholarly pursuits of a fellow/junior faculty member. Remember that, while deficiencies can be hidden, one should find the successes clearly on display.

In addition to this establishment of a supportive, mentored environment, it was further recommended that a curriculum be established that provides fellows *an in-depth understanding of biostatistics, clinical and laboratory research study design, critical literature review, principles of evidence-based medicine, ethical principles involving clinical research, and the achievement of satisfactory teaching skills.* Earlier recommendations had also included an introduction to *the process of preparation of grants for peer review.* It is hoped that, in this context, the extent and magnitude of research experience should allow trainees to submit their research findings for publication in refereed journals during their period of training or soon thereafter. In addition to creatively designing a curriculum to fulfill these goals, the subsequent challenge to the fellowship training programs will be to determine the manner by which one can assess if these goals are achieved that has continued to not be well-defined by the accreditation council for graduate medical education (ACGME) or residency review committees (RRC).

What Specifics to Look for in a Program or Position

Perhaps the most crucial challenge a junior investigator faces is to identify the optimal environment that allows him or her to attain independence. In the evaluation of the environment several factors need to be considered. Of utmost importance is the presence of a senior, established, funded investigator (or group of investigators) who is willing to serve as mentor and advisor. These adjectives are not chosen randomly. *Senior* implies this individual has been around the academic environment for years and thus knows the *ins and outs* of both the local and national research culture. The experiences of having written grants, of knowing the best places to apply for funding, and of networking with collaborative investigators are important attributes of the senior researcher. *Established* implies that the individual has already established a promising reputation. As a result, he or she will be more willing to provide direction toward and freedom to pursue projects that are tangential to his or her main focus and not be overly possessive of every aspect of the research endeavors. The ability to develop an independent line of inquiry in this setting is easier. The established investigator usually has more time available for mentoring; however, how well established they are may negatively impact on their availability, as they may be traveling frequently to invited lectureships and meetings. This *availability* should easily be gleaned from interviews with other staff/faculty within the laboratory setting. Finally, it is most likely that start-up funds for a junior researcher will be limited. Often, completion of developed aims will be dependent on the ability of a mentor to provide the necessary resources to do so. Worrying about funding sources early on can be a stressful situation.

If one examines the senior faculty at academic institutions across the country, it is easy to identify several investigators fulfilling these criteria. Nevertheless, not all of them will serve as good mentors. Thus, in addition to these characteristics, it remains imperative for the junior researcher to know the track record of the mentor with regard to junior faculty career development. Has he or she mentored trainees in either the past or at present? Have the previous trainees been productive in terms of a publication record? Have the trainees gone on to establish independent careers with established funding? These questions are important to answer

TABLE 9.2. Costs of supporting initial academic careers.

	Faculty description		
	Lab based	Clinical based	Clinician/ teacher
Salary + benefits			
Yearly ($ × 1,000)	120 ± 20	124 ± 18	128 ± 20
Period of full support (yrs)	3.1 ± 0.6	3.1 ± 0.8	
Equipment ($ × 1,000)	97 ± 73	35 ± 29	
Technical/supplies			
Yearly ($ × 1,000)	49 ± 18	37 ± 18	
Period of support (yrs)	3.0 ± 0.5	3.0 ± 0.7	
Research space (ft²)	540 ± 175	306 ± 194	
Time to achieve extramural support (yrs)	3.3 ± 0.7	3.3 ± 0.7	

Source: Adapted from Jobe et al. [8].

affirmatively if one is to hope to identify a supportive mentor for one's career training.

In addition to the individual mentor, one must evaluate the whole department to assess if the necessary resources are present that will allow for successful development of academic pediatricians engaging in either basic or clinical research. A useful summation of such resources is elucidated in the recent report from the Work Group on Research of the American Pediatric Society [8]. Along with the mentoring reviewed above, the Work Group listed additional resources the junior researcher should evaluate. Perhaps the most underappreciated factor is the initial financial commitment. The costs of an initial start-up package for a laboratory-based investigator are substantial. In a survey of 20 academic institutions, the average estimate of initial financial commitment for the first 3 years of appointment was $650,000. Average research space was estimated to be 540 square feet plus additional office space (Table 9.2). It is useful to consider strategies to defray some of these initial costs by applying for intramural funds set aside for junior faculty or mentored grants from sources such as the NIH in the form of a National Research Service Award (NRSA) or a KO8 grant. The group was explicit in noting that skimping on supplies and technical support impedes successful progress of a junior faculty member [8].

The next consideration is the division of time commitment between clinical responsibilities, administrative duties, and research time. Provision of protected time is key to allowing the young investigator ample opportunity for establishing himself or herself. Reasonable guidelines would allow 70%–80% protected research time in the context of 8–12 weeks attending coverage. Fortunately for the pediatric intensivist, consultative service and outpatient clinic coverage are often nonexistent, yet in this heavily technical subspecialty, clinical time cannot be truncated too minimally without risking a loss of clinical skills. More easily achieved is the ability of chairpersons or section chiefs to excuse young investigators from administrative duties in the early years of establishing their careers. In their report, the Work Group also estimated that the departmental financial commitment to develop one independent investigator will be upwards of $1.5 million, assuming a success rate of 50% [8]. Therefore, it behooves the individual to be certain that the department has the resources, mentors, and patience to support him or her through an estimated 3–5-year time frame. By examining the track record of an institution's capacity to successfully assist its junior faculty attain independence, one can ascertain one's own chances of gaining independence in that environment.

For those interested in clinical research, the necessary resources and timing of career development may differ. Because of the longer time to successfully complete clinical studies or generate databases used for hypothesis testing, establishment of a publication record and preliminary data may be slower than it takes for a laboratory-based researcher. Thus, departments need to use creative ways for designing faculty appointments and titles that can regulate the time allowed for career establishment and not risk the loss of support to promising individuals. Excepting the costs related to start-up equipment and space allocation, the resources necessary for salary, equipment, and staff support for the clinical investigator were estimated to be similar to those of the laboratory-based one (see Table 9.2).

With these resources in place, in the context of a supportive environment, a few specific strategies for fostering independence have been suggested [8]. First, it is important for the junior investigator to develop a publication record. Therefore, young researchers should be the first and corresponding authors. They should be encouraged to seek independent, supplemental funding (see sources below) and aim to develop lines of investigation independent from the mentor(s). In approaching nonmentored grants, they should utilize mentors as consultants rather than co-investigators. Finally, young investigators should seek out and be provided interactions with the research world outside of their immediate contact group. Taking advantage of both intra- and extramural opportunities to present their work allows junior faculty the chance to develop both good communication skills and collaborations with additional researchers. A polling of emergency department fellows reported a substantial absence of these factors in their training and was associated with increased stress related to research training [9]. Instead, by striving to attain these goals, departmental chairpersons and section chiefs will maximize the chances of motivated, talented junior faculty to achieve successful, independent research careers and reap the benefits of their long-term investment.

Where Can One Find Funding Opportunities?

Available research funding has ridden on the rails of a roller coaster over the past several years. Decreased private philanthropy and charitable giving has at times decreased private and intramural funds. Similarly, federal budget deficits and a slowing economy have impacted on the budget assigned to the NIH in current times. As a result, the previously generous budget with steady annual increases has waned again, with current federally allocated research funding at a suboptimal level. Despite this worrisome trend, the breadth of information provided by Internet use gives investigators several accessible resources for identifying funding opportunities. Although the available resources are too numerous to list here, an attempt is made to summarize some general sites commonly used by successful investigators.

As mentioned, two general types of funding are available—intra- and extramural. Intramural funding sources are those monetary resources set aside by one's own academic institution that are internally allocated by self-determined rules. In many instances, institutions that enjoy the greatest success with research career development have utilized such funds to provide that support necessary to transition trainees to independent funding. It is important to realize that in addition to being available to junior faculty, many internal funding programs are also available for retaining talented fellows for a transitional time period. Potential advantages

to this approach include a continuation of incomplete projects initiated as fellows, minimization of clinical time demands, maintenance of mentor relationships, and delaying of the tenure "clock" if the position is designed for instructor-level appointments. It is often in this time frame that preliminary data for extramural supplemental funding, mentored grants, or independent grant applications can be successfully generated.

Extramural funding is provided by numerous private and public sources, including private philanthropic organizations, industry, private contracts, and government sources. The evolution of the economic power of the United States since World War II is what has allowed for ongoing funding of numerous federal agencies. Those funds allocated to the NIH have allowed this agency to become the primary sponsor of extramurally funded research (~50%) in the United States [10]. The downside of this growth has been the inevitable politicization of research such that government perception of important research areas may not always mesh with that of the scientific community [11]. In addition, the dependency of these allocation funds on the current fiscal and economic environment of the country has resulted in the problematic *ups and downs* of NIH budget limitations.

Several useful sources are available to direct one to extramural opportunities. Deans' offices or sponsored program offices should possess exhaustive lists. Networking among colleagues within the academic setting, at national society meetings, or with scientific collaborators can identify starting points. In this age of Internet-accessible information, investigators have a plethora of useful sites for identifying funding sources. The following list includes several starting sites that can provide easy and mostly free access to numerous biomedical-funding opportunities. A particularly useful starting site is "A Grant Seeker's Guide to the Internet: Revised and Revisited," by Andrew J. Grant, PhD, and Suzy D. Sonenberg, MSW; see http://www.mindspring.com/~ajgrant/guide.htm. In reviewing the history of the Internet as a source of information, these authors proceed to provide brief outlines of funding opportunities listed at several other sites with direct links.

Additional sites that provide a tremendous breadth of extramural funding opportunities include the following: GrantsNet, co-sponsored by the Howard Hughes Medical Institute and the American Association for the Advancement of Science (http://www.grantsnet.org/); and The Grant Advisor Plus (http://grantadvisor.com), which provides grant examples, editorial assistance, as well as funding options but requires a 1-year subscription fee of approximately $400. The site administrators argue that this is a small investment for a large (i.e., funded grant) return. The are also the Community of Science Funding Opportunity site (http://fundingopps2.cos.com/), which boasts the world's largest funding database (400,000 funding opportunities totaling $33 billion); the Agency for Healthcare Research and Quality site (http://www.ahrq.gov/fund/), particularly apropos to clinical investigators; and the TRAM Web site (http://tram.east.asu.edu/fund/), initially developed by the Texas Research Administrators Group in 1995 and moved to Arizona State University East in 1999. Finally, any young investigator pursuing an independent, academic career needs to familiarize himself or herself with the NIH web site: http://grants.nih.gov/grants/index.cfm. Regardless of the sites used, it is important to remember that both the administrators of one's institutionally sponsored programs section as well as senior investigators should be judged capable of providing ongoing advice and information regarding the most practical funding opportunities available to the trainee and junior faculty.

Features that Characterize the Successful Researcher

Finally, what can the young physician–scientist bring to the table? There are several characteristics that have been noted by the world's greatest investigative minds over the course of history that are espoused to predict success in research. In his 2001 Joseph W. St. Geme Address, Dr. Russell Chesney provided an eloquent summary of those features that are indispensable toward developing a successful academic pediatric career [12]. "*Curiosity* is one of the permanent and certain characteristics of a vigorous mind" [13]. *Inquiry* is equally important. Quoting Thucydides, who wrote, "With reference to the narrative of events, far from permitting myself to derive it from the first source that came to hand, I did not even trust my own impressions, but it rests partly on what I saw myself, partly on what others saw for me, the accuracy of the report being always tried by the most severe and detailed tests possible" [14], Chesney stressed the importance of CONSTANT QUESTIONING. One must maintain an interest in advancing knowledge. One must display the capacity to see the connections between seemingly unrelated observations, to question dogma and thoughtless authority, and to engage in inquiry-based research. It is important to recognize that this is a life-long endeavor, and, thus, one must maintain an open mind and the ability to reinterpret old ideas in the context of modern technology. One must possess a lively, imaginative, creative, and energetic mind, for *Imagination is more important than knowledge*. As Abe Rudolph said, we do not want *tired old men and women on completion of fellowship*.

Finally, good research always depends on a good question, and good questions always come from the frustrations of a bedside, clinical challenge. Remember that the aim of research is to advance the care that can be provided to our patients at the bedside. By being observant in one's clinical work, an endless number of hypotheses can be generated and tested by vigorous experimental design. In this manner, our future physician–scientists will enjoy the fulfillment of having made a difference in their patients' lives.

References

1. McPherson JD, Marra M, Hillier L, et al. A physical map of the human genome. Nature 2001;409:934.
2. The human genome. Science genome map. Science 2001;291:1218.
3. Gruskin A, Williams RG, McCabe ER, et al. Final report of the FOPE II Pediatric Subspecialists of the Future Workgroup. Pediatrics 2000; 106:1224.
4. Moskowitz J, Thompson JN. Enhancing the clinical research pipeline: training approaches for a new century Acad Med 2001;76: 307.
5. Task Force on the Future of Pediatric Education. The Future of Pediatric Education II. Organizing pediatric education to meet the needs of infants, children, adolescents, and young adults in the 21st century. A collaborative project of the pediatric community. Pediatrics 2000;105:157.
6. Mulvey HJ, Alden ER, Simon JL, et al. The Future of Pediatric Education II: Reports from the project's five workgroups—a collaborative project of the pediatric community. Pediatrics 2000;106: 1173.
7. Federation of Pediatric Organizations. Pediatrics 2004;114:295–296.
8. Jobe AH, Abramson JS, Batshaw M, et al. Recruitment and development of academic pediatricians: departmental commitments to promote success. Pediatr Res 2002;51:662.
9. Hostetler MA, Davis CO. Research training among pediatric emergency medicine fellows. Am J Emerg Med 2002;20:222.
10. Wetzel RC. Research in pediatric critical care. In: Fuhrman BP, Zimmerman JJ, eds. Pediatric Critical Care. St. Louis: Mosby; 1998: 162.
11. Nicholson RS. Congressional pork versus peer review. Science 1992; 256:1497.
12. Chesney RW. Joseph W. St. Geme, Jr address 2001: can one have a successful academic career in 2001? Pediatrics 2001;108:1349.
13. Johnson S. On curiosity. In: Beck EM, ed. The Rambler, March 12, 1751, Bartlett's Familiar Quotations. Boston: Little, Brown and Company; 1980.
14. Thucydides. On inquiry. In: Beck EM, ed. The History of the Peloponnesian War (431–413 B.C.), Bartlett's Familiar Quotations. Boston: Little, Brown and Company; 1980:80.

10

Resident and Nurse Education in the Pediatric Intensive Care Unit

Girish G. Deshpande, Gwen Lombard, and Adalberto Torres, Jr.

Introduction

Learning is a lifelong process; this is especially true in medicine, which continues to evolve each day. Dreyfus and Dreyfus [1] described the stages of learning that individuals go through during their professional lives. These five stages are novice, advanced beginner, competent, proficient, and expert (Figure 10.1). Brenner applied this model in a study of the nursing profession. *Expertise develops when the clinician tests and refines propositions, hypotheses, and principle-based expectations in actual practice situations* [2]. Hands-on experience is essential for the development of the physician or nurse. In professional education, learners grow into teachers and teachers continue to be learners. The medical student becomes the first-year resident and a teacher of medical students. More senior residents are responsible for the education of junior residents. The ever-changing practice of medicine requires physicians and nurses to engage in continued learning. One never stops being a learner.

Uniqueness of Pediatric Intensive Care Units

Pediatric intensive care units (PICUs) are unique learning environments in several respects, including (1) the wide range of patient ages, (2) the severity of patients' illnesses, (3) the need for a rapid response to destabilization of critically ill patients, (4) seasonal variations in workload and training opportunities, (5) continually changing technology and medications, and (6) the wide variety of experience levels of staff. The age range of patients admitted to PICUs varies from preterm neonate to adult. Adults undergoing heart surgery for repair of congenital heart disease may be admitted to the PICU, if preferred by the cardiovascular surgeon. Many adults with life-long pediatric illnesses or conditions (e.g., cystic

fibrosis, cerebral palsy) may also be admitted to the PICU because of their small size, familiarity with the PICU staff, or primary care physician's referral preference.

Seasonal variations of certain diseases, especially infectious illnesses, result in differences in workload and learning opportunities for residents and new nurses. For example, residents rotating through the PICU during respiratory syncytial virus season have more chances of performing tracheal intubations than residents rotating through in the summer, whereas residents rotating through the PICU during the summer months are more likely to see near-drowning or trauma cases.

Teaching PICUs are generally located in the regional referral institutions and, therefore, they attract more complex and severely ill patients from local community hospitals. The PICUs house the sickest patients in the hospital, and all have distinct pathophysiologies. Illnesses range from status asthmaticus to smoke inhalation, from diabetic ketoacidosis to adrenal crisis, from meningitis to head injury, and from sepsis to child abuse. Often a rapid deterioration in a patient's critical condition demands that the therapeutic response be delivered with almost equal speed, limiting time spent discussing therapeutic options with the resident or nurse.

The constantly evolving technology and endless introduction of new medications also makes PICUs more challenging for learners who have to learn the basic principles while trying to stay up to date with new information. Learners in the PICU face a daunting task of acquiring both new skills and knowledge while simultaneously caring for the sickest of patients. They are also expected to develop skills such as self-directed and life-long learning [3]. At any time in the PICU there are a wide variety of professionals in training, which adds to the complexity of the learning environment. Although to new residents or nurses the PICU may appear alarmingly chaotic, intimidating, unforgiving, and unnerving, it offers a unique learning experience where they can expand their knowledge base, sharpen their clinical skills, and learn the value of a good clinical team.

Resident Education Techniques

There are several formats used for teaching residents. Traditionally, residents may be educated during patient care rounds, morning reports, noon conferences, or grand rounds (i.e., didactic lectures), small group discussions, mock codes (e.g., simulated

D.S. Wheeler et al. (eds.), *Science and Practice of Pediatric Critical Care Medicine*,
DOI 10.1007/978-1-84800-921-9_10, © Springer-Verlag London Limited 2009

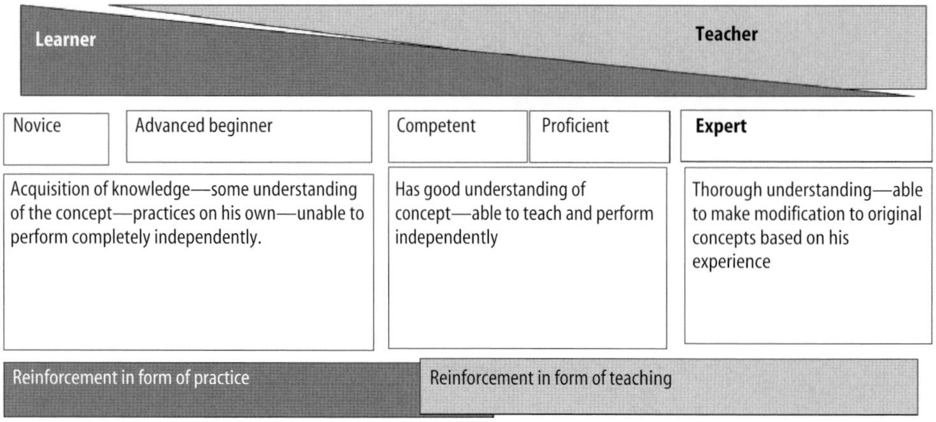

FIGURE 10.1. Five stages of skill acquisition.

cardiopulmonary arrest scenarios with mannequins), and in orga-nized, focused courses that use a combination of these techniques (e.g., Pediatric Advanced Life Support provider course). Novice nurses usually undergo orientation lecture series and learn while working with a preceptor.

Despite being the most widely used format, didactic lectures are well documented to be unsuccessful in changing physician perfor-mance and patient outcomes [4,5]. Hence, medical educators have begun to use more interactive education formats. Examples of medical education formats that have demonstrable success in influ-encing physician behavior and/or patient outcomes in inpatient pediatrics include problem-based learning (PBL) and computer-assisted learning (CAL).

Problem-based learning is a learner-oriented, instructor-facili-tated activity in which a specific case is presented from which learners must decide what information they need to seek to diag-nose or treat the problem. Problem-based learning was designed for small groups that work both together and independently on information gathering and problem solving. The instructor, who serves as a facilitator, selects the clinical scenario carefully to enhance the learners' cognitive and problem-solving abilities. Although PBL has been used in medicine for over 30 years and is a popular adult learning model, it is time consuming, and studies have shown that it has little long-term effect on self-directed learn-ing [6–8]. David and Patel provide an excellent review of PBL in pediatrics [9].

Advances in computer technology, increased accessibility to computers, and availability of medical resources on the Internet have pushed CAL to the forefront of medical education. One of the most informative and useful Web sites for pediatric intensive care is PedsCCM (http://pedsccm.org). Besides providing clinical tools, evidence-based reviews of applicable literature, and clinical guidelines useful in caring for critically ill children, it also gives links to other educational Web sites, such as the *PICU Course* (http://www.sccm.org/specialties/pediatrics/picu_course/).

The Pediatric Resident Committee, a subcommittee of the Pedi-atric Section of Society of Critical Care Medicine (SCCM), developed *PICU Course* to form a core curriculum for medical stu-dents and residents in pediatric critical care medicine. The slide presentations, authored by members of the Resident Education Committee, are available for download to a computer/server. The presentations were designed to provide a template for didactic ses-sions to be conducted by attending physicians or their designees.

Although *PICU Course* was intended to standardize PICU educa-tion, the presentations can be modified to incorporate variations in management, demographics, and so forth unique to the local area. The second phase of this site's development involves an *end of rotation* online test with case scenario–based questions. The examination is intended to evaluate resident performance and to compare it to peers locally and nationally, and to reinforce the principles of PICU care. Evaluation of the effectiveness of this resource on resident learning is lacking. Although there is insuffi-cient evidence to prove that CAL is better than traditional methods, learners have been shown to perform better when CAL supple-mented traditional methods [10]. Learners must possess basic com-puter literacy to take full advantage of this valuable and growing resource [11].

Mock codes offer a great opportunity to teach important critical thinking skills. Regular conduct of mock codes prepares the resident to perform in crisis situations when there is little time to discuss therapeutic options and assists with team building. Mock codes allow residents to participate not only in different roles but also in different settings. A successful mock code program has several benefits, one of which is working with nurses during a *crisis* when the stress of making a mistake is lowered [12].

Resident Education in Pediatric Critical Care

For more than 100 years, medical education occurred in commu-nity settings. In the mid-19th century, physicians were educated through preceptorships and apprenticeships. With introduction of the full-time university post-Flexner model (1910), education shifted to the universities and their teaching hospitals, where most pediatric education was teacher centered [13]. In 1987, in a summary of a report by the American Board of Pediatrics regarding the future training of pediatricians, Cleveland and Brownlee [14] com-mented that the current training programs did not adequately prepare pediatric residents for practice and recommended empha-sis on ambulatory or community-based training.

The *Final report of the FOPE II Pediatric Generalists of the Future Workgroup (2000)* describes the core attributes, skills, and compe-tencies of the future generalist pediatrician and outlines the impli-cations of these requirements for residency training and continuing medical education [15]. The authors state that

Residents must be assured excellent training in the stabilization of critically ill or injured children to manage their problems appropriately in acute care setting. This expectation requires sufficient experience in critical care medicine with older infants and children to be able to provide leadership to a team stabilizing a critically ill patient. A working knowledge of pediatric advanced life support and advanced pediatric life support techniques and algorithms, in addition to the knowledge base to construct a differential diagnosis for further care, is essential [15].

See Table 10.1 for the Residency Review Committee's current educational goals for the PICU [16].

In 1999, the Residency Review Committee published guidelines that permitted a total of 6 months of critical care training during pediatric residency, with a minimum of one rotation in the PICU and 3 months in the neonatal intensive care unit [17]. Since then, a large number of program directors have complained about the limited time residents are permitted to spend in intensive care settings. Directors of programs whose residents tend to practice in more rural areas have expressed the need for more intensive care unit (ICU) experience. The Residency Review Committee agreed that additional training in the ICU would be beneficial to residents and mandated an additional month of PICU experience. With the increase of 1 month in the required PICU experience, the minimum ICU time is now 5 months. The maximum time permitted in intensive care has changed from 6 to 7 months. The Residency Review Committee submitted its final version of the requirements to the Accreditation Council for Graduate Medical Education (ACGME) for approval at its meeting in February 2005 and requested an implementation date of July 1, 2005.

The increased proliferation of new ICUs and ICU beds in the United States has itself caused a shift in resident ICU rotation time. In their survey of program directors for the years 1982, 1987, and 1992, Carraccio and Berman [18] noted a significant increase in the number of PICU and neonatal intensive care unit (NICU) beds along with significant increases in the mean numbers of admissions to the PICU and NICU. During this period, 57% of program directors had increased PICU rotation time by a mean of 1.7 months from a previous mean of 2.5 months. This survey also showed that the number of residents entering primary care had stayed relatively constant, 60% in 1982 versus 56% in 1992. This increase in patient volume in the PICU requires well-trained primary care providers both for the initial stabilization and transportation to the PICU and for follow up after the discharge.

Education of the pediatric residents is even more difficult today for a number of reasons. The service needs for ICUs have been increasing over the past several decades, with advances in technology, earlier identification of potentially critical illnesses, and the survival of more and more premature infants and infants with congenital heart diseases and other technology-dependent illnesses. An emphasis on ambulatory pediatric rotations along with an increase in time spent in community pediatrics has also occurred, with pediatric residents spending less and less time caring for hospitalized patients. The new duty hours rule from the Residency Review Committee [19] limits residents to spend 80 hours per week (averaged over a 4-week period) in clinical and academic activities. Residents' continuity clinics also significantly reduce (10%–30%) inpatient care time. In addition, housestaff are expected to attend morning reports, didactic conferences, and grand rounds all of which require them to be relieved of patient care responsibilities. Other responsibilities of residents in the PICU consist of admitting patients with their history and physical examination, managing patients inclusive of procedures, collecting patient or clinical data (laboratory, imaging, and other tests), clarifying pharmacy data, participating in nursing discussions/clarifications, and making home care arrangements at the time of discharge of patients. Although these tasks teach residents about the inpatient health care system they are working in, they add very little to their knowledge of the patients or the illnesses and interfere with their formal education.

One approach taken to meet the service needs in the PICU and to relieve housestaff of their noneducational responsibilities has been the hiring of physician extenders such as advanced nurse practitioners and physician assistants. However, this alternative can be expensive, making hospitals reluctant to consider the educational needs of housestaff over service needs [18]. In addition, training these allied health professionals creates competition for learning opportunities between the housestaff and the physician extenders in smaller or slower PICUs.

Evaluation of Residents

Resident performance is assessed in six areas to the level expected of a new practitioner: patient care, medical knowledge, interpersonal skills and communication, practice-based learning and improvement, professionalism, and system-based practice. The ACGME website (http://www.acgme.org/acWebsite/RRC_320/320_gencomp.pdf) also provides several tools to evaluate the performance of residents. The expectations for the residents in these six areas are as follows:

Patient care: Residents must be able to provide family-centered patient care that is culturally effective, developmentally and age

TABLE 10.1. PICU educational goals of the residency review committee [16].

1. Residents rotating through the pediatric intensive care unit (PICU) must be familiar with the multidisciplinary and multiorgan implications of fluid, electrolyte, and metabolic disorders; trauma, nutrition, and cardiorespiratory management; infection control; and recognition and management of congenital anomalies.
2. The PICU rotation must be designed to teach the recognition and management of isolated and multiorgan system failure, assessment of its reversibility, and an understanding of the variations in organ system dysfunction by age of patient.
3. Residents must learn to integrate clinical assessment and laboratory data to formulate management plans for critically ill patients.
4. Residents must know and utilize the invasive and noninvasive techniques for monitoring and supporting pulmonary, cardiovascular, cerebral, and metabolic functions.
5. Residents must participate in decision making in the admitting, discharge, and transfer of patients in the ICUs; this includes resuscitation, stabilization, and transportation of patients to the ICUs and within the hospital.
6. Residents must understand the appropriate roles of the generalist pediatrician and the intensivist in these settings; participation in preoperative and postoperative management of surgical patients, including understanding the appropriate roles of the general pediatric practitioner and the intensivist in this setting; evaluation and management, during the pediatric intensive care experience, of patients following traumatic injury.
7. Residents are expected to learn several procedural skills, including training in basic and advanced life support, endotracheal intubation, placement of intraosseous lines (demonstration in a skills lab or PALS course is sufficient), placement of intravenous lines, arterial puncture, venipuncture, umbilical artery and vein catheterization, lumbar puncture, bladder catheterization, wound care and suturing of lacerations, procedural sedation, pain management, chest tube placement, and thoracentesis.

Source: From Donini-Lenhoff [16]. Reprinted with permission from the American Medical Association.

appropriate, compassionate, and effective for the treatment of disease and the promotion of health.

Medical knowledge: Residents must demonstrate knowledge of established and evolving biomedical, clinical, epidemiologic, and social–behavioral sciences and application of this knowledge to patient care.

Practice-based learning and improvement: This involves the investigation and evaluation of care of patients, the appraisal and assimilation of scientific evidence, and improvements in inpatient care.

Interpersonal and communication skills: Residents must be able to demonstrate interpersonal and communication skills that result in effective information exchange and teaming with patients, their families, and professional associates.

Professionalism: Residents must demonstrate a commitment to carrying out professional responsibilities, adherence to ethical principles, and sensitivity to diversity.

System-based practice: This is manifested by actions that demonstrate an awareness of and responsiveness to the larger context and system of health care, as well as the ability to call effectively on other resources in the system to provide optimal health care.

Educating New Graduate Nurses

Educating nurses in the PICU has its own unique challenges. Nurses often must learn while carrying a full clinical workload. New graduate nurses in the PICU have to simultaneously learn hospital policies and procedures and the pathophysiologies of the wide array of pediatric illnesses, while acquiring practical bedside skills (e.g., invasive catheter care). Clinical demands during periods of high census, high acuity, and/or inadequate staffing can disrupt the preceptor–novice relationship and create stress on the novice nurse that can be potentially detrimental to learning and to patient safety [20]. Strategies used to facilitate critical care learning by nurses include PBL, concept mapping, nursing narratives, learning contracts, and reflective practices [21,22]. The major limiting factor identified by PICU nurses as to which learning method they preferred was time constraints [23]. Students had a strong preference for courses in which theory and content were related to practice, making learning more relevant. A nurturing environment with knowledgeable preceptors, peer support, flexible work schedule, and multiformat educational approach (e.g., lectures, videos, case studies) has been successful in improving graduate nurse retention in the PICU [24]. Computer-assisted learning resources are available for critical care nurses [25] and can even facilitate learning critical nursing skills [26]. Interested readers are referred to excellent references that deal with conceptual [27,28] and practical [29–31] learning principles for critical care nurses.

Nursing care in the PICU requires meticulous attention to detail and good communication skills to provide the best care to the critically ill child. Patients are treated with a multitude of medications and infusions; a small error in calculation, composition, or administration could lead to disastrous results, potentially causing morbidity or mortality. The graduate nurse discovers early in her PICU education whether she or he possesses the ability to thrive in this highly challenging environment, which is often its own reward.

Use of Simulators in Medical Education

Experiential learning or learner-centered teaching has been accepted as the best strategy for educators in the PICU to employ. According to Kolb [32], it is through repeated learning experiences that learners' thoughts are formed and reformed. Guided practice allows learners to assimilate key concepts, attitudes, and skills. Skills to be learned in the PICU are either hands on, procedural, or problem solving. Problem-solving skills include making decisions when adequate information is not available or in the presence of conflicting information. Occasionally, clinical problems are encountered that come with little guidance from the literature or experience to help manage the case.

Medical education has been based on apprenticeship techniques since the era of Hippocrates. Medical simulation offers the potential for the evolution of new teaching paradigms for the new millennium [3]. The use of human patient simulators and reflective practice has recently come to the forefront of critical care education [3,11,33]. High-fidelity simulators are full-bodied mannequins that breathe, talk, blink, have a palpable pulse, make urine, and have audible bowel sounds similar to patients [33]. Simulators such as those made by METI (Medical Education Technology Inc., Sarasota, FL; www.meti.com) and Laerdal (Laerdal Medical Corp., Wappingers Falls, NY; www.laerdal.com) are becoming increasingly available in large academic medical centers. High-fidelity simulators provide ideal opportunities for experiential learning and hands-on practice with use of real instruments with real-time patient reactions to students' actions. The simulators provide a number of prescribed cases for students. In addition, real patient cases and data can be used to create scenarios that recreate what happened on the ward. Simulators can also be used to maintain skills that may be used rarely in the PICU, such as cardiopulmonary resuscitation [34]. Simulators can create adverse situations such as esophageal intubation or dislodged endotracheal tubes that in real life could be life threatening and hence cannot be deliberately created. It is mandatory that physicians recognize such situations immediately and manage them correctly and swiftly.

Simulators are educational tools that allow students to learn new skills in a safe environment. Scenarios can be played out so that learners can see the results of their actions without having the attending or instructors having to step in and correct their actions or decisions. The use of videotape provides an objective, time-coded record of trainee communication and actions and creates a powerful stimulus for learning during facilitated debriefing. Because the activities in the simulator pose no risk to patients or to professional liability, trainees are allowed to witness the natural evolutions of mistakes without the need for intervention by senior faculty [35]. Simulators can also be used for learner assessment and evaluation [36,37]. This is especially important for the competencies in residency education and being able to document a resident's ability to perform critical skills and procedures [38]. Thus, in a new era of exponentially increasing medical knowledge and ever-decreasing patient contact, simulation may offer an answer. According to Christine McGuire, professor of medical education at the University of Illinois, simulation offers an opportunity to leverage the advantages of experiential learning and reflective practices through three defining characteristics: simulation imitates but does not duplicate reality, offers almost limitless opportunities to *go wrong*, and provides corrective feedback as a guide to future action [37]. The Society of Critical Care Medicine has recently published *Simulators in Critical Care and Beyond* [3]. William Dunn, as editor, has compiled a series of articles on the history and use of high-fidelity simulators in medical education. This book is highly recommended reading for all residency directors and directors of PICU education.

Conclusion

The PICU offers a unique learning environment. There are several models for adult learning, and success depends on the stage of learner, method used, and skill of the instructor/facilitator. Teaching residents all the knowledge base and procedural skills required by ACGME during their limited work hours is a challenge being faced by intensivists across the country. A combination of the many available educational approaches should be tailored to meet local educational needs while conforming to national standards. High-fidelity simulators appear to be a safe and effective way to teach and evaluate residents, fellows, and nurses inside or outside of the PICU environment.

References

1. Dreyfus HL, Dreyfus SE. Mind over Machine: The Power of Human Intuition and Expertise in the Era of the Computer. New York: The Free Press; 1986.
2. Brenner P. From Novice to Expert: Excellence and Power in Clinical Nursing Practice. Upper Saddle River, NJ: Prentice Hall Health; 2001.
3. Dunn W, ed. Simulators in Critical Care and Beyond. Des Plaines, IL: Society of Critical Care Medicine; 2004.
4. Davis D, Thomson MA, Oxman A, Andrew D, Haynes RB. Changing physician performance: a systematic review of the effect of continuing medical education strategies. JAMA 1995;274:700–705.
5. Davis D, Thomson O'Brien MA, Freemantle N, Wolf F, Mazmanian P, Taylor-Vaisey A. Impact of formal continuing medical education. Do conferences, workshops, rounds, and other traditional continuing education activities change physician behavior or health care outcomes? JAMA 1999;282:867–874.
6. Colliver JA. Effectiveness of problem-based learning curricula: research and theory. Acad Med 2000;75:259–266.
7. Colliver JA. Educational theory and medical education practice: a cautionary note for medical school faculty. Acad Med 2002;77:1217–1220.
8. Ozuah P, Curtis J, Stein R. Impact of problem-based learning on residents' self-directed learning. Arch Pediatr Adolesc Med 2001;155: 669–672.
9. David TJ, Patel L. Adult learning theory, problem based learning, and paediatrics. Arch Dis Child 1995;73:357–363.
10. Tegtmeyer K, Ibsen L, Goldstein B. Computer-assisted learning in critical care: from ENIAC to HAL. Crit Care Med 2001;29:N177–N182.
11. Vozenilek J, Huff S, Reznek M, Gordon J. See one, do one, teach one: advanced technology in medical education. Acad Emerg Med 2004; 11:1149–1154.
12. Tegtmeyer K. Education in the age of the 80-hour work week. In: Tegtmeyer K, ed. Current Concepts in Pediatric Critical Care. Des Plaines, IL: Society of Critical Care Medicine; 2005:135–142.
13. American Academy of Pediatrics, Committee on Community Health Services. Community Pediatrics: An Annotated Bibliography. Grove Village, IL: American Academy of Pediatrics; 2002.
14. Cleveland W, Brownlee R, American Board of Pediatrics. Future training of pediatricians: summary report of a series of conferences sponsored by the American Board of Pediatrics. Pediatrics 1987;80:451–457.
15. Leslie L, Rappo P, Abelson H, Jenkins R, Sewall S. Final report of the FOPE II Pediatric Generalists of the Future Workgroup. Pediatrics 2000;106:1199–1223.
16. Donini-Lenhoff F, ed. Program requirements for residency education in pediatrics. In: Graduate Medical Education Directory 2004–2005. Chicago: American Medical Association; 2005:283–291.
17. Program Requirements for Residency Education in Pediatrics. In: Graduate Medical Education Directory 1998–1999. Chicago: American Medical Association; 1999:211–220.
18. Carraccio C, Berman M. Intensive care: impact on resident education. Clin Pediatr 1994;Oct:625–627.
19. Donini-Lenhoff F, ed. Institutional requirements. In: Graduate Medical Education Directory 2004–2005. Chicago: American Medical Association; 2005:13–21.
20. Endacott R, Scholes J, Freeman M, Cooper S. The reality of clinical learning in critical care settings: a practioner: student gap? J Clin Nurs. 2003;12:778–785.
21. Dobbin K. Applying learning theories to develop teaching strategies for the critical care nurse. Don't limit yourself to the formal classroom lecture. Crit Care Nurs Clin North Am. 2001;13:1–11.
22. Dix G, Hughes SJ. Strategies to help students learn effectively. Nurs Standard 2004;18:39–42.
23. Hewitt-Taylor J, Gould D. Learning preferences of paediatric intensive care nurses. J Adv Nurs 2002;38:288–295.
24. Janvrin S. Introducing new graduates into pediatric intensive care. A thorough on-the-job program turns anxious graduates into confident beginning practitioners. Nurs Manag 1990;21.
25. Bove L. Computer-assisted education for critical care nurses. Crit Care Nurs Clin North Am 2001;13:73–81.
26. DeAmicis P. Interactive videodisc instruction is an alternative method for learning and performing a critical nursing skill. Comput Nurs 1997;15:155–158.
27. Kinney MR. Education for critical care nursing. Annu Rev Nurs Res 1990;8:161–176.
28. Kuiper R, Pesut D. Promoting cognitive and metacognitive reflective reasoning skills in nursing practice: self-regulated learning theory. J Adv Nurs 2004;45:381–391.
29. Dickerson P. 10 tips to help learning. J Nurses Staff Dev 2003;19: 240–246.
30. Hohler S. Creating an environment conductive to adult learning. AORN J 2003;77:833–835.
31. Campbell J, Bell-Scott W. Unique solutions in pediatric critical care. Pediatr Nurs 2001;27:483–491.
32. Kolb DA. Experiential Learning: Experience as the Source of Learning and Development. Englewood Cliff, NJ: Prentice Hall; 1984.
33. Friedrich MJ. Practice makes perfect: risk free medical training with patient simulators. JAMA 2002;288:2808–2812.
34. Fiedor M. Pediatric simulation: a valuable tool for pediatric medical education. Crit Care Med 2004;32(Suppl):S72–S74.
35. Halamek L, Kaegi DM, Gaba DM, et al. Time for a new paradigm in pediatric medical education: teaching neonatal resuscitation in a simulated delivery room environment. Pediatrics 2000;106:e45.
36. Boulet JR, Murray D, Kras J, Woodhouse J, McAllister J, Ziv A. Reliability and validity of a simulation-based acute care skills assessment for medical students and residents. Anesthesiology 2003;99:1270–1280.
37. Tekian A, McGuire CH, McGaghie WC. Innovative Simulations for Assessing Professional Competence: From Paper and Pencil to Virtual Reality. Chicago, IL: University of Illinois at Chicago, Department of Medical Education; 1999.
38. Hugh DJ, Kurrek MM, Cohen MM, Cleave-Hogg D. The validity of performance assessments using simulation. Anesthesiology 2001;95: 36–42.

11

Evidence-Based Medicine in the Pediatric Intensive Care Unit

Adrienne G. Randolph

Introduction

Evidence-based medicine (EBM) was highly controversial when advocated by Dr. Gordon Guyatt and colleagues in the first of a series of articles published in *JAMA* in the 1990s [1]. By 2005, it has become politically correct for clinicians to state that they are EBM supporters. Most of these clinicians, however, do not know the history of EBM or understand the systematic approach that the practice of EBM requires. This chapter starts at the very beginning of clinical research and then leads us up to the era of EBM, describing what EBM is and why it came about. An example of how to approach a clinical situation using EBM is given. Ways to keep up with the evidence and efficiently find evidence is also reviewed. Finally, I address challenges to practicing EBM in the pediatric intensive care unit (PICU).

The Growth of Clinical Research

Most of the illustrative examples of the history of clinical research given below are excerpted from a book titled *Clinical Trials* by Pocock [2] and the James Lind Library, created to introduce people to the characteristics of fair tests of treatments in health care (www.jameslindlibrary.org). Starting in 1753, one of the first published clinical studies was by Lind, titled *A Treatise of the Scurvy* [3]. Below is a modified excerpt of this study:

I took 12 patients in the scurvy on board the Salisbury at sea. The cases were as similar as I could have them . . . they lay together in one place . . . and had one diet common to all. Two of these were ordered one quart of cider a day. Two others took 25 gutts of elixir vitriol. . . . Two others took two spoonfuls of oranges and one lemon given to them each day. . . . Two others took the bigness of a nutmeg. The most sudden and visible good effects were perceived from the use of oranges and lemons, one of those who had

taken them being at the end of 6 days fit for duty. . . . The other . . . was appointed to nurse the sick.

This study is important for two reasons. One is that it was the first strong *evidence* that vitamin C could be used to treat and prevent scurvy. The other is that Lind understood some basic features of good study design. He controlled for differences between patients by identifying those at the same level of illness. He controlled for other influences on outcome by giving these patients the same diet, except for the interventions, and the same amount of sunlight and other environmental exposures. He also had two patients in each treatment arm because, although one patient could improve just by chance, the likelihood of two patients improving was lower. Interestingly, despite this evidence, it was over five decades before lemon juice became standard use on British naval ships. Delays in the application of evidence are still a major problem two and a half centuries later.

Another early clinical researcher was Louis, who established clinical trials and epidemiology on a scientific footing [2]. In the 1800s, bleeding was the standard treatment for numerous serious and minor ailments across the United States and Europe. In 1835, Louis highlighted the needs for exact observation of patient outcome, knowledge of the natural progression of untreated controls, precise definition of disease prior to treatment, and careful observation of deviations from intended treatment [4]. Louis' careful comparisons showing no differences in the outcomes of patients with a variety of disorders who were bled and not bled led to the slow but eventual decline of bleeding as a standard treatment [2]—even though this practice had strong support for over a century.

In the early days of many areas of clinical medicine, especially in surgery, anesthesia, and critical care, the procedures and therapies led to dramatic improvements. With such profoundly clear benefits, the need for large numbers and control groups went by the wayside. Lister in 1870 [5] published a before–after study of antiseptics for amputation operations, reporting a 43% rate of mortality in 35 cases before antiseptic use versus a 15% mortality rate in 40 cases afterwards. Although he was bothered by the small sample size and claimed it was not significant (actually, it is statistically significant), the real problem with before–after studies such as this one is that many other things could have changed in the interim such as newer anesthetic methods, newer surgical techniques, and better basic hygiene. All of these improvements that developed over

D.S. Wheeler et al. (eds.), *Science and Practice of Pediatric Critical Care Medicine*,
DOI 10.1007/978-1-84800-921-9_11, © Springer-Verlag London Limited 2009

time limited the ability to ascribe the improved surgical outcomes to the antiseptic use.

The first reported randomized controlled trial results were in 1948 [6], when streptomycin plus bed rest was compared with bed rest alone for the treatment of pulmonary tuberculosis [7]. The novel features of this trial, besides the randomized assignment to groups, were that outcome assessors were blinded to the treatment allocation and that multiple clinicians were used to assess outcome and had to come to agreement. This leads to what clinical trials are designed to control for, which is called *bias*. Bias is a systematic difference between the research question and the actual question answered by the study that causes the study to give a wrong answer [8]. Carefully designed studies minimize bias. Bias can come from patient variables (e.g., patients in one group being more ill at baseline than in the other group), predictor variables (e.g., patients in one group are treated differently, besides the intervention), outcome variables (e.g., outcome assessors know which arm the patients were assigned to, and their assessment is influenced by this), or the placebo effect. Evidence-based medicine focuses on the design of studies to ensure that steps are taken to minimize bias to allow the real answer to the question to emerge.

In the late 1950s through the 1960s, there was a rapid growth of clinical studies and especially of randomized controlled trials. For some therapies such as penicillin, the impact on disease was so great that observational studies on small numbers of patients showing dramatic recovery [9,10] led to widespread use at the end of World War II and saved thousands of soldiers' lives. It is also true, however, that dramatic-appearing results from clinician observation are often refuted by subsequent randomized trials and that randomized trials can reveal highly significant effects that are dampened by nonrandomized studies. An example of the first is the rise and fall of *gastric freeze* for duodenal ulcer [11]. This intervention rose to be the standard of care in the 1960s based on the clinical experience of major opinion leaders and published statements such as "Since April 1961 no patients with duodenal ulcer disease have been operated upon on the senior author's surgical service. This circumstance in itself bespeaks the confidence in the method by patients as well as surgeons" [12]. Thousands of gastric freezing machines were subsequently sold. A proper randomized trial finally led to the abolishment of gastric freeze for duodenal ulcers because there was no difference in subsequent surgery for ulcer disease, gastrointestinal hemorrhage, or hospitalization for intractable pain for patients randomized to the sham treatment versus the gastric freeze [13].

An example of how a randomized trial can lead to more rapid implementation of a promising intervention due to stronger results is from the Salk polio vaccine trial [2,14,15]. In 1954, the annual incidence of polio was 1 in 2,000. Polio was epidemic but hit some geographic areas harder than others. Because of this, studies of preventive interventions had to be done with the control groups within the same geographic regions. Two studies were planned. Some health care regional authorities opted for an observed control approach where second graders were vaccinated and first and third graders served as controls. One million children participated in this study. Health authorities in other regions were concerned that bias could be introduced if the physician diagnosing polio, a diagnosis not always made with certainty, could guess whether or not the child received the vaccine. These practitioners opted for a blinded randomized controlled trial in which 800,000 children participated. The results were clear in the randomized study that the polio vaccine was highly effective; there was a 70% reduction in

polio, and all four deaths occurred in the control group. The observed control study also showed better outcomes in the vaccinated group; however, children in both groups who were invited to participate but declined had better outcomes in both groups, making the results difficult to interpret.

The 1960s through 1980s were years of rapid growth of the clinical literature with the publication of many thousands of clinical trials. Advances in computerization facilitated management of large datasets, the growth of statistical methods, and searching for medical information. Medical practice was still based, however, on the expertise of the individual practitioner, and there was no systematic way for practitioners to assess and incorporate these published findings into their practice.

The Origins of Evidence-Based Medicine

The birthplace of EBM was in McMaster University in Canada. *Clinical Epidemiology: A Basic Science for Clinical Medicine* was authored by Drs. Sackett, Haynes, and Tugwell and published in 1985 [16]. This core text contains all of the principles of EBM. Unfortunately, the principles were not presented in digestible packets, and the book was not an immediate hit among clinicians. Dr. Gordon Guyatt later coined the term *evidence-based medicine* and put these principles in a series of articles in *JAMA* starting in 1992 entitled *Users' Guides to the Medical Literature* [17]. Each guide has the same structure: (1) Are the results valid? (with different validity criteria for different types of questions); (2) What are the results? (effect size and precision); and (3) Are these results applicable to my patient? Assessing the validity of a study as the initial step can save the reader time. Fancy statistics will not fix a weak study design. If the study is not valid, there is no reason to read further. If the study design is of high quality and the study reports a statistically significant result, the next step is to ensure that the confidence interval around the treatment effect increases our confidence that the treatment is beneficial. If the study reports no effect, it is important to ensure that the study had sufficient power to test the hypothesis. Even if the study is valid, the sample size was large enough, and the confidence interval narrow, the study may not be applicable to your specific patient's situation.

Table 11.1 lists the users' guides' primary validity criteria for questions about therapy or prevention [18,19], diagnosis [20,21], prognosis [22], and for risk or harm [23] to show how different the criteria can be. To practice EBM, it is important to focus the clinical question and to choose and apply the correct users' guide criteria. There are over 25 users' guides currently available for different topics. Each of these can currently be found online at the Centre for Health Evidence (http://www.cche.net/che/home.asp), and they are also available in textbooks [24] and pocket handbooks. In addition, there are series of articles edited by Dr. Deborah Cook that were published in *Critical Care Medicine* using critical care examples [25].

To practice EBM is more than accessing and understanding the users' guides. Evidence-based medicine is defined as the conscientious, explicit, and judicious application of current best evidence to the care of individual patients [26]. The practice of EBM requires the integration of clinical expertise and critical appraisal to determine the applicability and quality of available evidence. Although clinical expertise is hard to define, one cannot effectively practice EBM without sound clinical judgment that comes from a wealth of patient experience. Practitioners of EBM make a commitment to

TABLE 11.1. Primary validity criteria for articles addressing therapy or prevention, diagnosis, prognosis and risk, or harm.

Therapy or prevention [18,19]
- Was the assignment of patients to treatments randomized?
- Were all of the patients who entered the trial properly accounted for and attributed at its conclusion?
  - Was follow-up complete?
  - Were patients analyzed in the groups to which they were randomized?

Diagnosis [20,21]
- Was there an independent, blind comparison with a reference standard?
- Did the patient sample include an appropriate spectrum of the sort of patients to whom the diagnostic test will be applied in clinical practice?

Prognosis [22]
- Was there a representative and well-defined sample of patients at a similar point in the course of disease?
- Was follow-up sufficiently long and complete?

Harm [23]
- Were there clearly identified comparison groups that were similar with respect to important determinants of outcome, other than the one of interest?
- Were the outcomes and exposures measured in the same way in the groups being compared?
- Was follow-up sufficiently long and complete?

use a systematic approach to search for, critically appraise, synthesize, and apply evidence in their clinical practice [26]. To do this requires a five-step approach:

1. Focusing the clinical question
2. Efficiently tracking down the best evidence with which to answer the question
3. Critically appraising the evidence
4. Applying valid, useful evidence in clinical practice
5. Evaluating your performance

To better understand this approach, it is most useful to study a few clinical examples.

An Example of the Evidence-Based Medicine Approach

The subspecialty of critical care in the specialty of pediatrics is a relatively small field. Although the amount and quality of evidence is improving, practicing EBM in the PICU can be challenging and often requires assessing evidence collected in critically ill adult populations or noncritically ill children and then determining if this evidence is applicable to your critically ill pediatric patient. Therefore, I will give an example of one question where evidence exists that is specific to the PICU patient and another where evidence must be extrapolated from other populations.

You just came on service in the PICU and you are pre-rounding with the medical residents at 7 am. Just 2 hours ago, a 4 month old with bronchiolitis was tracheally intubated and placed on mechanical ventilatory support. The patient had a positive test for respiratory syncytial virus (RSV) yesterday when he was admitted to the ward. The patient has severe failure to thrive and has dropped from the 60th percentile for weight at birth to the 5th percentile and is being worked up for cystic fibrosis (CF). They were unable to obtain enough sweat, and the DNA tests for CF markers are pending. The baby has always had a cough and has had a previous admission for pneumonia at age 2 months. You worry that this infant could have a very bad clinical course given the failure to thrive and possible CF. The

pediatric resident asks if ribavirin, a drug that is approved by the Food and Drug Administration for use in RSV bronchiolitis, is indicated for this patient. You are not certain, but you have time before rounds to search the medical literature.

You know that there have been multiple randomized trials published on the efficacy of ribavirin in RSV bronchiolitis. Therefore, your first goal is to determine if someone already performed a systematic review of this topic. You go to the National Center for Biotechnology Information Web site (http://www.ncbi.nlm.nih.gov) on your computer, choose PubMed in the "Search" box, and enter "Ribavirin and Respiratory Syncytial Virus." You then click on the limits section and limit the articles to ages of "All Child 0–18 years" and to publication type of "Meta-Analysis." Your search retrieves two citations. One study was published in 1996 and the other was published in 2004 in the Cochrane Database of Systematic Reviews [27]. [Note: The Cochrane Collaboration is an international nonprofit and independent organization, dedicated to making up-to-date, accurate information about the effects of health care readily available worldwide (www. cochrane.org). It produces and disseminates systematic reviews of healthcare interventions and promotes the search for evidence in the form of clinical trials and other studies of interventions.]

Your institution subscribes to the Cochrane Database so you are able to retrieve the full review online. You retrieve the article. You need to ensure that the review is valid. The Cochrane Collaboration sets and maintains high standards for systematic reviews. It is an excellent place to search for evidence because almost all of the reviews will meet the validity criteria set out by the users' guide for how to use review articles [28] (see Table 11.2). After going through the validity criteria, ensuring the article is valid and that it addresses the focused clinical question that you want to answer, you move on to the results. Twelve randomized trials were included in the review. Because a thorough systematic review was available, you did not need to go through these 12 trials and try to synthesize their results. The reviewers report the following [27]: "In four trials with 158 patients, mortality with ribavirin was 5.8% compared with 9.7% with placebo (odds ratio [OR] 0.58; 95% confidence interval [CI] 0.18 to 1.85). In three trials with 116 patients the probability of respiratory deterioration with ribavirin was 7.1% compared with 18.3% with placebo (OR 0.37; 95% CI 0.12 to 1.18). In three studies with 104 ventilated patients, the weighted mean difference in days of hospitalization was 1.9 fewer days with ribavirin (95% CI −4.6 to +0.9) and the weighted mean difference in days of ventilation was 1.8 fewer days with ribavirin (95% CI −3.4 to −0.2). No statistically significant differences in long-term pulmonary function or in incidence of recurrent wheezing following RSV infection were associated with the use of ribavirin." You can quickly determine that the confidence intervals for mortality and the probability of respiratory deterioration cross one. In addition, no long-term

TABLE 11.2. Users' guides for how to use review articles.

I. Are the results of the study valid?
  A. Primary guides:
    1. Did the overview address a focused clinical question?
    2. Were the criteria used to select articles for inclusion appropriate?
  B. Secondary guides:
    1. Is it unlikely that important, relevant studies were missed?
    2. Was the validity of the included studies appraised?
    3. Were assessments of studies reproducible?
    4. Were the results similar from study to study?

II. What are the results?
  A. What are the overall results of the review?
  B. How precise were the results?

III. Will the results help me in caring for my patients?
  A. Can the results be applied to my patient care?
  B. Were all clinically important outcomes considered?
  C. Are the benefits worth the harms and costs?

Source: From Oxman et al. [28]. Copyright 1994 American Medical Association. All right reserved. Reprinted with permission.

benefits were found. It is clear from this review that there is not strong evidence to justify use of ribavirin in this patient.

One of the residents is trained jointly in adult internal medicine and pediatrics. She asks if the patient should be given heparin prophylaxis to prevent deep venous thrombosis (DVT). She points out that in the adult ICU patients are almost universally given prophylactic heparin for DVT unless they have a clear contraindication. Your infant with RSV bronchiolitis has a femoral central venous line in place, and you know this is a risk factor for thrombosis. The indications for prophylactic anticoagulation in children, however, are not so clear. You are on the Quality Improvement (QI) Committee for your ICU. You answer the resident that you recently reviewed the evidence and attempted to create a protocol for which pediatric patients should receive DVT prophylaxis. You found that systematic review of the incidence of DVT in adult ICU patients revealed that 10%–30% develop a DVT in the first 2 weeks in the ICU [29]. In children, the overall rate in the PICU was reported in a single center study to be markedly lower, at 4% (95% CI [0%–9%] in all patients) [30]. You identified four studies, however, reporting a rate of 8%–44% of DVT in PICU patients with a femoral venous catheter in place [31–34]. Although your patient has this risk factor, and dosing of subcutaneous prophylactic heparin is available for infants from pharmacokinetic studies [35], your QI group found no evidence that use of prophylactic subcutaneous heparin is beneficial in preventing catheter-related DVT in infants. In fact, you found one randomized trial comparing prophylactic low-molecular-weight heparin to placebo to prevent catheter-related DVT in children that was negative [36]. This does not rule out efficacy, however, because the trial was stopped early because of slow enrollment, and the rate of catheter-related DVT was 11/78 (14.1%) in the heparin group versus 12/80 (12.5%) in the placebo group. To find a 25% relative risk reduction with 80% statistical power and an alpha (risk of finding the same result by chance) of 0.05 would require over 1,600 patients per group or a 95% greater sample size. One study found that 84% of 383 randomized trials reporting negative results in major medical journals did not have sufficient power to rule out a 25% relative difference. Therefore, the word is clearly not out on whether low-molecular-weight heparin is effective. In sum, although your patient is at risk for DVT, you answer the resident that you will not be implementing standard DVT prophylaxis with subcutaneous heparin until there are data indicating efficacy in infants and young children with femoral venous catheters.

To answer the second question about use of DVT prophylaxis required a significant amount of time to review the literature and multiple searches using various search techniques. Questions like these that come up recurrently about patients in the PICU are best addressed using an evidence-based review with a multidisciplinary team, dissemination of the findings to colleagues, and annual updating because new evidence may need to be incorporated. Publication of critical appraisals of the evidence in specific topic areas (e.g., treatment of bronchiolitis in the PICU [37] or enteral nutrition in the critically ill patient [38]) and development of evidence-based guidelines (e.g., prevention of ventilator-associated pneumonia [39] or prevention of intravascular catheter-related infections[40]) are extremely helpful. In this way, clinical practice can move more efficiently toward an evidence-based approach.

Finding and Keeping up with the Evidence

As was shown in the example, high-quality systematic reviews of the evidence, when available, save an enormous amount of time. Although reviews that do not take the systematic approach with the goal of performing a meta-analysis can be helpful in describing the physiology and pathology of a problem, they can present data in ways that are slanted to support the opinion of the central author. Using a systematic approach to search for, critically appraise, synthesize, and present the results minimizes the potential for bias.

The Cochrane Collaboration has already been mentioned. Another broader resource for finding systematic reviews is the Database of Abstracts of Reviews of Effectiveness (DARE). The editors of DARE search the literature for newly published reviews from any source that apply systematic methods to appraise the evidence (http://www.york.ac.uk/inst/crd/info.htm). DARE is an excellent first choice to determine if a systematic review has been published in Cochrane or elsewhere.

Often in pediatric critical care, systematic reviews are not available. Efficiently finding evidence in online medical search engines such as PubMed, a National Library of Medicine platform for searching MEDLINE, requires using the right terminology such as Medical Subject Headings (MeSH). There are search criteria developed by Dr. Brian Haynes for using PubMed to identify relevant articles that will yield a higher sensitivity (retrieving all relevant articles) and specificity (not retrieving irrelevant articles) [41–44]. PubMed has a special search feature called Clinical Queries based on the work of Dr. Haynes (http://www.ncbi.nlm.nih.gov/entrez/query/static/clinical.shtml) that automatically filters searches on questions of therapy, diagnosis, prognosis, etiology, and clinical prediction guides by looking for the highest levels of evidence in the literature.

Information overload is a constant problem plaguing clinicians. Given that research relevant to the pediatric intensive care setting may be found in the areas of internal medicine, neurology, surgery, trauma, infectious disease and hospital epidemiology, neonatology, pediatrics, radiology, oncology, and many other specialties, it can seem impossible to keep up with the literature [45]. Journal clubs that critically appraise relevant studies can save you time. The PedsCCM Evidence-Based Journal Club (http://pedscom.org/EBJournal_club.intro.php) identifies articles across a range of medical journals, reviews them using the users' guide approach, and now publishes a select number of these reviews in *Pediatric Critical Care Medicine*. The *Intensive Care Monitor* is also an excellent source that selects and critically appraises high-quality articles relevant to critical care medicine [46].

Evidence-Based Medicine in Pediatric Critical Care: Some Challenges

With optimal care, the mortality risk for most critically ill children is much lower than it would be for older adults with the same severity of illness. Chipping away at the reported 10%–25% baseline average mortality rate for these disorders is still important. Given that most interventions have a modest effect, yielding a 25% or lower relative risk reduction, this means that clinical trials powered to identify a reduction in mortality requires enrollment of over 700 patients per group even if baseline mortality was as high as 25% (assuming alpha 0.05, 80% power, 25% risk reduction). That kind of enrollment is a challenge to achieve even across 30 or more pediatric centers [47]. To answer the majority of questions about patient management that we confront on a daily basis will require collaboration of at least 25 centers to ensure adequate statistical power and enrollment over a 2–3 year time frame. Forming research groups to focus on such issues as acute lung injury, sepsis, bronchiolitis, acute severe asthma, and traumatic brain injury could facilitate the conduct of trials. Pediatric critical care units are fewer in number than adult and neonatal units. The Pediatric Acute Lung Injury and Sepsis Investigator's (PALISI) Network is an example of one such collaboration that has completed three multicenter randomized trials answering clinically important questions [48,49].

Because of the challenges of relatively low mortality, lack of an accepted nonmortality outcome measure to substitute, and difficulties in finding a sufficient number of patients even across multiple centers for trial enrollment, lack of evidence of therapeutic efficacy is a frequent occurrence in pediatric critical care. Applicability of evidence is the third section of every users' guide and must be given substantial thought. In fact, at least three users' guides are focused specifically on the challenges of applying evidence to patient care [50–52]. Understanding the outcomes for untreated controls is paramount before exposing them to an intervention that may modify this outcome. This requires high-quality studies of prognosis, risk, and prevalence. If the risk of mortality or serious morbidity is low in a subgroup of critically ill children, and the risk of serious side effects of an intervention is known to be high, then it may be prudent to steer clear of the intervention in the face of lack of evidence of efficacy even if there is strong data of efficacy in adult populations. Finally, incorporation of a patient's and family's preferences and values is essential to the practice of EBM. How to elicit preferences and how to incorporate them into clinical encounters in the ICU represents an enormously challenging frontier for EBM [51].

References

1. Evidence-Based Medicine Working Group. Evidence-based medicine. A new approach to teaching the practice of medicine. JAMA 1992;268(17):2420–2425.
2. Pocock SJ. Clinical Trials: A Practical Approach. Chichester: John Wiley & Sons; 1983.
3. Lind J. A Treatise of the Scurvy. In Three Parts. Containing an Inquiry into The Nature, Causes and Cure, of that Disease. Together with a Critical and Chronological View of What Has Been Published on the Subject. Edinburgh: A Kincaid and A Donaldson; 1753.
4. Louis PCA. Recherches sur les effets de la saignée dans quelques maladies inflammatoires et sur l'action de l'émétique et des vésicatoires dans la pneumonie. Paris: Librairie de l'Académie royale de médecine; 1835.
5. Lister J. Effects of the antiseptic system of treatment upon the salubrity of a surgical hospital. Lancet 1870;1:40–42.
6. Doll R. Controlled trials: the 1948 watershed. BMJ 1998;317(7167):1217–1220.
7. Medical Research Council, Streptomycin in Tuberculosis Trials Committee. Streptomycin treatment of pulmonary tuberculosis. BMJ 1948;ii:769–782.
8. Newman TB, Browner WS, Hulley SB. Enhancing causal inference in observational studies. In: Hulley SB, Cummings SR, eds. Designing Clinical Research. Baltimore: Williams & Wilkins; 2005:98–109.
9. Mahoney JF, Arnold RC, Sterner BL, Harris A, Zwally MR. Landmark article Sept 9, 1944: Penicillin treatment of early syphilis: II. By J.F. Mahoney, R.C. Arnold, B.L. Sterner, A. Harris, and M.R. Zwally. JAMA 1984;251(15):2005–2010.
10. Rosenberg DH, Arling PA. Landmark article Aug 12, 1944: Penicillin in the treatment of meningitis. By D.H. Rosenberg and P.A. Arling. JAMA 1984;251(14):1870–1876.
11. Maio LL. Gastric freezing: an example of the evaluation and medicine therapy by randomized clinical trials. In: Bunker JP, Barnes BA, Mosteller F, eds. Costs, Risks and Benefits of Surgery. New York: Oxford University Press; 1977:198–211.
12. Wangensteen OH, Peter ET, Nicoloff DM, Walder AI, Sosin H, Bernstein EF. Achieving "physiological gastrectomy" by gastric freezing. A preliminary report of an experimental and clinical study. JAMA 1962;180:439–444.
13. Ruffin JM, Grizzle JE, Hightower NC, McHardy G, Shull H, Kirsner JB. A co-operative double-blind evaluation of gastric "freezing" in the treatment of duodenal ulcer. N Engl J Med 1969;281(1):16–19.
14. Francis T, Korns RF, Voight RB, Boisen M, Hemphill FM, Napier JA, et al. An evaluation of the 1954 poliomyelitis vaccine trials. Am J Public Health 1955;45(5, Part 2):1–63.
15. Meier P. The biggest public health experiment ever: the 1954 field trial of the Salk poliomyelitis vaccine. In: Tanur JM, ed. Statistics: A Guide to the Unknown. San Francisco: Holden-Day; 1972:2–13.
16. Sackett DL, Haynes RB, Tugwell P. Clinical Epidemiology: A Basic Science for Clinical Medicine. Toronto: Little Brown & Company; 1985.
17. Oxman AD, Sackett DL, Guyatt GH. Users' guides to the medical literature. I. How to get started. The Evidence-Based Medicine Working Group. JAMA 1993;270(17):2093–2095.
18. Guyatt GH, Sackett DL, Cook DJ. Users' guides to the medical literature. II. How to use an article about therapy or prevention. A. Are the results of the study valid? Evidence-Based Medicine Working Group. JAMA 1993;270(21):2598–2601.
19. Guyatt GH, Sackett DL, Cook DJ. Users' guides to the medical literature. II. How to use an article about therapy or prevention. B. What were the results and will they help me in caring for my patients? Evidence-Based Medicine Working Group. JAMA 1994;271(1):59–63.
20. Jaeschke R, Guyatt GH, Sackett DL. Users' guides to the medical literature. III. How to use an article about a diagnostic test. B. What are the results and will they help me in caring for my patients? The Evidence-Based Medicine Working Group. JAMA 1994;271(9):703–707.
21. Jaeschke R, Guyatt G, Sackett DL. Users' guides to the medical literature. III. How to use an article about a diagnostic test. A. Are the results of the study valid? Evidence-Based Medicine Working Group. JAMA 1994;271(5):389–391.
22. Laupacis A, Wells G, Richardson WS, Tugwell P. Users' guides to the medical literature. V. How to use an article about prognosis. Evidence-Based Medicine Working Group. JAMA 1994;272(3):234–237.
23. Levine M, Walter S, Lee H, Haines T, Holbrook A, Moyer V. Users' guides to the medical literature. IV. How to use an article about harm. Evidence-Based Medicine Working Group. JAMA 1994;271(20):1615–1619.
24. The Evidence-Based Medicine Working Group. Users' Guides to the Medical Literature. Chicago: AMA Press; 2002.
25. Cook DJ, Sibbald WJ, Vincent JL, Cerra FB. Evidence based critical care medicine; what is it and what can it do for us? Evidence Based Medicine in Critical Care Group. Crit Care Med 1996;24(2):334–337.
26. Sackett DL. Evidence-based medicine. Semin Perinatol 1997;21(1):3–5.
27. Ventre K, Randolph A. Ribavirin for respiratory syncytial virus infection of the lower respiratory tract in infants and young children. Cochrane Database Syst Rev 2004;(4):CD000181.
28. Oxman AD, Cook DJ, Guyatt GH. Users' guides to the medical literature. VI. How to use an overview. Evidence-Based Medicine Working Group. JAMA 1994;272(17):1367–1371.
29. Attia J, Ray JG, Cook DJ, Douketis J, Ginsberg JS, Geerts WH. Deep vein thrombosis and its prevention in critically ill adults. Arch Intern Med 2001;161(10):1268–1279.
30. DeAngelis GA, McIlhenny J, Willson DF, Vittone S, Dwyer SJ, III, Gibson JC, et al. Prevalence of deep venous thrombosis in the lower extremities of children in the intensive care unit. Pediatr Radiol 1996;26(11):821–824.
31. Beck C, Dubois J, Grignon A, Lacroix J, David M. Incidence and risk factors of catheter-related deep vein thrombosis in a pediatric intensive care unit: a prospective study. J Pediatr 1998;133(2):237–241.
32. Krafte-Jacobs B, Sivit CJ, Mejia R, Pollack MM. Catheter-related thrombosis in critically ill children: comparison of catheters with and without heparin bonding. J Pediatr 1995;126(1):50–54.
33. Pierce CM, Wade A, Mok Q. Heparin-bonded central venous lines reduce thrombotic and infective complications in critically ill children. Intensive Care Med 2000;26(7):967–972.

34. Talbott GA, Winters WD, Bratton SL, O'Rourke PP. A prospective study of femoral catheter-related thrombosis in children. Arch Pediatr Adolesc Med 1995;149(3):288–291.

35. Massicotte P, Adams M, Marzinotto V, Brooker LA, Andrew M. Low-molecular-weight heparin in pediatric patients with thrombotic disease: a dose finding study. J Pediatr 1996;128(3):313–318.

36. Massicotte P, Julian JA, Gent M, Shields K, Marzinotto V, Szechtman B, et al. An open-label randomized controlled trial of low molecular weight heparin for the prevention of central venous line-related thrombotic complications in children: the PROTEKT trial. Thromb Res 2003;109(2–3):101–108.

37. Davison C, Ventre KM, Luchetti M, Randolph AG. Efficacy of interventions for bronchiolitis in critically ill infants: a systematic review and meta-analysis. Pediatr Crit Care Med 2004;5(5):482–489.

38. Heyland DK, Cook DJ, Guyatt GH. Enteral nutrition in the critically ill patient: a critical review of the evidence. Intensive Care Med 1993;19(8):435–442.

39. Dodek P, Keenan S, Cook D, Heyland D, Jacka M, Hand L, et al. Evidence-based clinical practice guideline for the prevention of ventilator-associated pneumonia. Ann Intern Med 2004;141(4):305–313.

40. O'Grady NP, Alexander M, Dellinger EP, Gerberding JL, Heard SO, Maki DG, et al. Guidelines for the prevention of intravascular catheter-related infections. Centers for Disease Control and Prevention. MMWR Recomm Rep 2002;51(RR-10):1–29.

41. Haynes RB, McKibbon KA, Walker CJ, Mousseau J, Baker LM, Fitzgerald D, et al. Computer searching of the medical literature. An evaluation of MEDLINE searching systems. Ann Intern Med 1985;103(5):812–816.

42. Haynes RB, Wilczynski N, McKibbon KA, Walker CJ, Sinclair JC. Developing optimal search strategies for detecting clinically sound studies in MEDLINE. J Am Med Inform Assoc 1994;1(6):447–458.

43. Haynes RB, McKibbon KA, Wilczynski NL, Walter SD, Werre SR. Optimal search strategies for retrieving scientifically strong studies of treatment from Medline: analytical survey. BMJ 2005;330(7501):1179.

44. Haynes RB, Wilczynski N. Finding the gold in MEDLINE: clinical queries. ACP J Club 2005;142(1):A8–A9.

45. Cook DJ, Meade MO, Fink MP. How to keep up with the critical care literature and avoid being buried alive. Crit Care Med 1996;24(10):1757–1768.

46. Dobb G. An introduction to Intensive Care World Monitor. Intensive Care World Monitor 1994;1:1–2.

47. Randolph AG, Meert KL, O'Neil ME, Hanson JH, Luckett PM, Arnold JH, et al. The feasibility of conducting clinical trials in infants and children with acute respiratory failure. Am J Respir Crit Care Med 2003;167(10):1334–1340.

48. Randolph AG, Wypij D, Venkataraman ST, Hanson JH, Gedeit RG, Meert KL et al. Effect of mechanical ventilator weaning protocols on respiratory outcomes in infants and children: a randomized controlled trial. JAMA 2002;288(20):2561–2568.

49. Willson DF, Thomas NJ, Markovitz BP, Bauman LA, DiCarlo JV, Pon S, et al. Effect of exogenous surfactant (calfactant) in pediatric acute lung injury: a randomized controlled trial. JAMA 2005;293(4):470–476.

50. Dans AL, Dans LF, Guyatt GH, Richardson S. Users' guides to the medical literature: XIV. How to decide on the applicability of clinical trial results to your patient. Evidence-Based Medicine Working Group. JAMA 1998;279(7):545–549.

51. Guyatt GH, Haynes RB, Jaeschke RZ, Cook DJ, Green L, Naylor CD, et al. Users' guides to the medical literature: XXV. Evidence-based medicine: principles for applying the users' guides to patient care. Evidence-Based Medicine Working Group. JAMA 2000;284(10):1290–1296.

52. McAlister FA, Straus SE, Guyatt GH, Haynes RB. Users' guides to the medical literature: XX. Integrating research evidence with the care of the individual patient. Evidence-Based Medicine Working Group. JAMA 2000;283(21):2829–2836.

12

Patient Safety in the Pediatric Intensive Care Unit

David C. Stockwell and Anthony D. Slonim

Introduction

Patient safety is an important tenet of medical practice generally and of intensive care specifically. Over the past 5 years, safety has become an increasingly important topic because of the release of the Institute of Medicine's (IOM's) *To Err is Human* report, which highlighted the issue of patient safety for both the lay public and medical professionals [1]. The Society of Critical Care Medicine is also actively engaged in education and in improving patient safety for patients with critical illness. With this heightened awareness, the pediatric intensive care practitioner needs to understand the fundamental concepts of patient safety, where they fit within health care quality, and how they can be measured, studied, and improved upon for the benefit of critically ill children.

The Relationship Between Quality and Safety

Quality is a term that has a long and nonspecific history in health care. A recent attempt to characterize health care quality and the prevailing paradigm for evaluating clinical quality is detailed in the IOM's second report, *Crossing the Quality Chasm* [2]. The document recommends *six aims for improvement*—safety, effectiveness, equity, timeliness, patient-centeredness, and efficiency—which are intended to identify the fundamental domains that need to be addressed to improve health care services delivered to individuals and populations.

The President's Commission on Healthcare Quality used another classification schema to characterize health care quality

using the relationship between health care risks and benefits [3]. *Underuse* refers to a service in which the potential benefits outweigh the potential risks yet the service is not provided [2–5]. *Overuse* refers to a service in which the potential risks outweigh the potential benefits yet the service is still provided [2–5]. *Misuse* refers to variation in the provision of services as well as the potentially avoidable errors and complications that occur because of the manner in which a service is provided [2–5].

The characterization of variability in intensive care is not a new concept. The variable care provided in both pediatric and adult intensive care units (ICUs) has been realized for more than a decade [6,7]. This variability occurs with respect to ICU structures (e.g., environment), processes (e.g., preparation of the skin prior to central venous catheterization), and outcomes (e.g., mortality) and provides insight into opportunities to improve the safety and quality of care delivered in these settings.

Safety is an important foundational element and is often referred to as the first step in achieving health care quality. Safety is defined as the freedom from accidental injury. Alternatively stated, safe care is care that minimizes risks and optimizes benefits. This is important for two reasons. First, medical care, particularly intensive care, has inherent risks and benefits. The challenge for ICU providers is to optimize benefits and minimize the occurrence of risk. Second, patients and their families also have a role in safe care. The consent process is designed to provide information about the potential risks, benefits, and alternatives of treatments and to allow decisions that align with the family's personal interests. Together, providers, patients, and families can improve the safety of care in the ICU.

Classification of Safety and Medical Errors

A number of classification systems have been proposed to more fully understand patient safety. The IOM used a system that classified medical errors that jeopardize patient safety as diagnostic errors, procedural errors, treatment errors, prophylactic errors, and nosocomial infections. Table 12.1 provides examples of each of these types of medical errors in the pediatric ICU (PICU). This approach makes intuitive sense for ICU providers because it mirrors the clinical approach to patients.

D.S. Wheeler et al. (eds.), *Science and Practice of Pediatric Critical Care Medicine*,
DOI 10.1007/978-1-84800-921-9_12, © Springer-Verlag London Limited 2009

TABLE 12.1. A classification schema and examples for medical errors in the pediatric intensive care unit.

Category	Examples
Diagnostic errors	Wheezing attributed to asthma is really congestive heart failure
	Hypoxia is not recognized as a cause of agitation
	Signs of intracranial hypertension are not appropriately recognized
	Arterial blood gas values are inappropriately interpreted
Treatment errors	Treatment of intracranial hypertension without appropriate calibration of the monitor
	Failure to provide antipseudomonal coverage to neutropenic, febrile patients
	Renal failure during aminoglycoside treatment
Nosocomial infections	Bloodstream infections
	Ventilator-associated pneumonia
	Urinary tract infection
Procedural errors	Pneumothorax occurring during central venous catheterization
	Nasogastric feeding tube placed in the lung
	Unplanned extubation
Prophylactic errors	Failure to provide appropriate position changes with resulting decubitus ulcer formation
	Failure to provide appropriate stress ulcer prophylaxis
	Failure to provide appropriate deep venous thrombosis prophylaxis

The Pediatric Intensive Care Unit Environment: Complex and Tightly Coupled

The PICU is a complex and tightly coupled system. Complexity is the degree to which system components are specialized and interdependent. Complex systems are more prone to errors. *Coupling* is a term used to describe the interdependence of different components of the system. Tightly coupled systems have little *room for error*, whereas loosely coupled systems can tolerate delays or variations in sequencing [8]. As a result of its two system traits, the PICU environment is unique. This uniqueness has implications for the types of errors that occur (see Table 12.1) and the strategies that can be used to remediate them. For example, if variability contributes to error, one approach to improving safety would be to reduce

the variability in the structures and processes of these complex systems with the hope of improving outcomes. At the most fundamental level, this includes the use of policies and procedures to help guide practice, but a more sophisticated approach includes tactics such as leadership training, crew resource management training, clinical protocols, guidelines, and process analysis.

Methods to Improve Patient Safety in the Pediatric Intensive Care Unit

Processes are the steps by which patients and their care providers interact. A systematic analysis of these processes can highlight the variability occurring within these interactions and lead to opportunities to reduce risk points and improve the delivery of care. There are several methods to analyze processes; many of them are derived from industries other than health care, and each has its inherent limitations (Table 12.2). Managers in these industries utilize process analysis to ensure safety during production while simultaneously improving efficiency and quality. There are three standard approaches that are being used currently in health care and two newer techniques that are experiencing some success in this environment.

Performance Improvement Methods

Traditional performance improvement (PI) methods have been advanced within the industry under the total quality management (TQM) and continuous quality improvement (CQI) paradigms. For more than two decades, the value of these tools to medical practice and hospital operations has been apparent. These techniques aim to continually improve health care processes by reducing variability and streamlining care. There are several methodologies available for this purpose. One approach, known as the PDSA cycle, approach breaks the analysis of processes into four discrete steps: *Plan, Do, Study, Act*. This approach is administered in a repetitive fashion to a particular health care problem in a series of *cycles*. For example, if the initiative of interest is the reduction of bloodstream infections in the PICU, several PDSA cycles can be considered. The first cycle might focus on provider hand washing and hygiene. A second cycle might focus on standardizing skin preparation for invasive procedures. Each cycle should be short in duration (2–4 weeks) and be accompanied by the collection of data to monitor

TABLE 12.2. Comparison of process analysis techniques.

	Root cause analysis	Failure mode and effects analysis	Probabilistic risk assessment
Timing	Retrospective	Prospective	Prospective
Description	Multidisciplinary team sequentially asks what happened and why it happened	Defines what can fail and the way it can fail (failure modes), determines the effect of each failure mode on the system, classifies each potential failure mode according to its severity, and determines the response to the failure	Calculates the conditional probabilities associated with health outcomes in complex systems with multiple interactions and dependencies as occurs in health care
Scope	Local	Local	Multiinstitutional
Benefits	Typically able to identify the source of error	Proactively identifies sources of errors, able to address "near-miss" events	Provides an assessment of risks by prioritizing those events, based on the probabilities of occurrence, that are needed most to improve the system's reliability
Limitations	May miss a larger organizational error, focuses on one-time incidents, no attention to "near misses"	Unable to incorporate impact of additive errors	More complex to construct

improvements. This approach can be quite effective in improving health care outcomes. Although a number of newer methods with different names exist, the PI approach remains the fundamental underpinning for process analysis techniques.

Root Cause Analysis

Root Cause Analysis (RCA) is a standardized process analysis technique that is used by hospitals to understand the circumstances of a bad event. The technique is used to investigate and analyze serious and sentinel events after their occurrence. It is a process that is required by the Joint Commission for Accreditation of Healthcare Organizations (JCAHO) to maintain continuous accreditation [9]. The RCA is a multidisciplinary method used to retrospectively identify those aberrant processes that contributed to the adverse event. In a stepwise process, a multidisciplinary team sequentially asks, *what happened* and *why it happened* to determine the fundamental reasons or *root causes* for the event's occurrence. The root causes generally fall into multiple themes, including human factors (e.g., fatigue), organizational factors (e.g., workplace policies and procedures), and technical factors (e.g., missing or inappropriate equipment) [10].

Although RCA is useful in its approach to the evaluation of an adverse event, the inherent disadvantages of the RCA method diminish its applicability to a continuous error reduction strategy in health care generally and the PICU specifically. Perhaps, most important, RCA is a *retrospective* method of process analysis, performed after the occurrence of an event (see Table 12.2). In addition, RCA groups generally focus only on sentinel events resulting in patient death or serious morbidity. It is increasingly recognized that the fundamental epidemiology of errors (incidence, severity) is complicated by the fact that one also needs to consider prevented errors (near misses) and errors that occurred but from which no harm resulted (absorbed events) [11]. These events are particularly important in the PICU. Medical directors in the PICU would be expected to maintain vigilance over their nosocomial infection rates, for example, and not wait until a child's death from a nosocomial infection before undertaking an analysis.

Failure Mode and Effects Analysis

The Failure Mode and Effects Analysis (FMEA) methodology is used in the automotive industry to identify problems in product design and manufacture (e.g., of shock absorbers) before a potential failure in production occurs [12]. It consists of defining what can fail and the way it can fail (failure modes), determining the effect of each failure mode on the system, classifying each potential failure mode according to its severity, and determining the response to the failure. Steps can then be taken to change the design or process to eliminate the failure, reduce its impact, or compensate for the failure should it occur.

Prospective process identification methods such as FMEA may be more appropriate applications for promoting safety in high-risk health care settings. In fact, the JCAHO now requires the incorporation of *prospective* process analysis methods (FMEA specifically) into organizational patient safety plans [13]. This approach can be applied to the PICU as well. For example, the PICU may decide to prioritize those processes that occur commonly, are high risk, or are problem prone. The administration of vasoactive infusions in the PICU would meet this definition. Prospectively a team could map out the process of vasoactive infusion administration from

prescribing, through processing, dispensing, and administration to the patient. The team would then be able to review the steps in their process, identifying the risk points where dosage calculations, preparation of infusions, and mediation administration may be variable. The team would then be able to review the steps in their processes to reduce errors and improve safety. Some examples of safety improvements related to this process in several PICUs include the elimination of the rule of six calculation, the use of standardized infusion concentrations, and the use of central venous catheters for the administration of these medications to eliminate events related to caustic intravenous infiltration.

Limitations of Root Cause Analysis and Failure Mode and Effects Analysis

There are reasons to believe that the RCA and FMEA methods, by themselves, will fall short in being able to produce meaningful results in terms of patient safety interventions for the health care industry. First, the methods are used on a local level without the benefit of multiinstitutional experiences to help guide the model [1,13–15]. Second, individual health care institutions often focus on their own safety problems and inadequacies. As a result, the institutions are concerned about allowing their data to become transparent to the public or to other professionals because they may be exposing themselves to litigation or further public scrutiny [1,2]. For example, if Hospital X has had two serious events related to blood product transfusions administered during trauma in the past year, it might choose to improve the processes surrounding the administration of rapid-release blood products using an RCA or FMEA. However, even if the hospital discovers important information that can assist other institutions and prevent duplication of effort, it is neither obliged to nor likely interested in sharing that information publicly to improve blood product safety more broadly [1].

Currently, patient safety efforts are viewed negatively as inadequacies in care and as potential opportunities for litigation rather than as opportunities to share information that can improve safety in the industry [1,2]. Hence, patient safety interventions need to provide a broader view that takes into account the efforts of multiple institutions' ideas and strategies [1,13–15]. Even when FMEA and RCA are performed flawlessly, these qualitative tools are not designed to assist in identifying risk point combinations in complex systems that are more likely to lead to errors [16]. For example, FMEA may identify both sleep deprivation and the lack of experience by residents as contributors to medication-prescribing errors in the PICU. However, it does not allow one to account for the distinction caused by the independent or combined effects of sleep deprivation *and* the lack of experience in contributing to the prescribing error. Fourth, these tools do not assist in identifying risk reduction strategies, which may be helpful in reducing the number of errors. Finally, these qualitative tools do not assist the institution in prioritizing interventions based on quantitative risk. If the members of the RCA team inappropriately assess the risk associated with a particular process, the institution may expend considerable resources correcting a problem that in fact may have little to do with the risk of a recurrent event.

Six Sigma

Six Sigma is a process analysis technique that is being increasingly used in many health care organizations. It is a disciplined approach that is prospective, like FMEA. However, Six Sigma sets specification limits by aiming to eliminate defects or drive them to an occurrence rate that is at a level below six standard deviations from the mean occurrence rate. Failure Mode and Effects Analysis simply describes the process without measuring or specifying the limits of acceptance.

Six Sigma methodology can be used to measure and improve both operational and service-related performance. For example, in health care Six Sigma has been used to improve many common processes such as emergency department to bed wait times, resource use per patient, and market growth. It could also be used in the PICU to improve events such as unintended extubations, bloodstream infections, or even the timeliness of transfers from the PICU to the ward [17]. An example of Six Sigma improvements in a situation that is analogous to the PICU is the use of system design decisions in anesthesia. With this approach, anesthesia-related deaths have been dramatically reduced [18].

Probabilistic Risk Assessment

Probabilistic Risk Assessment (PRA) is another tool that is used in industry that may have applications to health care (see Table 12.2) [19]. Probabilistic Risk Assessment provides probabilistic assessments of risk associated with events particularly at the tail of risk distributions where the estimates may be as rare as 1 in 1,000,000 or 1 in 10,000,000. The reduction of adverse events to the level of 1 in 1,000,000 is the dogma behind the Six Sigma methodology described earlier and highlights the attention being applied by the health care industry to these low-frequency, high-impact events [20]. There are many examples of low-frequency high-risk events in the PICU, such as complications from extracorporeal membrane oxygenation, blood product transfusion reactions, and procedural complications.

Probabilistic Risk Assessment significantly improves on FMEA by calculating the conditional probabilities associated with health outcomes in complex systems with multiple interactions and dependencies as occurs in health care [21,22]. It uses the techniques of process analysis, decision support, and statistical modeling to determine the relationships between components of complex systems. These models detail all of the steps of a particular process prospectively like FMEA described above. In fact, an FMEA is a byproduct of the PRA process. The model is informed by the addition of probabilities of occurrence for faulty processes within the system that lead to that bad outcome (see Table 12.2). This allows the model to provide an assessment of risks by prioritizing those events, based on the probabilities of occurrence, that are needed most to improve the system's reliability.

An example of medication errors can demonstrate the robustness of PRA. Failure Mode and Effects Analysis may identify a process that requires a double check of a medication by a nurse before its administration to a patient. Failure Mode and Effects Analysis provides neither the likelihood that the nurse will perform the double check nor the probability that the double check will prevent a medication administration error. Like FMEA, PRA also identifies the process as a particular risk point. However, PRA additionally provides an estimate of how often a nurse will double check the medication, an estimate of the confidence in that prediction, and a sensitivity analysis that allows an assessment of the risk associated with the medication administration across the range of probabilities of having a nurse double check the medication before its administration. With this probabilistic information,

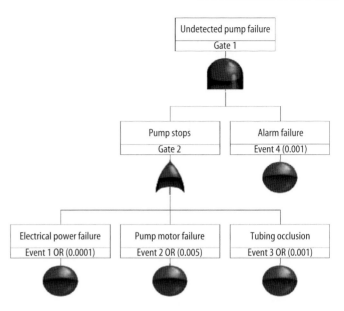

Figure 12.1. A simple Fault Tree depicting an undetected medication pump failure.

a determination of how important this double check process is to an institution's overall medication safety program can be made. Alternatively, other strategies that pose higher risks may be addressed first.

Figure 12.1 is an example of a Fault Tree, which provides a pictorial representation of different process steps and event combinations. In this case, the event is a medication pump malfunction. The circles represent basic events associated with this outcome and their occurrence rates. These events are grouped by two different types of *gates*, which allow for the combination of these basic events and their probabilities in contributing to the risk of the outcome of interest. The model can be informed by both quantitative and qualitative risk estimates. The quantitative estimates can be drawn from large administrative databases and epidemiologic studies. The qualitative estimates are specific to particular institutions and can be assessed by using frontline staff that directly interact with a particular process. Understanding these qualitative elements is essential to fully appreciating the risk of adverse outcomes in health care.

This example also highlights a very important opportunity provided by PRA. Medical errors depend on systems of care that require redundancy in order to achieve reliability and improve patient safety [23,24]. Health care is in many ways different from other industries and in no other practice is this as apparent as in the PICU. It depends on human interaction between a patient and a practitioner during illness and recovery [23–25]. This interaction is emotional, significant, and some would argue essential for recovery. However, it is this "humanness" in health care that is also responsible for some of the safety problems [1,23–25]. Practitioners are not computers and have a limited ability to process multiple pieces of often-contradictory information. Practitioners need to eat, drink, sleep, and have bathroom breaks. They also have personal lives and stresses that may alter their focus or influence their attention while they are caring for patients. These *human factors* are important to consider when mapping patient safety problems, and PRA is a useful tool to allow this to occur [26–35].

A Practical Guide to Improving Safety

Improving the Culture

A programmatic approach to patient safety is important in preventing medical errors in the PICU. The program begins at the time of employment and ensures that the employee is aware of potential risks to safety in the PICU. Workplace cultural issues are important to providing a PICU environment that promotes quality generally and patient safety more specifically. Providers need to believe that the provision of quality health care is aligned with the goals of their unit and their organization [36]. Success in patient safety in the PICU depends on the ability to understand a systems approach in analyzing the innumerable patient care processes that contribute to bad outcomes. This starts with a blame-free environment in which providers are given incentives for reporting adverse occurrences but one that also holds providers accountable for the care that they deliver.

Engaging the Frontline Staff

Achieving an understanding of the types of medical errors and the methods for quantifying their existence at a system level does not, by itself, assist the PICU provider in improving patient safety at the bedside. Real steps to improve patient safety require improvements in the structures and processes that go into delivering the care. This begins with an understanding of patient safety at the provider level. Health care providers may fail to use very simple care practices such as appropriate hand hygiene and barrier precautions when caring for a child to prevent the inadvertent transmission of an infectious agent. The health care provider may not fully appreciate how equipment such as monitors, ventilators, or defibrillators can interact with patients or staff to create safety problems. If success in the improvement of quality for patients is to be achieved, opportunities to capitalize on the knowledge and tools provided by other industries as described earlier should be utilized. Risk assessment techniques coupled with process analysis strategies to prioritize initiatives, formulate a plan, and redesign clinical practices, based on the evidence-based literature, will produce the best outcomes and can readily be communicated to and understood by bedside clinicians.

Fostering a Team

The IOM has also called for promoting *effective team functioning* [1,2]. In part deficiencies in the health care system may be due to the lack of coordinated care and communication both within and among members of the health care team. Even routine PICU care is complex care. Intensivists manage patients who typically require a team of multiple disciplines, specialists, and consultants. It involves numerous resources within the hospital and several departments. Engaging all of these participants into strategies aimed at improving the patient's health requires effective leadership. Critical care trainees may be relatively unprepared in their training to meet the demands of team leadership in the complex environment of the PICU without specific and focused training [37].

Getting the Job Done

The growing enthusiasm for interventions to improve quality for patients, such as reducing the variability in organizational struc-

ture and the patient care process [38,39], has resulted in numerous suggestions for improvement. An example of reducing variability in structure is the use of ICU physician directors and the 24-hour intensivist model of coverage [38,39]. The Leapfrog Group has suggested that improved ICU outcomes depend on intensivists providing care within a closed ICU system [40]. Opportunities to reduce the variability in clinical processes can be achieved by using clinical practice guidelines and pathways. Opportunities and approaches to assess and communicate directly about specific situations in the complex ICU environment also need to be considered [41]. For example, the *SBAR* technique, which addresses *S*ituation, *B*ackground, *A*ssessment, and *R*ecommendation in a critical situation, may be a useful approach for the PICU team to adopt [41].

Conclusion

This overview of patient safety provides a starting point for understanding the context of patient safety in the PICU. Understanding the types of errors, how to analyze them, and what to do to ameliorate them are important components of any PICU safety program.

Acknowledgments. Dr. Slonim is supported in part by the Agency for Healthcare Research and by Quality Grant: KO-8 HS-14009.

References

1. Kohn LT, Corrigan JM, Donaldson MS, eds., and Institute of Medicine, Committee on Quality of Health Care in America: To Err is Human: Building a Safer Health System. Washington, DC: National Academy Press; 2000.
2. Institute of Medicine, Committee on Quality of Health Care in America: Crossing the Quality Chasm: A New Health System for the 21st Century. Washington, DC: National Academy Press; 2001.
3. Lohr KN, ed. Medicare: A Strategy for Quality Assurance. Washington, DC: National Academy Press; 1990.
4. Donabedian A. Explorations in Quality Assessment and Monitoring, Volume 1. The Definitions of Quality and Approaches to its Assessment. Ann Arbor, MI: Health Administration Press; 1980.
5. Ginzberg E. Health Services Research: Key to Health Policy. Cambridge, MA: Harvard University Press; 1991.
6. Pollack MM, Cuerdon TC, Getson PR. Pediatric intensive care units: results of a national study. Crit Care Med 1993;21:607–614.
7. Groger JS, Strosberg MA, Halpern NA, et al: Descriptive analysis of critical care units in the United States. Crit Care Med 1992;20:846–863.
8. Perrow C. Normal Accidents. New York: Basic Books; 1984.
9. The Joint Commission on Accreditation of Healthcare Organizations online. Hospitals, Policy and Procedure. Available at: http://www.jcaho.org/accredited+organizations/hospitals/sentinel+events/se_pp.htm. Accessed April 5, 2005.
10. McNutt RA, Abrams R, Aron DC. Patient safety efforts should focus on medical errors. JAMA 2002;287:1997–2001.
11. Wears RL, Janiak B, Moorhead JC, et al. Human error in medicine: promise and pitfalls, part 2. Ann Emerg Med 2000;36:142–144.
12. FMEA Info Centre. Available at: http://www.fmeainfocentre.com. Accessed April 5, 2005.
13. The Joint Commission on Accreditation of Healthcare Organizations: Medical Errors, Sentinel Events, and Accreditation. A Report to the Association of Anesthesia Program Directors, October 28, 2000. Oakbrook Terrace, IL: JCAHO.
14. Leape LL, Bates DW, Cullen DJ, et al. Systems analysis of adverse drug events. JAMA 1995;274:35–43.

15. Roos NP, Black CD, Roos LL, et al. A population-based approach to monitoring adverse outcomes of medical care. Med Care 1995;33: 127–138.
16. Linerooth-Bayer J, Wahlstroem B. Applications of probabilistic risk assessments: the selection of appropriate tools. Risk Anal 1991;11: 239–248.
17. iSix Sigma. Available at: http://www.isixsigma.com/sixsigma/six_ sigma.asp. Accessed April 5, 2005.
18. Gaba D, Howard SK, Fish KJ. Crisis Management in Anesthesiology. New York: Churchill Livingstone; 1994.
19. Marx D, Slonim AD. Assessing patient safety risk before the injury occurs: An introduction to Socio-Technical Probabilistic Risk Assessment. Qual Saf Healthcare 2003;12(Suppl 2):33–38.
20. www.6-sigma.com. Accessed January 27, 2003.
21. Hamed MM. First order reliability analysis of public health risk assessment. Risk Anal 1997;17:177–185.
22. Van Otterloo RW. Probabilistic risk assessment: An historic overview from determinism to probabilism. Microelectron Reliab 1995;35: 1357–1362.
23. Vincent C, Taylor Adams SE, Stanhope N. A framework for the analysis of risk and safety in medicine. BMJ 1998;316:1154–1157.
24. Marx D. Patient Safety and the Just Culture: A Primer for Health Care Executives. Report prepared for MERS-TM, Columbia University, New York, New York, April 2001.
25. Rechard RP. Historical relationship between performance assessment for radioactive waste disposal and other types of risk assessment. Risk Anal 1999;19:763–808.
26. Moore DRJ, Sample BE, Suter GW, et al. Risk based decision making: The East Fork Poplar Creek case study. Environ Toxicol Chem 1999;18: 2954–2958.
27. Forester JA, Whitehead DW, Kolaczkowski AM, et al. Results of nuclear power plant application of a new technique for human error analysis. Paper presented of OECD/NEA specialists meeting on human performance in operational events; October 13–17, 1997; Chattanooga, TN.
28. Hsueh KS, Mosleh A. The development and application of the accident dynamic simulator for dynamic probabilistic risk assessment of nuclear power plants. Reliab Eng Syst Saf 1996;52:297–314.
29. Sues RH, Chen HC, Oswald EA, et al. Integrating internal events in an external probabilistic risk assessment: Tornado PRA case study. Reliab Eng Syst Saf 1993;40:173–176.
30. Morris SC, Meinhold AF. Probabilistic risk assessment of nephrotoxic effects of uranium in drinking water. Health Phys 1995; 69:897–908.
31. Chang SS. Implementing probabilistic risk assessment in USEPA Superfund program. Hum Ecol Risk Assess 1999;5:737–754.
32. Bowers TS. The concentration term and derivation of cleanup goals using probabilistic risk assessment. Hum Ecol Risk Assess 1999;5: 809–821.
33. Simon TW. Two dimensional Monte Carlo simulation and beyond: a comparison of several probabilistic risk assessment methods applied to a superfund site. Hum Ecol Risk Assess 1999;5:823–843.
34. Yu D. A realistic cancer risk assessment of inorganic arsenic. J Environ Sci Health 1998;33:1149–1170.
35. Cullen AC. The sensitivity of probabilistic risk assessment results to alternative model structures: a case study of municipal waste incineration. J Air Waste Manage Assoc 1995;45:538–546.
36. Beckman U, Bohringer C, Carless R, et al. Evaluation of two methods for quality improvement in intensive care: facilitated incident monitoring and retrospective medical chart review. Crit Care Med 2003;31: 1006–1011.
37. Stockwell DC, Pollock MM, Turenne W, Slonim AD. Leadership and management training of pediatric intensivists: how do we gain our skills?" Pediatr Crit Care Med 2005;6:665–670.
38. Nipshagen MD, Polderman KH, DeVictor D, Gemke RJ. Pediatric intensive care: results of European study. Intensive Care Med 2002;28:1797–1803.
39. Pearson G, Shann F, Barry P, et al. Should paediatric intensive care be centralized? Trent Versus Victoria. Lancet 1997;26:1213–1217.
40. The Leapfrog Group. http://www.leapfroggroup.org. Accessed April 5, 2005.
41. SBAR technique for communication: a situational briefing model. http://www.ihi.org/IHI/Topics/PatientSafety/SafetyGeneral/Tools/ SBARTechniqueforCommunicationASituationalBriefingModel.htm Accessed April 5th, 2005.

13
Pediatric Critical Care in Developing Countries

Gregory L. Stidham and William M. Novick

Introduction

Globalization is a term heard frequently in recent years, so much so that it has become something of a *sound bite*. Strictly speaking, globalization is the process of denationalization of business markets, politics, and legal systems, and the term is an entry portal into discussions of the *global economy*. This process has consequences that affect local economies, human welfare, and environment, all of which have led to considerable debate about whether this process is a good thing or bad, with sound arguments on both sides.

The term *third world* was first coined by the French demographer Alfred Sauvy. The term derives from conceptual similarity to the term *third estate*, which referred to the commoners of France before and during the French Revolution, as opposed to the priests and nobles, who made up the first and second estates, respectively. Sauvy wrote that, like the third estate, the third world is *nothing*, and it *wants to be something*. This concept implies that the third world is exploited in much the same way as the third estate was. The analogy was carried further by likening the first estate to the developed, industrialized western nations (first world), and the second to the industrialized Soviet Union. The terms have survived the dissolution of the Soviet Union. The underdevelopment of the third world is characterized by a number of traits: (1) their economies are devoted to producing primary products for the developed world and to providing markets for their finished goods; (2) traditional, rural social structures are predominant; (3) high population growth is present; and (4) poverty is widespread. Despite these commonalities, the third world is still diverse, as it comprises countries at many different levels of economic development. In addition, even in the poorest of countries there is often a wealthy elite, with large amounts of wealth concentrated in the hands of a small minority, creating great disparities between rich and poor.

As economies in the third world became more absorbed into and subservient to the economies of the developed first world, a world market was created in which the third world countries became dominated by the West. Traditional economies and societies were disrupted, leading to and furthering continued underdevelopment. Confounding these unbalanced economic relationships is the rate of population growth. In 1980, the world's population was estimated at 4.4 billion, with 72% in the third world. At present the world population exceeds 6.5 billion, with more than 80% in the third world. The challenges to third world countries are enormous and the road to escape this underdevelopment difficult. These challenges extend to health care, and the plight of these countries should not escape the attention of health care workers in developed nations.

In a more general sense not limited to business enterprises and economics, the term *globalization* may be seen as the general interconnectedness of our world today. Events in even the most remote places on our planet instantly become the news in most other places. Details of the fight against the AIDS epidemic in Africa are instantly available to anyone with Internet access. News of the effects of the December 2004 tsunami in the southwest Pacific was instantly available, and the Internet provided a way to coordinate relief efforts more quickly and efficiently than ever before.

In this more general sense, *globalization* also includes the networking of those practicing pediatric critical care in developing countries with those in developed countries. Practitioners in developing countries are more aware of the scientific substrates that underpin our subspecialty, as well as more aware of the resources that are available to their counterparts in the more privileged countries on our globe. In addition, practitioners in developed countries have become, over the past quarter century, more aware of the plight of their counterparts in the third world. Many have become interested in helping these colleagues, but most have been unsure how their skills can be best put to use to the advantage of their counterparts and the children they serve.

This chapter is an attempt to analyze the many complex factors that influence critical care in developing countries, to propose a model for increased collaboration between intensivists in the two worlds that does not ignore the overriding health care priorities in the third world, and finally to present information about resources, including volunteer opportunities.

D.S. Wheeler et al. (eds.), *Science and Practice of Pediatric Critical Care Medicine*,
DOI 10.1007/978-1-84800-921-9_13, © Springer-Verlag London Limited 2009

TABLE 13.1. Relationship between country income status and child mortality rates.

Country income status	Under-5 mortality (Deaths/1,000 live births)
Low	121
Lower middle	40
Upper middle	22
High	<7

General Issues in International Child Health

Efforts to improve care in international health traditionally have focused on one of two areas: disaster relief and general health care. These two strategies to assist developing countries are vastly different, but equally important. Disaster relief is not the focus of this chapter, but brief mention is appropriate.

Developing countries are especially vulnerable to unexpected tragedies—war and political conflict, with resultant refugee needs; and environmental crises, such as earthquakes, hurricanes, and tsunamis. Such tragedies have obvious implications for pediatric critical care practitioners, and, although they are not the emphasis of this chapter, failure to mention two resources directed toward disaster relief would be remiss. First, the American Academy of Pediatrics has created the CHILDisaster Network (http://www.aap.org/disaster/), a database of pediatricians who have volunteered their short-notice availability to organizations involved in disaster relief efforts. Second, Case Western Reserve University and Rainbow Babies and Children's Hospital host an annual course on "Management of Humanitarian Emergencies." 2005 marks the ninth offering of this course (http://cme.cwru.edu/brochures/2005/humanitarian_management/default.htm).

Very little is published about the state of pediatric critical care in undeveloped countries, while a modicum of information has been published pertaining to adult and neonatal critical care. Scientific critique of the problems facing pediatric intensive care units (PICUs) in developing countries is therefore lacking, as are proposed solutions. Furthermore, if outcomes research is in its infancy in developed countries, it is virtually nonexistent in developing ones.

More than 10 million children under the age of 5 years die each year in the developing world [1]. One child in 10 dies before the age of 5 years compared with 1 in 143 in developed countries. The vast majority of these deaths are from causes considered preventable with good overall care, good nutrition, and access to medical treatment. This child mortality rate is clearly linked to poverty (Table 13.1). In 2002, 48 countries had mortality rates for those under 5 years of greater than 100 per 1,000 live births. Fifteen countries (14 of them in sub-Saharan Africa) had rates greater than 200. Of the 10 million annual third world child deaths, 70% result from a disease or a combination of disease and malnutrition, including acute respiratory infections, diarrhea, measles, and malaria, that would be preventable in a high-income country (Table 13.2 and Figure 13.1). Malnutrition is an important factor in more than half of these

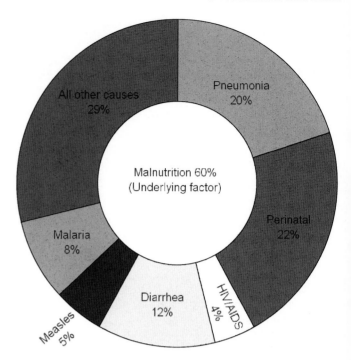

FIGURE 13.1. Leading causes of death in children under 5 years of age in undeveloped countries. (Modified from Bryce J, Boschi-Pinto C, Shibuya K, Black RE, WHO Child Health Epidemiology Reference Group. WHO estimates of the causes of death in children. Lancet 2005;365:1147–1152.)

deaths. A recent publication by UNICEF reported that more than half of the world's children are suffering from severe deprivations because of poverty, war, and HIV/AIDS. This report offers a detailed analysis of the seven basic "deprivations" that doom children's futures as a result of severe poverty (Table 13.3) [2].

Although a relationship between child mortality and poverty would seem obvious, a review of data supporting this relationship provides important background for understanding the nature of the problems faced in these countries and potential solutions. In 2002, the average under-5 mortality rate was 121 deaths per 1,000 live births in low-income countries. In lower middle-income countries, the rate was 40 per 1,000, 22 in upper middle-income countries, and <7 in high income countries. Table 13.4 lists the 11 poorest countries in the world. Ten of these 11 countries are on the African continent, most of them sub-Saharan [1,2].

Existing Knowledge about Critical Care in Developing Countries

Critical care in developing countries tends to be, of necessity, extremely regionalized. Most developing countries have large metropolitan centers that have given rise to some degree of tertiary

TABLE 13.2. Causes of mortality in children under 5 years of age.

Cause of death	Annual deaths
Pneumonia	2 million
Diarrheal disease	2.2 million
Preventable infection	5 million
Measles	0.5 million

Source: World Health Organizaiton [1].

TABLE 13.3. The seven basic "deprivations" of poverty and their effects on the world's children.

- 640 million children lack adequate shelter
- 500 million children lack access to sanitation
- 400 million children lack access to safe water
- 300 million children lack access to information
- 270 million children lack access to health care
- 140 million children have never been to school
- 90 million children are severely food deprived

TABLE 13.4. The 11 poorest countries in the world, in descending order.

1. Ethiopia
2. Democratic Republic of Congo
3. Burundi
4. Sierra Leone
5. Guinea-Bissau
6. Niger
7. Eritrea
8. Malawi
9. Mozambique
10. Nepal
11. Tanzania

care, including critical care. However, the capabilities of these "referral centers" are extremely variable and entirely dependent on resources available. Moreover, no two developing countries are alike in their approach to critical care, which, along with the paucity of published information, makes generalization difficult. Finally, examination of published experiences in developing countries is limited by a selection bias in that only the most developed PICUs in these developing countries will have the resources or motivation to publish their experiences, leaving little or no information about the conditions in PICUs in the least developed countries. Despite these limitations, examination of some of the relevant published information does give some idea of the challenges facing critical care practitioners and some approaches to their solution. Some of these papers are reviewed here.

One of the few reports of demographics and outcomes in a PICU in a developing country was published by Khilnani et al. [3]. The investigators prospectively gathered data on 948 children admitted over a 3-year period to the 10-bed PICU at the Apollo Hospital in New Delhi. Mean age was 42.5 months, and mean Pediatric Risk of Mortality (PRISM III) score was 18.5. Average length of PICU stay was 4.5 days, and overall mortality rate was 6.7%. Nearly 21% required mechanical ventilation for an average duration of 6.4 days. Diagnoses included, in descending order of frequency, respiratory, cardiac, neurologic, infectious, trauma, and other surgical. The authors underscore the similarity of their demographic, outcome, and complication data to those published by PICUs in the developed world.

Zar et al. [4] reported their experience with children admitted with pneumonia in two PICUs in Cape Town, South Africa, during the calendar year of 1998. Of 103 consecutively admitted patients, 76 were enrolled, with 27 not enrolled because of death, parental refusal of consent, or >48 hours elapsed after admission. Of the 76 enrolled children, 21 (27.6%) were HIV positive, 15 (71.4%) not previously diagnosed. In 8 (38.1%) of the HIV-positive patients, *Pneumocystis carinii* (PCP) was the causative organism. Overall in-hospital mortality rate was 18.4%, 28.6% in HIV-positive patients, and 44% in PCP-infected patients. This study is important for several reasons. First, it documents the growing importance of HIV in children, including those admitted for intensive care, reflecting a change in the demographics of these patients over the past two decades. Second, it demonstrates the efficacy of treatment for PCP pneumonia in this population, a population with more advanced disease at diagnosis than is usually seen in developed countries, with results that are comparable. Finally, a comment by the authors in the conclusion of their paper raises important questions faced by PICU practitioners in developing countries: "Some hospitals . . . have implemented a policy that excludes children known to be infected with HIV from the ICU. Set in this context, the observation in this article that effective ICU management can contribute to a satisfactory outcome from pneumonia . . . highlight[s] yet another

dilemma presented to health care providers in developing countries experiencing the HIV epidemic."

The Zar study also highlights the impossibility of extrapolating from the experience of one *developing* country to another. South Africa is still considered a developing country, but it is far different from its northern neighbors of Ethiopia, Republic of Congo, and Burundi. Critical care has existed in South Africa since the late 1960s and 1970s [5]. The Critical Care Society of South Africa was established in the 1980s, and extensive regionalization and organization has occurred, with units graded from Level I to Level IV. A severe shortage of ICU beds continues to dictate strict admission criteria, but in more undeveloped *developing countries*, the beds are practically nonexistent. The concept of *developing countries* is, therefore, a continuum, and each country and its needs must be assessed specifically.

In a retrospective study of diabetic ketoacidosis in a PICU in Chandigarh, India, Jayashree and Singhi reviewed 68 patients admitted between 1993 and 2000 [6]. Mortality rate was 13.2% (9 patients), and deaths were caused by septic shock (4/9), cerebral edema (2/9), cerebral edema with pulmonary edema (2/9), and hypokalemic dysrhythmias (1/9).

Kanafani et al. [7] have described their experience with ventilator-associated pneumonia at the American University of Beirut Medical Center, finding that their incidence was higher than usual reported incidences. In addition, they found a greater preponderance of resistant organisms.

Goh et al. [8] have reported some surprising results of a prospective study comparing *limited-access* admissions with direct admissions to their PICU at University Malaya Medical Center in Lumpur, Malaysia. Limited-access patients were transported from rural hospitals by nonspecialty teams, and although younger and with a higher prevalence of respiratory disease, did not differ in PRISM score from those with direct access (admitted from hospital ward or emergency room). Despite the initial poor accessibility to advanced care, the outcomes were no different between the two groups. These results conflict with those of Hatherill et al. [9]. Trevor Duke, in a thoughtful accompanying editorial [10], commented, "Whether . . . developing and transitional countries should have a paediatric ICU transport service is a balance of overall health priorities. . . . Errors in the transport of a minority of children . . . would be minimized, but it might not lead to an overall fall in . . . child mortality if scarce financial and human resources were channeled away from improving the quality of paediatric care in rural and district hospitals."

A paper of significant historical and practical importance was published by Dayal in 1980 [11]. In Agra, India, a low-cost, experimental unit was developed for caring for low-birth-weight infants. The unit did not have incubators, much less ventilators, but consisted primarily of a unit in which mothers were requested to stay after their babies' birth. Breast feeding was taught and encouraged. Warming was accomplished with blankets and hot water bottles in winter and cooling in summer with inexpensive room coolers available at the time. The study demonstrated that with these modest interventions, survival of a substantial number of infants between 1,000 and 2,000 g could be accomplished without the use of expensive and sophisticated equipment. The historical and practical importance of this article lies in the numbers of developing countries whose resources are the same as or less than those available in Agra a quarter of a century ago, making these interventions as relevant in these countries today as they were in Agra then.

Ameh et al. [12] reported their 10-year experience with 154 neonates who underwent emergency surgery in their institution in

Zaria, Nigeria. Surgical emergencies represented 40% of all surgical procedures performed in neonates over that period. Overall mortality rate was 30.5%, with two thirds of the deaths caused by overwhelming infection and most of the remainder caused by respiratory insufficiency. The authors identified as important factors contributing to mortality and morbidity (1) delayed referral from outlying rural health centers or from home (representing nearly 95% of the referrals) and (2) the lack of neonatal ICU (NICU) resources for postoperative care.

Even in more advanced NICUs mortality rate is high. Kambarami et al. [13] reviewed their experience with all neonates admitted to their NICU in Zair, Zimbabwe, during 1998. A total of 234 neonates with a median birth weight of 1,730 g were admitted, 73% for medical (mostly respiratory distress) and 26% for surgical indications. Mortality rate was 46.4% and was unrelated to continuous positive airway pressure use, age at admission, sex, or duration of stay. Need for positive pressure ventilation was associated with mortality. The authors underscore the difficulty of drawing conclusions about risk factors in the face of suboptimal care in general.

Jeena et al. [14] reported in 1999 their 25-year experience in a PICU in Durban, South Africa. The PICU admissions as a percentage of general pediatric admissions increased from 1.5% to 7%, with an average of >300 admissions per year. More than 90% of the 7,580 children were tracheally intubated, 80% requiring mechanical ventilation. Vaccine-preventable diseases such as measles and tetanus declined over the time period, largely being replaced by HIV-related syndromes. Mortality rate was 35%, with nearly 24% of the deaths occurring within the first 24 hours of admission.

Nouira et al. [15] compared utilization and outcome of an adult ICU in a developing country (Tunisia) with that in a developed one (France). Tunisian patients were younger, in better baseline health, and less ill upon admission than patients admitted to the French unit. However, French patients had a lower mortality rate (17.2% vs. 22.5%) than Tunisians and received more treatment. In the highest and lowest severity groups, mortality rates were comparable between the two units, despite the fact that the French patients received more treatment; in the mid-range of severity, the Tunisians had a higher mortality rate. The authors observe that the Tunisian unit appears more cost-effective for the high-severity group of patients and less so for the mid-severity group and speculate that such observations might improve how resources are allocated in units with severe resource constraints.

One of the few articles profiling the state of pediatric critical care in a developing country was published in 1993 by Schnitzler [16]. In Argentina at that time, 8.2% of the gross national product was spent on health care for a population of 32 million. Infant mortality rate was higher than that in developed nations (24.5 per 1,000 live births). The distribution of PICU beds was typical for that of a developing country: of 244 beds nationally at that time, more than 60% were located within or near the capital. The authors cite bed shortages as important challenges, forcing premature discharges from PICUs, poor coordination with emergency services, poor organization and regionalization of services, and manpower shortages.

Review of the available literature leads to several conclusions and observations:

1. The most common causes of childhood mortality in developing countries are not those associated with PICU deaths in developed countries, but rather are the result of failures of primary care and public health efforts, such as sanitation, immunization, and access to health care.

2. The *resource steal* phenomenon caused by the expense of critical care and its benefits for a comparatively small number of children creates an ethical dilemma for PICU practitioners in these countries and for colleagues from developing countries desiring to be of assistance.

3. Most developing countries have some form of critical care for children, even the poorest. However, a common pattern is usually seen in which whatever PICU resources that exist are concentrated in one or two centers, and even these centers are invariably lacking to some degree in equipment, supplies, manpower, and training.

4. Because of this geographic distribution of PICU resources, transportation of children from outlying areas to these centers is an important challenge.

Ethical Issues and Child Health Priorities in Developing Countries

In wealthy countries of the world, although resource constraints and allocation are commonly discussed issues, these concepts are vastly different from those in similar discussions that take place in poor countries. In the United States, for example, *resource allocation* usually means competition for somewhat limited numbers of available intensive care beds. It certainly does not imply utilization of large portions of available health care dollars at the expense of far more cost-effective initiatives, such as development of and access to basic health care, sanitation, immunizations, nutrition, and so forth. The ethical principle of *distributive justice* would imply that resources be allocated fairly among beneficiaries. Furthermore, it would also imply that the use of large amounts of limited resources to benefit a small number of individuals, while depriving large numbers of individuals of potentially striking benefits, cannot be justified. Sachdeva has explored the complexity of these issues in a thoughtful editorial [17].

What role, then, can and should pediatric critical care medicine play in the health care of developing countries? The answer is not easy and, recognizing that each developing country is probably in its own phase of development, the answer may very well be unique for each country. For a country that has not accomplished basic sanitation or developed a successful immunization program, or that lacks even basic pediatric inpatient resources, development of critical care can hardly be justified. On the other hand, countries that have made progress in more basic care, including even some degree of critical care, might justifiably look toward the development of *assisted* critical care resources. It is here that the altruistic contributions of individuals and organizations from wealthier countries can make all the difference, allowing the developing countries to concentrate their own resources on more basic care, without having to ignore totally, for example, children dying for lack of congenital heart surgery.

Many of these countries will have some form of intensive care services, which can serve as a foundation for further *assisted* development. Through the formation of relationships with programs in wealthier, developed countries, these PICUs can benefit in a number of ways—access to donated equipment and supplies currently lacking; basic critical care training on site; intermittent training that elevates the level of services provided for short periods of time, building sequentially on each learning experience; development of "intellectual connections" that provide an immediate source of telephone consultation, and perhaps even in the future, with some modest development, telecommunication via computer and Internet; training experiences of various lengths of time in the developed host country for selected individuals; and contacts for needed resources that extend beyond critical care.

There are many organizations that sponsor volunteer opportunities in developing countries of varying lengths of time for pediatricians. Most of these involve primary care, and many pediatric intensivists who engage in such volunteer work actually do so as primary care pediatricians. A relatively small portion of these volunteer opportunities involve projects actually requiring the skills of an intensivist, and some of these are listed at the conclusion of this chapter. Volunteer assignments can be as short as 2 weeks or as long as 2 years. However, most pediatric intensivists are not in a position to volunteer for periods longer than a few weeks to a few months (see Tables 13.5 and 13.6 for further information on volunteer opportunities and organizations).

TABLE 13.5. Organizations with potential need for general pediatric or pediatric critical care expertise.

Name & contact info	Duration	Expenses covered	Description
Doctors of the World Maria Dugan 212-226-9890, ext. 230 duganm@dowusa.org www.doctorsoftheworld.org	1–12 months	Transportation, lodging	Affiliated with Doctors Without Borders. Programs in war-torn or disaster-stricken regions
Doctors Without Borders (Medecins sans Frontieres) 212-679-6800 doctors@newyork.msf.org www.doctorswithoutborders.org	6–12 months, career	Transportation, lodging, food	The largest independent international voluntary emergency relief service. Serves areas of conflict, famine, and natural disasters
Health Volunteers Overseas Kate Skillman 202-296-0928 hvo@aol.com www.hvousa.org	2 weeks to 3 months	Variable by individual project; volunteer usually pays transportation	Strong, nearly but not quite exclusive, emphasis on teaching. HVO Pediatrics Division sponsored by AAP. Current projects in Cambodia, Guyana, Malawi, St. Lucia, Uganda-Kampala. Well organized
International Medical Corps Jennifer Crawford 310-826-7800 imc@imc-la.com www.imc-la.org	2–4 weeks to 1 year	Transportation, housing, food	Emphasis on disaster relief with restoration of independence. Site updated frequently
Interplast, Inc. Beverly Kent 650-934-3312 IPNews@interplast.org www.interplast.org	2 weeks	Volunteer pays for food and $350 toward other expenses; other transportation, lodging and food expenses covered	Free reconstructive surgery to children with additional emphasis on teaching. Desires pediatricians, but does not specify intensivists
Lalmba Association Bob Roark 303-420-1810 lalmba@lalmba.org www.lalmba.org	1–3 years	Transportation, housing, food	Operative over 40 years; focuses on the poorest countries in Africa, with primary care needs foremost. Other nonmedical children-related programs co-existent
Minnesota International Health Volunteers 612-871-3759 http://www.mihv.org expenses	3 months to 1 year	Transportation, housing, food; shorter term assignments available but vounteer assumes more expenses	Strong emphasis on primary care. Emphasizes education. Strong presence in Thailand, Haiti, Kenya, Nicaragua, and Uganda
Operation Rainbow Sue Ellen Ruggles 281-980-0088 rainbow@compass.net www.compassnet.com/rainbow	10 days to 3 weeks	All expenses paid by volunteer	Provides reconstructive surgery to poor children through surgical trips; also emphasizes teaching; focuses on Latin America, China, Philippines. No specific mention of pediatricians, but most do have need
Operation Smile Patricia Daigle 757-321-7645 alisandrelli@operationsmile.org www.operationsmile.org	1–3 weeks	Volunteer contributes $350 to trip and food; lodging and transportation provided	Reconstructive surgery trips around the world. Specifically utilizes pediatric intensivists
Physicians for Peace Foundation, Inc. 757-625-7569 adm@physiciansforpeace.org www.physicians-for-peace.org	4–18 days	Transportation, housing, food	Organizes various types of surgical trips with emphasis on teaching. Check Web site

TABLE 13.5. *Continued*

Name & contact info	Duration	Expenses covered	Description
Project HOPE Cindy Marino 800-544-4673 recruit@projhope.org www.projhope.org	Variable: few days to career	Varies with specific project	Sponsors wide variety of programs in most parts of the world. Needs vary with specific program or project. Check Web site
Healing the Children 800-992-0324 or 509-327-4281 (National headquarters) administrator@healingthech ildren.org www.healingthechildren.org	1–2 weeks	Housing and food	Variety of surgical trips in manyparts of the world. National headquarters Web site has links to each of the 15 chapters, each of which sponsors projects
HBS Foundation, Inc./Hopital Bon Samaritain Rienke van Hall 561-493-3113 hbsfl@bellsouth.net www.hbslimbe.org	2 weeks to 6 months	Housing and food	Runs and staffs small inpatient hospital in rural Haiti with surgical services supplied by rotating visiting teams. Large outpatient service; 45-bed ward for handicapped and abandoned children. Uses volunteers with all sorts of backgrounds
International Children's Heart Foundation Sandy McMahan 901-869-4243 skmcmahan@aol.com www.babyheart.org	2 weeks	Transportation, housing, food.	Organizes and conducts 10 to 12 2-week trips per year, 15 to 30 congenital heart surgeries per trip. Size and composition of team vary with site, but almost always includes pediatric intensivist(s)
Medicine for Peace Dr. Michael Viola 202-362-9121 mviola@msn.com www.medpeace.org	2–4 weeks	Transportation and housing	Dedicated to provision of medical and other assistance to children who are victims of war. Current projects include Iraq, Bosnia, and Haiti. Needs pediatricians. See Web site
Palestine Children's Relief Fund Stephen Sosebee 330-678-2645 ThePCRF@aol.com www.pcrf.net	Varies	Transportation, housing and food	Organizes surgical trips to a variety of sites in Middle East; surgeries include plastic, orthopedic, ophthalmic, and cardiac
Medical Training Worldwide Ramon Berguer, M.D. 916-863-0940 info@med-training- worldwide.org www.med-training- worldwide.org	1–2 weeks	Housing and food	Organizes various surgical trips with emphasis on teaching. Programs in Latin America, India, Ukraine, and elsewhere. See Web site
Friends Without a Border Kumru Aruz 212-691-0909 fwab@interport.net www.fwab.org	6 months	Housing and food	Funds and operates the new Angkor Hospital for Children in Siem Reap, an impoverished province of Cambodia. Needs pediatricians and subspecialists to teach local staff
Surgicorps International Bonnie Skavo 412-231-2069, ext. 544, or 720-565-6505 info@surgicorps.org www.surgicorps.org	1–3 weeks	All expenses by volunteer	Organizes two to three plastic surgery trips per year to Tanzania, Vietnam, Brazil, Paraguay, and Guatemala. See Web site for upcoming trips and possible pediatric needs
Children's Cross Connection Pamela Rundle 770-716-1926 cccprundle@earthlink.net www.cccinternational.org	1–2 weeks	Varies with different programs	Organizes surgical team visits for orthopedic, craniofacial, plastic, and cardiac surgery and renal transplantations in El Salvador and Ethiopia.

Note: The information in this table was obtained mainly from the database available online at the American Academy of Pediatrics' Web site. A few additional organizations not in the database are also included. Organizations with denomination-specific religious requirements for volunteers were excluded, along with those with explicit evangelization goals. Information is thought to be current and accurate as of the time of this writing.

www.rainbowbabies.org/services/centers/InternationalChildHealth
This page, on the Web site of Rainbow Babies and Children's Hospital and Case Western Reserve University, describes the institution's Center on International Health, one of a kind in the United States

www.who.int
The home page for the website of the World Health Organization, this is the entryway into an enormous amount of information, much of it having to do with maternal and child health

www.developmentgoals.org
This site offers detailed data analysis, up to date, on progress made toward accomplishment of the Millennium Development Goals, the roadmap agreed upon by all members of the United Nations in a commitment to eliminate poverty

www.paris21org/betterworld
Another site offering current statistics on aspects of world poverty, with a large section on infant and child health

www.volunteersforprosperity.gov/
Web site that maintains an extensive database of organizations that use professional volunteers

www.internationalhealthvolunteers.org
Another independent database of volunteers and projects needing them

www.ama-assn.org/ama/pub/category/1529.html
Web page of the American Medical Association concerning international health and volunteerism

How meaningful can short-term volunteer experiences be? Most who have partaken in such projects will testify to the importance of the experiences in their own lives, but such testimony begs the question of what is accomplished for the programs being served in the developing countries. I would like to propose a model for the development of pediatric critical care resources in certain types of developing countries that does not conflict with public health and primary care priorities, does provide value to the beneficiary programs by elevating their capabilities, and finally provides services to children who would not otherwise receive them. I will use as an example of such an enterprise the International Children's Heart Foundation and, in particular, the experience of that organization in Nicaragua.

International Children's Heart Foundation and Project Open Heart, Managua

The International Children's Heart Foundation (ICHF) was founded in 1993 to help provide cardiac services—medical and surgical, diagnostic and therapeutic—to children in developing countries. The type of involvement of ICHF in different countries depends on existing resources and is tailored in such a way as to best meet the needs in the individual country. Many of the sites where ICHF has had a presence have had some sort of congenital heart program in existence (e.g., Zagreb, Croatia; Lima, Peru), but cases were previously limited to straightforward diagnoses and procedures. The role of ICHF in these centers has been to build upon existing resources and skills to allow local caregivers to provide more complicated care. In other centers, no program exists whatsoever. Here the role of ICHF is to help local caregivers develop and implement a program.

The modus operandi of ICHF is to sponsor teams of volunteers for 2-week stints at the host center. The composition of the team depends, again, on the local resources. In some of the more advanced centers that are capable of much of the diagnostic and postoperative care, the team may be composed of as few as three or four individuals, including an experienced surgeon. In the less advanced centers, the team may comprise the entire spectrum of caregivers, including surgeon, anesthesiologist, intensivist(s), cardiologist, perfusionist, scrub technician, and ICU nurses. Occasionally the team may also include a respiratory therapist or a bioengineer. In all cases, team members work closely and individually with their local counterparts, as important primary goals include increasing their education and their skills. In the 10 years between April 1993 and March 2003, ICHF organized and conducted 83 surgical trips to 14 countries, operating on a total of 1,580 children for an average of 158 per year, but witnessing considerable growth in numbers in the latter portion of those years [18]. Overall survival rate is 90.5% and is comparable with rates in U.S. centers when adjusted for RACH-1 [19].

Nicaragua, with a population of 5.4 million, is second to Haiti as the poorest country in the Western Hemisphere. The average yearly income is the equivalent of $730 per capita. Nurses' salaries average $800 per year, and 48% of the population is considered to be living below the national poverty level. Unemployment/underemployment exceeds 50%. Infant mortality rate is 36 and the under-5 mortality rate is 45 per 1,000 live births.

The Children's Hospital in Managua, Nicaragua, *Hospital Infantil de Jesus Manuel Rivera*, is a 220-bed facility located in the heart of the capital and is the major teaching facility for pediatrics in the country. For more than 15 years, the medical staff has included both pediatric cardiologists and pediatric intensivists, but no cardiac surgeon. Indeed, before the first ICHF trip to Managua, no open-heart procedure had ever been performed in the country on any age patient.

During the 1970s and early 1980s, children with congenital heart disease were flown to Cuba for corrective or palliative surgery, which was provided without charge to the families or to the Nicaraguan government. This arrangement ceased to be available by the late 1980s and early 1990s. With an estimated birth rate of 25 per 1,000 population in 2005, a population of 5.4 million, and a congenital heart disease incidence of ~5 per 1,000 live births, just under an estimated 700 children would be born every year with congenital heart disease. With >90% of these needing surgery, the backlog of untreated children was growing rapidly in the early 1990s, and the medical staff soon identified the lack of surgical resources as a major problem and for their institution one of their highest priorities. This led to the creation of *Proyecto Corazon Abierto* (Project Open Heart).

After two preliminary preparatory trips, the first surgical trip to Managua took place in 1994. The procedures were *simple* ones, limited to atrial septal defect and ventricular septal defect repairs, as these were thought to be the first types of procedures needing to be learned by the local surgeons. Initially, one trip was made annually. However, it soon became clear that optimal learning could only occur with more frequent opportunities, and the number was increased to three per year. In addition, the complexity of cases has been able to be increased somewhat to include tetralogy of Fallot, Glenn procedures, and some valve replacements.

Between that first trip in 1994 and the summer of 2005, a total of 14 trips have been accomplished, and 274 patients have received surgeries they would not otherwise have had. Of equal importance, although still short of the goal of independence, the physicians and nurses have become increasingly competent in their ability to care for these children. Five children died during these trips, leading to an overall mortality rate of <2%—a mortality rate for these lesions that is comparable with those in large centers in the United States.

Disposable supplies and medicines for these trips have all been donated. The personnel have all been volunteers. Transportation of supplies and equipment from the United States to Nicaragua has been donated by commercial carriers. Transportation of volunteers has been provided by a variety of donors, including a number of local Rotary Clubs in the United States, Variety International, and others. Some lodging has been provided by the same donors and some by donations raised locally in Managua. Local transportation for the team was provided by the Ministry of Health. Thus, all of these surgical trips were accomplished with virtually no "stealing" of local funds allocated to primary care or public health efforts. The actual cost of these trips—not including donated medicine and supplies—is less than $20,000, which includes the money raised in the United States and the cost of lodging in Managua. This amount would barely cover the cost of care for two children with uncomplicated VSD repair in the United States.

In addition to the donation of disposable supplies and medicines, the project has been able to provide a donated echocardiogram machine, a cardiopulmonary bypass machine, a variety of ventilators and monitors, and, through the participation of bioengineers, the ongoing maintenance of existing equipment. All of these donations have had a significant impact on the care of critically ill or injured children well beyond those specifically treated by the project for congenital heart disease.

The enhanced ability of nursing and physician staffs to provide care for more severely ill or injured children, achieved through the tutelage that occurs during these trips, is yet another *ripple effect* of these teaching-oriented missions. At the beginning of the program, invasive monitoring was not performed in the PICU. Beginning with the first surgical trip, nursing and medical staffs were instructed in the placement, maintenance, and interpretation of arterial and central venous pressure lines, monitoring that has now become routine for the sicker patients admitted to the unit.

Two final benefits of programs such as this deserve mention, although they are the most intangible of all. First are the effects of such programs on morale in the involved institutions and even their countries. Most developing and impoverished countries and programs are burdened by the realization that their path is challenging and difficult. The immediate successes achieved by programs such as the one in Managua, although ultimately far less important than the long-term importance of creating an independent program, help engender motivation, hope, and pride in those who are struggling against what seem insurmountable odds. Second are the effects of the programs on volunteers. Many PICU physicians, nurses, respiratory therapists, surgeons, and more, have a desire to donate their time, services, and skills to their colleagues in less privileged countries and to their patients. Programs that not only allow but depend on volunteers who are not able to donate more than small periods of time can tap into an enormous resource of altruistic individuals. These short-term volunteer projects can become part of longer term programs, which ultimately can enhance the capabilities of colleagues in developing countries to provide better care to their critically ill and injured children.

References

1. World Health Organization. The World Health Report, 2005: make every mother and child count. Geneva: World Health Organization, 2005.
2. UNICEF. The State of the World's Children, 2005: childhood under threat. New York: UNICEF, 2004.
3. Khilnani P, Sarma D, Singh R, Uttam R, Rajdev S, Makkar A, et al. Demographic profile and outcome analysis of a tertiary level pediatric intensive care unit. Indian J Pediatr 2004;71:587–591.
4. Zar HJ, Apolles P, Argent A, Klein M, Burgess J, Hanslod, et al. The etiology and outcome of pneumonia in human immunodeficiency virus-infected children admitted to intensive care in a developing country. Pediatr Crit Care Med 2001;2:108–112.
5. Mathivhal LR. ICU's worldwide: an overview of critical care medicine in South Africa. Crit Care 2002;6:22–23
6. Jayashree M, Singhi S. Diabetic ketoacidosis: predictors of outcome in a pediatric intensive care unit in a developing country. Pediatr Crit Care Med 2004;5:427–433.
7. Kanafani ZA, Kara L, Hayek S, Kanj SS. Ventilator-associated pneumonia at a tertiary-care center in a developing country: incidence, microbiology, and susceptibility patterns of isolated microorganisms. Infect Control Hosp Epidemiol 2003;24:864–869.
8. Goh AY, Abdel-Latif M-A, Lum LC, Abu-Bakar MN. Outcome of children with different accessibility to tertiary pediatric intensive care in a developing country—a prospective cohort study. Intensive Care Med 2003;29:97–102.
9. Hatherill M, Waggie Z, Reynolds L, Argent A. Transport of critically ill children in a resource-limited setting. Intensive Care Med 2003;29:1547–1554.
10. Duke T. Transport of seriously ill children: a neglected global issue. Intensive Care Med 2003;29:1414–1416.
11. Dayal RS. Problems and management of low birth weight babies in an improvised neonatal unit of a developing country. Bull Int Pediatr Assoc 1980;3:36–46.
12. Ameh EA, Dogo PM, Nmadu PT. Emergency neonatal surgery in a developing country. Pediatr Surg Int 2001;17:448–451.
13. Kambarami R, Chidede O, Chirisa M. Neonatal intensive care in a developing country: outcome and factors associated with mortality. Cent Afr J Med 2000;46:205–207.
14. Jeena PM, Wesley AG, Coovadia H. Admission patterns and outcomes in a paediatric intensive care unit in South Africa over a 25-year period (1971–1995). Intensive Care Med 1999;25:88–94.
15. Nouira S, Roupie E, El Atrouss S, Durand-Zaleski I, Brun-Buisson C, Lemaire F, et al. Intensive care use in a developing country: a comparison between a Tunisian and a French unit. Intensive Care Med 1998;24:1144–1151.
16. Schnitzler EJ. Pediatric intensive care in Argentina. Crit Care Med 1993;21:s403–s404.
17. Sachdeva RC. Intensive care-a cost effective option for developing countries? Indian J Pediatr 2001;68:339–342.
18. Novick WM, Stidham GL, Karl TR, Guillory KL, Ivancan V, Malcic I, et al. Are we improving after 10 years of humanitarian paediatric cardiac assistance? Cardiol Young 2005;15:379–384.
19. Jenkins KJ. Risk adjustment for congenital heart surgery: the RACHS-1 method. Semin Thorac Cardiovasc Surg 2004;7:180–184.

14

The Pediatric Intensive Care Unit of the Future: Technological Advances in Pediatric Critical Care Medicine

Kenneth Tegtmeyer

Introduction

There are numerous factors that affect the ability of a pediatric intensive care unit (PICU) to remain *modern*. Much of what is discussed in this chapter may be out of the reach of most PICUs because of issues related to cost. Limitations of the return on investment (ROI) may make seemingly indispensable upgrades in equipment unobtainable, and challenges related to the small market that is pediatric critical care may also limit development. That being said, this chapter summarizes the current *state of the art* of the PICU in the early 21st century that may be available but not widely employed and then discusses future possibilities that may come to exist in an idealized, well-supported (and well-funded) PICU.

Today's Modern Pediatric Intensive Care Unit

Monitoring

One of the primary advantages of admitting a critically ill or injured child to the PICU is the ability to monitor more closely the moment-to-moment changes that he or she is going through and thus be able to respond and react quickly to these changes and initiate treatment in a timely and expeditious manner. Most PICUs now have systems to allow remote monitoring of multiple critically ill patients at one or more central monitoring locations within the PICU. This obviates the need for a nurse or aide to be physically present at the bedside at all times and allows for simultaneous monitoring of several patients by multiple members of the health care team. Current technology exists to have alarm or other data transmitted remotely to a pager or other computer/ monitor system so that a clinician at a distance can have access to the data [1–3].

Data Collection and Management

The Flow Sheet

Each individual patient in the PICU generates reams of data (e.g., vital signs, including heart rate, respiratory rate, temperature, blood pressure, and oxygen saturation; results of invasive monitoring, including measurement of central venous pressure, arterial blood pressure, end-tidal CO_2; laboratory data, including results of arterial blood gas analysis; hourly intake and output; nursing assessments; and so forth). The challenge that these data present has been recognized for a long time, and it is an ideal role for computerization to play to ease the collection and management of this volume of data. Computerized information systems (CISs) have been present in the PICU for more than 20 years but are still well short of their potential. Early systems and even most systems in place today are unable to match the paper flowchart for either speed of perusal or ease of use. Because of issues of resolution and readability, as well as cost and space restrictions regarding large monitors, no CIS can present the same amount of data in one space that a well-designed and completed patient flowsheet can. However, where the CIS excels is in the accuracy, precision, and granularity of the data that it can collect. Whereas the paper record is limited to the ability of the nurses to directly observe or obtain the measurement and transcribe it to paper, most CISs will automatically extract and store data from the monitors. To ensure that the data entered into the record have been at least glanced at by a member of the health care team, the nurse generally *signs* the data.

Granularity refers to the resolution of the data. The spectrum of granularity can be appreciated if one looks at the different levels of care. In the outpatient clinic, data are collected at a very coarse level of granularity. Periodic measurements of height, weight, and blood pressure over periods of months to years would be an example of the most coarse data collection health care practitioners employ. On the inpatient wards, vital sign measurements every 4 to 8 hours are obviously finer than those of the outpatient clinic but yet still more coarse than the data collected in the PICU. The CIS then allows practitioners an edge to the next level of fineness of granularity by automating data collection at an even shorter interval than realistically feasible using a paper record. Although most CISs will collect all information generated, there is still a coarseness to the data collection. Vital sign recordings may occur even as frequent as every minute with current CISs, but there are still data in the middle that may yet prove useful. There are experimental systems

D.S. Wheeler et al. (eds.), *Science and Practice of Pediatric Critical Care Medicine*,
DOI 10.1007/978-1-84800-921-9_14, © Springer-Verlag London Limited 2009

in place that allow true continuous recording of vital sign data, giving access to such information as beat-to-beat variability of heart rate and blood pressure. One clinical example where this fineness of granularity of data is currently clinically important is with regard to pulsus paradoxus. Pulsus paradoxus is a state in which arterial blood pressure has an exaggerated drop during inspiration compared with exhalation [4]. Pulsus paradoxus can be a sign of pericardial tamponade as well as an indicator of severity of respiratory illness in children [5]. Because blood pressure varies with the phase of a patient's ventilatory cycle, standard data collection, and even data collection with most CISs, would not be able to pick up the variations that happen just seconds apart. Currently it takes a clinician to observe the oscillations in blood pressure, and documentation of this state must be done either separately in the progress record or in a side note to the flowsheet. A fine granular CIS will be able to incorporate such data into the clinical record.

The Electronic Medical Record

The concept of the electronic medical record (EMR) has been around for a long time. References to using computers for an EMR appear as early as the early 1960s [6,7], but penetration of a complete EMR is still quite variable. Clinical data as discussed in the previous section are one component of the EMR. Laboratory data have long been stored electronically. Radiologic data are nearly completely electronically stored at this date, but incorporating all aspects of the medical record into one comprehensive medical record is still rare to find. There are numerous arguments in support of an EMR. Storage space necessitated by an ever-expanding patient population and that population's medical record is a constant challenge for hospitals and clinics. Intensive care units are particularly problematic in terms of the quantity of paper generated for a medical record, as discussed above. It is not uncommon for pediatric patients to be discharged from the PICU with charts that weigh many times more than the patients themselves. An EMR also increases the availability of the chart. Gone are the waits for the chart to arrive from medical records or storage.

Portability is a long-term goal but with some current-day implications. In 1994, during his State of the Union Address, then President Bill Clinton proposed a series of changes to health care that included the portability of medical information [8]. Although the original concept suggested that patients could carry their record around on a wallet-sized card, technological advancements, particularly with regard to the World Wide Web and secure data networks, may obviate the need for this kind of portability. In reality, the Health Insurance Portability and Accountability Act (HIPAA) has added challenges to the sharing of medical data without the express knowledge or consent of the patient. Some hospital systems and large health maintenance organizations have been able to generate EMRs that are accessible across network hospitals and clinics [9,10], but currently there is no system for cross portability among hospital networks or clinics.

Physician documentation is one of the slowest aspects of the EMR to develop. It is still uncommon today for physician notes to be directly incorporated into the EMR, let alone be electronically generated in the first place. Increasing demands of payers, particularly Medicare and Medicaid, have made physician documentation both more crucial and more complicated. Physician notes are now intimately connected to billing [11]. The more data that need to be included in the physician note, the more time it will take to produce the note. A well-constructed EMR can decrease the time required for appropriate documentation through the use of templates, standard language sets, and the automated incorporation of ancillary data via integration with the CIS. The goal thus is to increase the amount of time available for direct patient care by decreasing the time spent documenting direct patient care.

Another advantage of the EMR though is that it can help avoid fraud by incorporating the rules regarding billing and documentation into the note generation software to ensure that the level of the note supports the level of billing. This is the one aspect, of everything discussed in this chapter, that actually pays for itself. Possibly the biggest challenge that has kept this practice from being more widespread in the PICU is that, by the nature of being multidisciplinary, the data or documentation needed for one patient, for example, a tracheally intubated 2-month-old child with respiratory syncytial virus (RSV) bronchiolitis is dramatically different from that needed for a 14-year-old tracheally intubated child with a severe closed head injury. Creating an EMR that is flexible enough to incorporate both of these patients, while not generating large areas of blank space or requesting superfluous data, such as the intracranial pressure (ICP) of the RSV patient, can be challenging. Standardized EMRs are even harder to generate across disciplines and specialties, as each group has its own unique needs and styles of documentation.

One of the primary limitations of instituting an EMR is determining what to do with the old paper medical record. The current standard is to optically scan the entire contents of the paper medical record and incorporate it electronically into the EMR. There are obvious limitations to this. One is that optical images of pages take substantially larger amounts of memory space than do electronically generated records, let alone the time and cost of scanning all of the past medical records. This makes the system needed to store the data relatively large, but more importantly slows the access of the data. Granted, with every passing month computer processor speed gets faster, and this will make it easier to scan through larger quantities of pages. The other challenge is that there is no simple way to search the data. Although optical character recognition (OCR) software programs can readily identify typed and some hand printed words, they are still far off from being able to recognize the most challenging of written words, those of a physician. Another limitation, as previously mentioned, is that of portability. In the earlier stages of EMR generation, great effort was generated in developing a standard nomenclature for data. Health Level 7 (HL-7) is the standard for data interchange in health care. The bottom line is that HL-7 is what allows vendors to develop software that can both tap the various data generators, such as the clinical laboratory, and develop clinical information systems and monitors to work with the same data set. Essentially, regardless of the makers of the equipment, the monitors, or the laboratory machinery, the data generated will be labeled in a consistent manner that can then be used to manipulate, store, and present the data. This is what would allow data to be transported from one hospital system to another, without the need for an expansive paper record. Currently there are no systems in place for cross network transfer of data, but, when they are developed, they will depend on having a uniform data structure. Currently, some systems are being developed that would even allow transfer from a transport team en route to and from a referring institution [12].

One of the early limitations to EMRs was that hospitals were not originally designed to have multiple computer terminals spread throughout the wards and units to allow ready access to a computerized medical record. Fortunately, technology such as flat screen monitors, secure wireless data transmission, and the ever-shrinking size of the PC has allowed even older hospitals to set up multiple computer stations without taking up all available desktop space with the necessary equipment or undergoing extensive remodeling. In fact, all PICUs should have access to multiple workstations that also allow the user to connect to PubMed and other on-line educational resources.

Wireless technology in particular has made it easier for clinicians to carry information with them throughout the hospital and even to the bedside. There are a variety of techniques for doing this, the smallest of which is the handheld personal digital assistant (PDA). The two primary operating systems, PalmOS™ and Microsoft PocketPC™ are both capable of interacting with the CIS through a wireless connection. These small devices are best suited to retrieval of text-based data such as recent vital sign information or the most recent laboratory data. Several functions of the palm-sized devices can make them convenient, particularly to nursing staff. Despite their small size they can store large quantities of reference data. Storing drug references is a particularly useful function of the PDA, but there is a myriad of other educational references available. Other functions that have been used in the hospital and clinical settings are collecting research data and entering patient data into a CIS. PDAs could easily be programmed to deliver reminders as to when medications or treatments are due and have been successfully implemented to manage respiratory care protocols [13,14].

Larger portable devices such as laptops or tablet computers have the advantage over PDAs of larger screen sizes and resolutions, as well as more powerful processors. Tablet PCs and laptops can offer reasonably good presentation of visual data such as radiologic studies, which can be taken to the patient's bedside and discussed with the patient and/or the family. Although they may not have high enough resolution to reliably allow interpretation by the radiologist, they can be used as an effective communication tool. The tablet or laptop connected to a wireless information system within the PICU can serve multiple functions, including accessing laboratory and other CIS data, generating physician documentation, and communicating with referring physicians and remote family members. This has been demonstrated in at least one institution as a way to allow displaced families to communicate with friends and relatives about their child's illness, as well as allowing the intensivist to keep the referring physician up to date on the patient's progress in the PICU [15].

Patient Care

Patient safety is the driving force behind many of the more recent innovations in patient care. Numerous national organizations, ranging from the federal regulatory level, such as the Joint Council on Accreditation of Healthcare Organizations (JCAHO), think-tank groups such as the Institute of Medicine, and consumer-based organizations such as the Leapfrog Group are all putting pressure on hospitals to improve patient safety. The Leapfrog Group, a group of large employers and health insurance purchasers that have joined together to improve the quality of patient care, in particular has put pressure on ICUs because of their disproportionately large share of the health care costs in the United States, to improve patient care, and likewise to improve outcomes and efficiency. Standardization of drip concentrations and elimination of the use of the *rule of six* has been one of the more contentious changes. The

JCAHO has requested this change to try to decrease the incidence of preventable medication errors in the PICU. Other technological changes have come into play to try to minimize serious medical errors. Programmable intravenous and syringe pumps that will calculate appropriate fluid rates based on concentration and patient weight are the standard in PICUs today. These devices add a level of safety at the terminal point, just before the medication is administered to the patient, but should not completely replace human double checking and calculations.

Computerized Provider Order Entry (CPOE) is rapidly becoming the primary mechanism by which orders get entered in the hospital setting, and the PICU is certainly no exception. Groups such as Leapfrog Group that are seeking to raise the level of care in ICUs across the country are contributing to the push for items like CPOE to help decrease the incidence of errors in the hospital. A good CPOE system has a collection of features that help to minimize medical errors related to ordering. Ordering should be weight based and tied to the baseline weight of the patient. It should be cross referenced to standard recommended dosing for the medications being ordered, although some reasonable level of override can be allowed, such as when patients develop tachyphylaxis to medications after long-term administration. The orders should be cross referenced to the patient's other medications to ensure there are no problematic compatibility or allergy issues.

One of the biggest concerns regarding the implementation of CPOE in the PICU is the speed at which it can be performed. In a PICU that is already facing time constraints related to decreased resident staffing and increased demands for documentation, the CPOE system needs to be efficient enough and user friendly enough that it does not increase the amount of time needed to write orders. Despite more than 15 years of exponential growth in the use of computers, there are still many among us who are not the most facile with computer use. Systems must remain in place for acute needs to be met, such as in resuscitations, that allow for bypassing of the CPOE system. Templates for admission orders, specific to the service, procedure, or diagnosis can make order writing much simpler. Additional templates for daily orders, grouped by systems or problems, such as cardiac, renal, and respiratory, can also expedite the order writing process. The bottom line is that CPOE, like all other physician/provider computer interfaces in the PICU, needs to be supported in such a way that the providers can suggest modifications to fit their needs that will be met in a timely fashion.

Staffing

There are a wide variety of models currently in play to staff PICUs. Neither academic units nor private units have a single standard for staffing by physicians and other advanced practice personnel [16]. Pediatric residents have traditionally played a major role in the *round the clock function* of academic PICUs, but work-hour restrictions instituted in July 2003 have limited residents to 80 hours per week [17,18]. In some PICUs this has meant that large portions of the week are left uncovered by residents. Pediatric critical care fellows, also considered as residents in the eyes of the Accreditation Council for Graduate Medical Education (ACGME) are also subject to the same 80-hour work-week restrictions. Pediatric ICUs have found varying ways to cope with this dilemma. One approach is the incorporation of advanced practice nurses and physician assistants into the coverage team. In these models the pediatric nurse practitioner or physician assistant takes on the role traditionally covered by residents, including data collection, presentation on rounds, and documentation in the medical record. They will perform common procedures, including tracheal intubation and central line placement. They may also participate in and coordinate clinical research, as well as educational activities both for nurses and for residents in the PICU. However, they are universally working under the guidance of an attending physician; they cannot currently cover the unit independently.

Another trend in PICU coverage has been the growing number of units that are covered by *24/7 in-house* attending pediatric intensivists. The reasons for moving toward this level of coverage vary from location to location, but prominent reasons include work-load demands, an increasingly sicker patient population, and formalizing work hours. The biggest challenge of adapting an in-house model is the need for additional critical care physicians. Currently, the rate of training of fellows is just meeting or slightly exceeding the rate of retirement of practicing intensivists. The transition to in-house coverage will create a further demand for new practitioners or perhaps additional models of coverage for the PICU.

Regionalization and Specialization

The concept of regionalization of pediatric critical care services was highly touted in the 1980s and early 1990s. The idea that larger PICUs had better outcomes and that critically ill children would benefit from pooled resources has been well supported in the literature. However, this concept of regionalization and specialization does not appear to be affecting public policy. In the years between 1995 and 2001, there were increases in the numbers of both PICU beds per pediatric population and PICUs in general [19–21]. There are increasing numbers of PICUs in this country of all sizes. While urban populations continue to grow, the number of large PICUs is growing rapidly. Meanwhile, there are a growing number of moderate-sized communities that previously were considered too small to support a PICU that are now finding the patient population to be large enough to justify a small PICU. Politically these smaller units can create many challenges for larger urban units. In general, many urban PICUs draw patients from around the region. The establishment of a small PICU within their traditional market can result in a decrease in patients and therefore revenues.

The local PICUs face several challenges. One is the desire for families to be able to stay close to home when their child is critically ill, which is one of the leading reasons for the development of the PICU in the first place. Another issue is how to maintain skills in nurses who may have only episodic exposure to critically ill patients.

A major concern with regard to the development of smaller PICUs is the suggestion by a series of studies that outcomes are better in larger PICUs. The evidence is suggestive that it is actually in the lower risk mortality group that the most substantial improvement in mortality occurs [21]. In general, it would be this lower risk group of relatively less sick children that would be more likely to stay in the local PICU. Further complicating the picture are more recent data that suggest that it is moderate- to large-sized PICUs that do better than the very largest PICUs [20]. What these data may suggest is that some units are better than others with particular diagnoses and conditions. Further research needs to be done to help discern whether there are characteristics of the low-risk patients that make them actually higher risk or if there are identifiable characteristics of the PICUs that increase the risk of mortality.

The Future: Practical Resolutions to Current Problems, Logical Next Steps Following Current Trends, and Hypothetical Idealized Possibilities

Monitoring

Wireless/Cableless Monitors

The improved miniaturization and higher fidelity wireless communications, combined with well-shielded medical equipment should allow the relatively short-term implementation of patient-based monitoring systems that wirelessly communicate with the health care team, wherever they are located in the hospital. Storage will be done in a continuous, high-fidelity manner. Current standards such as Bluetooth and 802.11(x) wireless communications have varying roles for data transmission in the PICU. Early tests of Bluetooth with intensive care and operating room equipment suggest that there is not a problem with interference [22], which was originally a concern with cellular phone technology [23]. The primary limitation of Bluetooth is its limited rate of data transmission and the relatively shorter distance over which Bluetooth maintains its optimal transmission rate. Bluetooth, or some future generation, will be the most likely technology to be incorporated into wireless monitor techniques primarily because of the ability to uniquely identify each individual piece of equipment and therefore tie each piece of equipment to the specific patient. For higher rates of data transmission, such as that necessary for high-resolution images, however, Bluetooth is profoundly limited.

The 802.11(x) technology is much better suited to high-speed high-volume data transmission. The 802.11b and 802.11g systems are the original standards for wireless transmission. They are based on the 2.4 GHz radiofrequency and allow speeds of up to 20 MB per second of data transmission. However, these systems have been slow to be implemented in hospitals because of concerns regarding security of data transmission. The 802.11i is the most likely candidate for heavy penetration in the health care market because of its increased emphasis on encryption and security, which has been the major limitation of earlier generations of this wireless technology [24].

Newer Monitoring Modalities

Newer monitoring modalities focus on either further refinements of data that are currently collected or on development and refinement of new monitoring modalities that will enhance our understanding of critical illnesses. Researchers are currently looking to employ artificial intelligence to analyze the minutiae of data for clues of early signs of deterioration or recovery so that interventions can be started or weaned earlier. Elements of currently collected data such as beat-to-beat variations in electrocardiographic tracing [25,26] or overall variability of parameters such as heart rate, blood pressure, and respiratory rate will receive a greater level of scrutiny to help identify early signs of either deterioration or recovery [27–29]. Monitoring of the central nervous system is likely to get much more sophisticated. Multiple technologies have been employed in the past to assess brain function and health in the critically ill patient, including jugular venous bulb saturations, transcranial oxygenation, subanalysis of electroencephalographic leads (Neurotrac, BIS), and microdialysis. The most prominent technologies have looked at either brain electrical activity or brain tissue oxygenation. In all likelihood it will be some newer modality that is used to monitor brain electrical activity or tissue oxygen delivery or consumption, such as is only currently available using microdialysis techniques or metabolic magnetic resonance imaging technology [30] that will be used to generate a global picture as well as a local picture of brain health.

Noninvasive Monitoring

Techniques of interpreting noninvasively collected data to generate data only previously available through implanted invasive catheters should be able to provide a much greater level of understanding of factors such as cardiac output.

Interactivity Between Monitors and Patient Care Devices

An even more intriguing concept is whether monitoring and support equipment can communicate in a manner that optimizes patient care. Imagine a ventilator that is able to monitor not only oxygenation and ventilation but also the degree of airway recruitment, intrapulmonary shunting, pulmonary compliance, lung stretch, pulmonary cytokine production, airway obstruction, and so forth. With this information the ventilator could go through algorithms that would optimize the ventilator strategy for the individual patient, find the optimal positive end-expiratory pressure, inspiratory rate, mode, and tidal volume (or pressure control), minimizing the risk of ventilator-induced lung injury and minimizing the duration of time the patient spent on the ventilator. A cardiac monitor tracking systemic vascular resistance, volume status, contractility, cardiac output, and urine output could titrate specific agents such as volume administration, inotropic agents, vasoconstrictors, or vasodilators as is merited by the data obtained.

Data Collection and Management

The Electronic Medical Record

A fully integrated EMR, transferable or accessible from location to location as the patient moves, should be the primary goal. In addition, it should be additive; as the patient is seen at different institutions, the medical record from that institution becomes incorporated into a global medical record for the patient. Compliance with HIPAA-type regulations will be much greater because the patients will be the ones with ultimate control of who has access to their EMR. Issues related to litigation and medical malpractice will need to be addressed before the widespread portability becomes available. The integrated medical record will automatically incorporate both clinical and laboratory information, including radiology reports, so that the patient's most current information is available wherever the patient is or where the physician who is treating the patient needs the data to be. The medical record will require a minimum of additional time from the clinician to complete, but it will be useful in both patient care and billing. Out of this EMR the PICU will be able to automatically extract stripped data for the purpose of maintaining a database for evaluation of PICU performance. Large-volume, highly granular data collection will allow more accurate models for prediction of survival based on the patient's condition at presentation or at various steps along the way [31–34]. The EMR should also coordinate with clinical study protocols for easy prospective collection of data with minimal manipulation of the record.

Computerized Physician Order Entry

The combination of increasing use of care pathways and, hopefully, a greater dataset of well-designed pediatric critical care clinical studies should allow the development of both protocol-driven orders and automated prompts and suggestions for possible care improvements. In order to function well, each practitioner will need to have instant access to any patient and be able to write orders that are instantly transmitted to the central receiving site. A wireless PDA-type device that is unique to each provider will be the best tool for this, as a unique identification number can be assigned to both the practitioner and the device and act as one level of safety and security. In teaching institutions, resident orders can result in instant notification to the attending physician, who could modify and send back the order or let it pass unchanged. Presumably there could be levels of risk associated with the orders so that some orders could either be directly approved without the attending physician's input or be passed through a risk filter so that only high-risk orders would need independent confirmation.

Staffing

There will likely continue to be a wide variety of staffing models in PICUs around the country. Academic institutions are likely to see the biggest change, because duty hour restrictions and the continuing shift toward outpatient training will decrease the number of residents available to staff PICUs. Changes will need to occur in pediatrics, as in other specialties, to ensure that physicians in training receive adequate exposure to an adequate number of patients during training. There will probably be a shift toward either longer residencies or earlier specialization within pediatrics such that those residents who wish to pursue critical care can focus their training at an earlier point in time.

Advanced practice nurses are heading toward requiring a doctoral degree for practice. This Doctorate in Clinical Nursing will recognize the advanced level of training and standardize advanced practice nursing education around the country. What is truly hard to predict is what impact this will have on the staffing of PICUs. Currently there is a shortage of nurses to work in their traditional role [35,36], and limitations in space in nursing schools would seem to suggest that there is a finite number of nurses available and that the pool from which Doctorates in Clinical Nursing might be drawn is shallow. In all likelihood, given the limitations in the numbers of pediatric intensivists in training, the number of residents available, the number of nurses available, and so forth, there will need to be some sort of compromise in how PICUs are staffed.

Incorporation of hospitalists into the critical care team is one possible answer. With more emphasis on outpatient experience in residency, general pediatricians will have less experience taking care of hospitalized patients. Hospitalists are already playing an increasing role in the management of hospitalized patients, a trend that started in internal medicine but is becoming increasingly popular in pediatrics. Hospitalists are able to become more experienced and more comfortable in managing the increasing complexities of the hospitalized pediatric patient. This trend allows clinical pediatricians to spend more time in the office as well. As experts in inpatient care, hospitalists could play the logical bridge in PICU coverage. Enabling nurses to be more independent thinkers within a team framework will be essential to any future care model.

Regionalization and Specialization

If current trends continue, there will be a larger number of smaller PICUs distributed between a mixture of suburban and moderate-sized cities across the country. An increase in the number of PICUs without a substantial increase in the number of pediatric intensivists will lead to a need for innovative methods of providing critical care services to these smaller units while maintaining the large volumes and unique expertise that come with larger regional PICUs. One of the logical steps would be to partner smaller outlying PICUs with larger regional PICUs through telemedicine connections. High-speed data networks offer the opportunity for an intensivist to observe both clinical data collected from the patient monitor as well as video and audio data from the patient. In this scenario, moderately critically ill patients such as children needing continuous nebulization therapy, low-level trauma patients, and others who need a moderate level of intervention but higher level of monitoring could stay in a local PICU but still have the benefits of input from a pediatric intensivist, who in turn would have a better grasp of the clinical status of the patient by being able to both visibly see the patient and have real-time vital sign information. In the event that the patient's clinical condition deteriorated or necessitated a higher level of care, the transport team could be dispatched to bring the child to the larger PICU. This has been employed successfully in several locations already [37–40] and has the potential to expand PICU consultation and collaboration beyond current borders.

The major limitation in the regionalized, telemedicine-directed PICU is that there is still a need for procedural skills at the local site. Although robotic remote surgery has been performed even at distances of 7,000 km or more [41–43], it is not clear that procedures such as central line placement or tracheal intubation will ever be amenable to remote robotic assistance. How these units could be adequately staffed to ensure that someone skilled in invasive procedures on children were available 24 hours per day is not known. Potential sources for this skill level are adult intensivists, CRNAs, or perhaps advanced practice nurses or physician assistants who had additional training in the care of critically ill and injured children. These advanced practitioners could periodically spend time at the home institution to gain additional experience in procedures.

Conclusion

The physical structure and configuration of the PICU of the future is largely unknown. Logical extensions of current research and practice suggest that the future PICU will become even more data dependent, but hopefully our understanding of what to do with the data will be greatly expanded as improved collaborative efforts in pediatric critical care continue to push the envelope of our understanding. New equipment, new monitors, sicker patients, and improved outcomes will all rely on what is probably the most unclear picture of the future—that of who will be around to staff the units and what roles will be played by which provider.

References

1. Breslow MJ, et al. Effect of a multiple-site intensive care unit telemedicine program on clinical and economic outcomes: an alternative paradigm for intensivist staffing. Crit Care Med 2004;32(1):31–38.

2. Celi LA, et al. The eICU: it's not just telemedicine. Crit Care Med 2001;29(8 Suppl):N183–N189.

3. Rosenfeld BA, et al. Intensive care unit telemedicine: alternate paradigm for providing continuous intensivist care. Crit Care Med 2000;28(12):3925–3931.

4. Park M. Pediatric Cardiology for Practitioners, 2nd ed. St. Louis, MO: Mosby-Year Book; 1988:370.

5. Steele DW, et al. Pulsus paradoxus: an objective measure of severity in croup. Am J Respir Crit Care Med 1998;157(1):331–334.

6. Ledley RS, Lusted LB The use of electronic computers in medical data processing: aids in diagnosis, current information retrieval, and medical record keeping. Ire Trans Biomed Electron 1960;ME-7:31–47.

7. Schenthal JE. The electronic medical record. Bull School Med Univ MD 1962;47:53–55.

8. Braithwaite J, Westbrook J. America's health care reforms. Health Inform Manag 1994;24(1):32–33.

9. Marshall PD, Chin HL. The effects of an electronic medical record on patient care: clinician attitudes in a large HMO. Proc AMIA Symp 1998:150–154.

10. O'Connor K. Computerized records gain ground. Infocare 1997;22:24–25.

11. Miller DD, Getsey CL. Impact of a compliance program for billing on internal medicine faculty's documentation practices and productivity. Acad Med 2001;76(3):266–272.

12. Gandsas A, et al. Wireless vital sign telemetry to hand held computers. Stud Health Technol Inform 2001;81:153–157.

13. Volsko TA. Portable computers and applications in respiratory care. Respir Care 2004;49(5):497–506.

14. Iregui M, et al. Use of a handheld computer by respiratory care practitioners to improve the efficiency of weaning patients from mechanical ventilation. Crit Care Med 2002;30(9):2038–2043.

15. Braner DA, et al. Interactive Web sites for families and physicians of pediatric intensive care unit patients: a preliminary report. Pediatr Crit Care Med 2004;5(5):434–439.

16. Reynolds G. Economics of in-house call. In: Tegtmeyer K, ed. Current Concepts in Pediatric Critical Care Course. Des Plaines, IL: Society of Critical Care Medicine; 205:83–103.

17. ACGME. Work hours language. For insertion into the Common Program Requirements for all Core and Subspecialty Programs by July 1, 2003. Chicago: Accreditation Council for Graduate Medical Education; 2004.

18. Gelfand DV, et al. Effect of the 80-hour workweek on resident burnout. Arch Surg 2004;139(9):933–940.

19. Randolph AG, et al. Growth of pediatric intensive care units in the United States from 1995 to 2001. J Pediatr 2004;144(6):792–798.

20. Marcin JP, Song J, Leigh JP. The impact of pediatric intensive care unit volume on mortality: a hierarchical instrumental variable analysis. Pediatr Crit Care Med 2005;6(2):136–141.

21. Tilford JM, et al. Volume–outcome relationships in pediatric intensive care units. Pediatrics 2000;106(2 Pt 1):289–294.

22. Wallin MK, Wajntraub S. Evaluation of Bluetooth as a replacement for cables in intensive care and surgery. Anesth Analg 2004;98(3):763–767.

23. Yeolekar ME, Sharma A. Use of mobile phones in ICU—why not ban? J Assoc Physicians India 2004;52:311–313.

24. IEEE 802 Standard. Institute of Electrical and Electronics Engineers, 2004.

25. Glass TF, et al. Use of artificial intelligence to identify cardiovascular compromise in a model of hemorrhagic shock. Crit Care Med 2004;32(2):450–456.

26. Tegtmeyer K, Massey B, Goldstein B. Diagnosing shock via artificial intelligence: applying machine learning techniques to medicine. Crit Care Med 2004;32(2):602–603.

27. Goldstein B, et al. Decomplexification in critical illness and injury: relationship between heart rate variability, severity of illness, and outcome. Crit Care Med 1998;26(2):352–357.

28. Pontet J, et al. Heart rate variability as early marker of multiple organ dysfunction syndrome in septic patients. J Crit Care 2003;18(3):156–163.

29. Stein PK, et al. Association between heart rate variability recorded on postoperative day 1 and length of stay in abdominal aortic surgery patients. Crit Care Med 2001;29(9):1738–1743.

30. Macmillan CS, et al. Traumatic brain injury and subarachnoid hemorrhage: in vivo occult pathology demonstrated by magnetic resonance spectroscopy may not be "ischaemic." A primary study and review of the literature. Acta Neurochir (Wien) 2002;144(9):853–862.

31. Gemke RJ, van Vught J. Scoring systems in pediatric intensive care: PRISM III versus PIM. Intensive Care Med 2002;28(2):204–207.

32. Heard CM, Fletcher JE, Papo MC. A report of the use of the Dynamic Objective Risk Assessment (DORA) score in the changing pediatric intensive care environment. Crit Care Med 1998;26(9):1593–1595.

33. Marcin JP, et al. Prognostication and certainty in the pediatric intensive care unit. Pediatrics 1999; 104(4 Pt 1):868–873.

34. Pearson GA, Stickley J, Shann F. Calibration of the paediatric index of mortality in UK paediatric intensive care units. Arch Dis Child 2001;84(2):125–128.

35. Buerhaus PI, Staiger DO, Auerbach DI. Why are shortages of hospital RNs concentrated in specialty care units? Nurs Econ 2000;18(3): 111–116.

36. Diehl-Oplinger L, Kaminski MF. Need critical care nurses? Inquire within. Nurs Manage 2000;31(3):44, 46.

37. Marcin JP, et al. Using telemedicine to provide pediatric subspecialty care to children with special health care needs in an underserved rural community. Pediatrics 2004;113(1 Pt 1):1–6.

38. Marcin JP, et al. Use of telemedicine to provide pediatric critical care inpatient consultations to underserved rural Northern California. J Pediatr 2004;144(3):375–380.

39. Marcin JP, et al. The use of telemedicine to provide pediatric critical care consultations to pediatric trauma patients admitted to a remote trauma intensive care unit: a preliminary report. Pediatr Crit Care Med 2004;5(3):251–256.

40. Wetzel RC. The virtual pediatric intensive care unit. Practice in the new millennium. Pediatr Clin North Am 2001;48(3):795–814.

41. Bauer J, et al. Remote percutaneous renal access using a new automated telesurgical robotic system. Telemed J E Health 2001;7(4): 341–346.

42. Lee BR, et al. Laparoscopic telesurgery between the United States and Singapore. Ann Acad Med Singapore 2000; 29(5):665–668.

43. Marescaux J, Rubino F. Robot-assisted remote surgery: technological advances, potential complications, and solutions. Surg Technol Int 2004;12:23–26.

15
Molecular Biology in the Pediatric Intensive Care Unit

Lesley A. Doughty

Introduction

The translation of bench research to bedside clinical practice in pediatric critical care medicine has been broadly aimed and slowly paced. Although research in pediatric critical care is still in its infancy, some important progress has been made specific to critical illness in neonates and children. Mostly, however, findings from adult research have been extrapolated to pediatric critical illness when applicable. The progression from clinical observation with pathologic correlates to a sophisticated understanding of organ pathophysiology has been continuous over many decades. Currently research in critical illness is occurring on many fronts, ranging from improvements in supportive care (reducing ventilator-associated pneumonia), to iatrogenic contributions to disease (ventilator-induced lung injury), as well as disease-specific molecular mechanisms and therapies. Within each of these areas investigation is also being aimed at epidemiologic questions, organ function, and survival assessment using in vivo animal models, as well as intense molecular biologic dissection of the mediators, signaling pathways, and diverse cell–cell interactions present in complex diseases. Recently, a new area of focus has evolved: the genomic/proteomic assessment of gene activation and protein expression during critical illness by high throughput microarray technology. Having been conducted with animals, these studies are now being conducted with humans suffering from a variety of illnesses with the hope of expanding our knowledge of disease mechanisms, understanding genetic predispositions, and hopefully discovering new targets for pharmacologic manipulation.

Much of what forms our understanding of the physiology/pathophysiology of the body has come from bench to bedside work done over several decades in whole-animal models as well as models designed to simulate whole-organ function (e.g., the Langendorf isolated rat heart model). More recently the term *bench to bedside* has been used with reference to molecular pathophysiology of critical illness. However, models used for the study of whole-animal and organ physiology by contributors such as F. Starling, A.C. Guyton, J.B. West, J.L. Robotham, S. Permutt, T. Starzl, and P. Safar, to name a few, have built the foundation of our understanding of physiology and identified targets for therapy that continue to be refined.

Little of this research has been focused specifically on pediatric pathophysiology. Some phenomena have been reproduced in pediatric models, and clinical correlative data and some phenomena have simply been accepted without specific confirmation of shared pathophysiology between adults and children. Clearly some features unique to the newborn population have been specifically investigated—for instance, persistent pulmonary hypertension of the newborn (PPHN), hyaline membrane disease (respiratory distress syndrome [RDS]), and congenital heart disease. More recently, large prospective randomized clinical trials have been carried out in children as well as adults in disease entities where pathophysiology is assumed to be similar (e.g., activated protein C for septic shock and surfactant for acute respiratory distress syndrome [ARDS]). Some have yielded similar results, confirming shared pathology, and some have not. Benefit in adult studies but not in pediatric studies such as the results with activated protein C, may be caused by a skewed risk/benefit ratio on the basis of lower septic shock mortality rates for children than adults (10% vs. 30%) [1,2]. Alternatively and less likely is the idea that the pathophysiology is age dependent. The translation of scientific discovery to the exploration of new therapies and bedside use for children with critical illness will continue to require rigorous evaluation and continued community commitment to participate in clinical trials.

Scientific discovery is revealing new candidates for therapeutic targeting in critical illness at a rapid pace. Our ability to assess these targets clinically when adequate preclinical data exist must keep pace. Study design and patient inclusion difficulties from prior trials must be examined in order to select patients most likely to benefit from unconventional therapies that may pose some risk. This is an exciting time in the critical care community given the plethora of pathways being explored for disease intervention. Preclinical models are being continuously refined to better reproduce human injuries, disease states, and timing of interventions. In addition, over time the scientific community has come to a much better understanding of the natural history and the evolution of the host response to our worst disease entities, allowing further

D.S. Wheeler et al. (eds.), *Science and Practice of Pediatric Critical Care Medicine*,
DOI 10.1007/978-1-84800-921-9_15, © Springer-Verlag London Limited 2009

refinement of preclinical models. As this work continues, the potential therapies brought to clinical trials may in fact be more likely to succeed than previous failed attempts.

Several lines of research currently promise to bridge the gap between molecular concepts and understanding of human disease with anticipation that this work will add to therapeutic strategies in critical illness. Below are some examples of promising work in the fields of traumatic brain injury, septic shock, and acute lung injury. There are countless examples and as such, and this is by no means a complete list.

Traumatic Brain Injury

The scope of research in traumatic brain injury (TBI) today is vast, with rodent models permitting molecular biologic, histopathologic, physiologic, and behavioral consequences of TBI. In addition, large animal models are being used with continued monitoring of intracranial pressure, cerebral perfusion pressure (CPP), cerebral metabolic rate (CMRO$_2$), cerebral blood flow (CBF), as well as neurochemical changes by cerebral microdialysis after traumatic insult [3]. Many of the identified pathologic mediators have been examined in the clinical setting in cerebrospinal fluid (CSF) or brain tissue from brain-injured patients. In addition, cerebral microdialysis and functional magnetic resonance imaging/positron emission tomography scanning have been used to explore physiologic findings in patients that derive from experimental models (Figure 15.1).

Experimental models have continued to improve with respect to simulation of the spectrum of variables encountered in clinical TBI scenarios. Rodent models provide the opportunity for dissection of important mediators and signal transduction pathways resulting in neurotoxicity, inflammatory responses, and cell death pathways. Many of these models also incorporate pathway inhibitors and genetic knockout animals to analyze the contribution of specific molecules. The endpoints of these models can provide histopatho-

logic evidence of lesion volume, survival, and some neurodevelopmental sequelae; however, significantly less physiologic data can be obtained. Larger animal models provide much of the physiologic data involving intracranial pressure (ICP), CPP, and CBF monitoring [3]. Because the small animals do not receive ongoing intensive care–like medical support, the result of supportive interventions on physiologic endpoints as well as outcomes cannot be evaluated. Despite the fact that more *intensive care* support can be provided for large animal models, the time frame postinjury over which this care is provided is much shorter than critical care of the brain-injured patient whose most intense support is generally required over the first several days [3,4].

Primary brain injury occurs at the time of trauma and as such is not subject to medical/surgical interventions. After that time, continued injury can occur from secondary brain insults. Supportive critical care of the brain-injured patient is largely aimed at preventing secondary insults, which are known to worsen outcome. These additive events include hypotension, hypoxia, fever, increased ICP, and cerebral herniation. Creating models that replicate the variety of types of primary brain injury and the spectrum of secondary insults has been very difficult and limiting. Examples of primary injuries that have been difficult to simulate are induction of coma, diffuse axonal injury (DAI), and brainstem injury in contrast to those employing focal cortical injury such as fluid percussion and controlled cortical impact [3]. Fewer still are models involving angular acceleration or angular rotational injury without impact to simulate DAI. Sustained post-traumatic coma has been very difficult to reproduce, although recently models including lateral acceleration and angular rotation to produce DAI in swine have succeeded in producing coma with reproducibility [3]. Translation of this model to rats has been extremely difficult despite the ability of models to produce DAI. Again, unlike large animal models, mass lesions in rodents do not induce coma. Another significant limitation to current models is that they focus largely on adult animals with little investigation of neonatal/juvenile animals. The data that do exist importantly demonstrate significant differ-

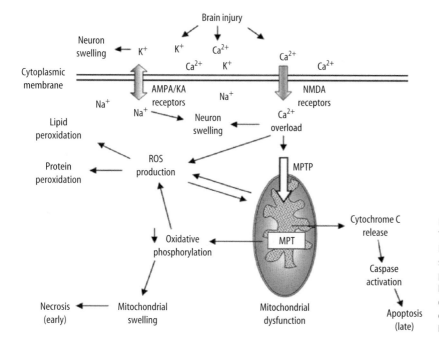

FIGURE 15.1. Molecular mechanisms of traumatic brain injury (TBI). The pathways activated in severe TBI include excitotoxicity via the N-methyl D-aspartate receptor leading to Ca overload, neuronal swelling, generation of reactive oxygen species (ROS), mitochondrial permeability transition (MPT) pore (MPTP) activation, Ca influx, and loss of mitochondrial transmembrane potential leading to impaired oxidative phosphorylation, cytochrome c release, and finally cell death via necrosis/apoptosis. (Adapted from Enriquez and Bullock [11].)

ences between neonatal, juvenile, and adult vasomotor responsiveness and mitochondrial dysfunction, indicating that vulnerability to TBI and its sequelae are different in the developing brain when compared with mature animals [3].

Secondary insults such as hypotension and hypoxemia are extremely important to outcomes as demonstrated in animal models as well as with human data. Some animal models have added these insults following focal TBI and shown that the addition of hypoxia resulted in worsened neurologic functional outcomes as well as relative amounts of excitotoxicity and cell death [3–5]. Hypotension added to these models resulted in depletion of intracellular energy sources and worsened intracellular acidosis. In an elegant rat model [6], investigators found that hypotension and hypoxia after TBI worsened ICP, cerebral edema, and neuronal death. Unfortunately, in part because of some of the inherent difficulties described above, few studies have extended these questions to simultaneous changes in neurochemical mediators, signaling pathways, and cellular changes with or without pathway inhibitors or to reflect the impact of supportive neurointensive care strategies.

Continued improvements in modeling, especially incorporating primary injury types, secondary insults, and supportive care interventions, with monitoring of molecular alterations will continue to advance our knowledge of TBI mechanisms, allowing more thorough assessment of putative interventions. Exciting advances that have the potential to contribute to transitioning from the experimental model to clinical care soon involve both therapeutic advances as well as improved modeling.

Alterations in Cerebral Blood Flow

Ischemic injury is a common secondary insult after severe TBI [7]. Many mechanisms can contribute, including diminished CBF early after TBI from vasospasm from increased release of vasoconstricting mediators and diminished vasodilator release, vascular occlusion/injury, compression from high ICP resulting from mass effect or diffuse cerebral edema, and systemic hypotension with impaired cerebral autoregulation [8–13]. Much work has been done to clarify the evolution of CBF abnormalities and to define critical mediators with the hope of identifying key mediators for pharmacologic intervention to improve outcome.

Many studies have demonstrated diminished CBF in infants, children, and adults within the first 24 hours after focal or diffuse TBI [8–14]. Post-traumatic hypoperfusion may be an important contributor to secondary brain injury and therefore is an exciting therapeutic target. Alterations in both vasodilators and vasoconstricting mediators have been demonstrated early after TBI. Although there are some conflicting reports, many discrepancies may be accounted for by different injury models, time points, different animal species, and/or different endpoint analyses.

Cerebrovascular tone is maintained by a balance of vasodilators and vasoconstrictors that are constitutively present. In pathologic situations, the balance of production or function of these molecules may be altered. Others may be induced and become major contributors. An enormous body of literature demonstrates alteration of function and/or expression after TBI of many common cerebrovascular vasodilators such as nitric oxide (NO), adenosine, cyclic guanosine monophosphate (cGMP), cyclic adenosine monophosphate, prostanoids, and bradykinin, and some of these alterations are associated temporally with alterations in CBF after TBI [reviewed in 11].

Nitric Oxide

Given that NO is a potent cerebrovascular vasodilator, its production, time course, and potential risk/benefit ratio after TBI have been studied. Nitric oxide vasodilates by increasing cGMP, causing smooth muscle relaxation locally. There are many functions attributed to NO in both physiologic and pathologic states. In many pathologic models of multiple diseases, inducible nitric oxide synthase (iNOS) and NO are increased and correlate with severity of pathology. Interestingly, inhibitors of iNOS do not consistently improve outcome across all inflammatory and/or hypoxia-ischemia models. After TBI, the data are much the same and similarly confusing [15–18]. Inducible nitric oxide synthase, however, is induced by many stimuli such as hypoxia/ischemia, inflammatory insults, and tissue injury [15–18]. Production of NO by iNOS can result in vasodilation of many vascular beds, including the cerebrovasculature, and may be a very important regulator of CBF after TBI [15–18]. In addition, NO is also highly reactive with free radicals such as superoxide leading to the production of peroxynitrite with resultant protein nitrosylation, lipid peroxidation, and tissue damage. Alternatively, NO can be oxidized to nitrite then nitrate by myeloperoxidase in neutrophils and macrophages [15–18]. Because of this reactivity with free radicals, it has been suggested that NO has antioxidant properties. It is not clear which function of NO is the most important after TBI, although its impact on CBF, neurologic sequelae, and oxidant stress after TBI have been investigated.

Shortly after TBI, a transient increase in tissue NO occurs followed by a sustained early decrease in levels for up to 4 hours as seen by monitoring with a cortical intraparenchymal NO electrode after TBI. Coincident with this decrease in NO was a drop in CBF as measured by laser Doppler flow [19,20]. Oxygen free radicals are generated after TBI and can rapidly react with NO to form peroxynitrite. Decreased NO and CBF early after TBI is related to reaction of NO with oxidative free radicals generated by TBI [21,22]. By pretreating with the exogenous free radical scavengers superoxide dismutase and catalase to reduce oxidant stress, NO tissue levels and CBF are increased [23]. To further support the concept that NO is serving as an antioxidant, administration of L-arginine, the immediate precursor of NO, also increased tissue NO levels and improved CBF after TBI [22,24], indicating that NO consumption may outstrip its supply of precursors. Inducible nitric oxide synthase mRNA, protein content, and enzymatic activity are induced within hours following TBI. These data support an imbalance between production of NO and consumption by reaction with free radicals with a net balance of low NO tissue levels leading to decreased CBF early after TBI. Theoretically, severely low NO levels could contribute to ischemia by decreasing CBF. If so, this mechanism could potentially contribute to secondary brain injury early after TBI.

In contrast to low NO early after TBI, other authors have reported upregulated tissue NO and iNOS protein and activity compared with uninjured animals later after TBI (24–72 hours) [25]. Also in iNOS-/- mice, increased oxidative stress as well as depletion of the antioxidant ascorbate were seen at 24–72 hours after TBI, supporting the antioxidant role of NO and its consumption early after TBI, which resolves after 24 hours [22,26]. Most reports examining NO later after TBI (24–72 hours) showed increased NO but did not examine coincident CBF [27,28]. As a consequence, only supplementation of L-arginine very early after TBI (when CBF is diminished) has demonstrated simultaneous increases in NO and CBF associated with improved histopathologic outcome [22,23]. Minimal experimental data exist examining pharmacologic alterations of NO at later time points (after the first 24 hours) to assess whether the evolution of depressed to exaggerated NO content is physiologic or pathologic and whether CBF follows this evolution.

Controversy exists regarding whether NO is beneficial or detrimental to TBI outcome. Several authors have documented outcome improvement from specific iNOS inhibitors administered after TBI based on histopathologic outcome (lesion volume, reduced cortical neuronal necrosis) and neurologic function (contralateral sensorimotor function) [27,29]. In different studies, inhibitors were administered intraperitoneally once, twice per day for 3 days, or by continuous infusion over 3 days [30]. The TBI model was fluid percussion (FP) in all studies. No CBF or oxidant stress markers were evaluated during these experiments. Another report demonstrated similar results using iNOS−/− mice with a cryogenic brain injury model [31]. In contrast to these data, a neuroprotective role for NO has been demonstrated by several authors using iNOS inhibitors administered both at the time of TBI and by continuous infusion for 5 days in rats [32]. These data were confirmed using iNOS−/− mice [32,33]. Furthermore, administration of L-arginine to augment tissue NO also was neuroprotective [22,23]. The endpoints measured were histopathologic (contusion volume and neuronal loss) and neurologic (motor performance and spatial memory performance) functions. Traumatic brain injury was induced by a controlled cortical impact model (CCI) [22,32,33]. It is unclear whether the contradictory data represent differences in models (FP vs. CCI), endpoint analyses, or iNOS inhibitor administration technique or timing (single injection vs. continued infusion).

Human data can often provide correlative data to support experimental animal data. Examples of such include demonstration of enhanced end products of NO metabolism such as nitrite/nitrates and S nitrosoalbumin in human CSF peaking several days after TBI [33,34]. Further data supporting an antioxidant role for NO are demonstrated by reduced levels of endogenous antioxidants coincident with increased levels of markers of oxidant stress in human CSF days after TBI [25]. These data support animal data, showing increased evidence of NO and free radical formation in the brain days after TBI; however, these data cannot resolve conflicting animal outcome data given the descriptive nature of such evidence.

This detailed description of the controversial role of NO in TBI exemplifies the difficulty in translating research findings from the bench to the bedside. As is often the case, pursuing the transition from bench to bedside with interesting and promising mediators, pathways, and potential therapies is difficult because of contradicting animal data. Efforts to clarify these contradictions by controlling variables would be helpful in assessing a possible therapeutic role for such mediators. Consistent effects of alterations of NO (inhibition or augmentation) across several models of TBI would strengthen the conclusion about NO. Experiments using consistent timing and method of administration as well as dose of inhibitors/enhancers would also strengthen conclusions about mediator benefit or harmful impact. In addition, the use of consistent endpoints histologically and with regard to neurologic function is important. Furthermore, demonstrating the impact of these strategies on the putative mechanisms of NO, (e.g., alteration of CBF and oxidant stress after treatment with inhibitors or enhancers) would lend further credibility to conclusions regarding benefit of mediator manipulation. Because evidence exists to suggest that detrimental versus beneficial effects of NO may be

critically governed by timing and cellular localization and linked to the level of oxidative stress in the injured tissue after TBI, optimal timing and duration for NO-related therapies also need to be assessed [26]. Now that conflicting results exist regarding the role and impact of NO, hopefully investigators will make efforts to explore these issues to clarify the controversy particularly prior to human trials.

Vasoconstrictors

The vasoconstricting peptide endothelin (ET) has three known subtypes (ET-1, -2, and -3). Endothelin-1 is produced by numerous cell types, including aortic endothelium. In addition, it is expressed in neurons, glial cells, choroid plexus cells, hypothalamic tissue, and macrophages capable of crossing the blood–brain barrier during injury [17,35]. Multiple stimuli can induce ET-1, such as tissue hypoxia, hematoma/hemoglobin, thrombin, transforming growth factor-β (TGF-β), angiotensin II, vasopressin, and interleukin-1 (IL-1). Many reports have demonstrated increased ET-1 levels in human CSF after subarachnoid hemorrhage. Animal models of subarachnoid hemorrhage confirm this, and the timing of this increase is coincident with ischemia-induced vasospasm [36]. Inhibitors of ET-1 and ET receptor antagonists are capable of preventing vasospasm, demonstrating the importance of ET-1 in cerebral vasomotor tone in ischemia [17,35]. Fewer studies have examined the role of ET-1 after TBI, although similar data are accumulating [37–39]. Like cerebrovascular disease, ET-1 CSF levels are increased after TBI in humans and in animal models such as CCI and FP [17,35]. Administration of ET receptor antagonists, especially to subtype ET_A, known to mediate vasoconstriction, reduced edema and postinjury neurologic deficits in a rat CCI model [40]. After TBI, cerebral autoregulation, specifically vasodilation, in response to systemic hypotension is impaired in animal models [35]. Several reports demonstrate ET-1–mediated impairment of vasodilation of pial arteries in response to systemic hypotension after TBI (piglet FP, rat weight drop closed head trauma [CHT]) [35,41–43]. The potential mechanisms described involved ET-1–mediated induction of superoxide with impairment of vasodilation. To date ET remains a promising target for increasing CBF early after TBI in the hypoperfused phase, and the fact that Food and Drug Administration–approved ET antagonists exist and are being studied in other disease states, including subarachnoid hemorrhage, raises the possibility that this target may reach the bedside for therapy of post-TBI early hypoperfusion [44].

Glutamate

Glutamate, an important excitatory neurotransmitter, is hypothesized to be important in the pathophysiology of TBI. There are several types of receptors for glutamate in the brain, including the ionotropic class, members of which are named based on their ligands. The best known are the N-methyl D-aspartate (NMDA) receptors, which when activated allow calcium to enter neurons [11]. In addition, the alpha-amino-3-hydroxy-5-methyl-4-isoxazolepropionic acid receptors (AMPA) and kainate receptors are both important in Na^+ and K^+ exchange [11]. Metabotropic glutamate receptors also exist on astrocytes and activate other complex intracellular signaling cascades. Multiple antagonists to glutamate receptors have provided neuroprotection in experimental TBI. The best studied is the NMDA pathway with antagonist/inhibitors aimed at multiple binding sites, ion channels, and subunits (i.e.,

NR2B); however, efforts aimed at blocking AMPA, kainate receptors, and metabotropic receptors are ongoing [11].

Evidence for glutamate neurotoxicity derives originally from the fact that it is toxic to neurons in culture via excess influx of calcium and sodium into cells with swelling, apoptosis, and/or necrosis [11,45–47]. In addition, glutamate levels after human TBI were increased and remained increased for several days, with the highest levels correlating with severity [11,12]. Antagonists to multiple types and multiple subunits of glutamate receptors have provided neuroprotective effects in experimental TBI. Unfortunately, such neuroprotection has not consistently been translated into clinical care [11,48–50]. There are multiple possible explanations for failure of neuroprotective effects in humans, including human study design, although a compelling issue concerning glutamate highlights an important difficulty in bringing therapies to the clinical arena. The reason for increased brain glutamate after TBI remains a controversial issue. Possible explanations range from nonspecific release from damaged cell membranes, to excessive release at the synaptic level, to diminished uptake from decreased receptor expression and/or decreased intracellular ATP [11]. Different models have contributed data to support all of these mechanisms, thereby maintaining the controversy.

In addition to the above controversy, the critical toxic mechanism of excess glutamate in TBI also remains poorly understood. Multiple lines of evidence support glutamate-induced neurotoxicity, including demonstration that excessive neuronal excitation mediated by extracellular sodium and toxic calcium flux into the cells can contribute to cell death [11,47,51,52]. Conflicting data exist, including the demonstration that synaptic NMDA receptors promote cell survival and that some NMDA antagonists can be harmful post-trauma compared with pre-trauma [52]. Despite enormous efforts using multiple NMDA antagonists in many trials, no consistent benefit has been demonstrated from NMDA antagonists after TBI [11,53–55]. Because much of the promising experimental evidence for beneficial effects in TBI were from the administration of NMDA antagonists pre-trauma rather than post-trauma, the possibility of a very short therapeutic window exists for this type of agent. Other explanations for NMDA antagonist failure include poor penetration into the penumbra area surrounding traumatic foci and a dose-dependent toxicity limiting the dose administered to humans to levels below those administered to animals in successful studies [53–57]. Given the possibility that synaptic and extrasynaptic NMDA receptor activation results in opposing cell survival effects, it is possible that glutamate, although present at high levels after trauma, can signal differently depending on time after injury and receptor availability [11]. To further complicate the potential clinical benefit of NMDA antagonists in TBI, by microdialysis technique, glutamate levels were more elevated in TBI patients with secondary ischemic events, focal contusions, and subdural hematomas, contrasting with only slight and transient elevation of glutamate levels in patients with DAI and epidural hematomas [12]. These data would predict that a role for NMDA antagonists may vary depending on lesion type. Obviously, there remains much to be learned about the role of glutamate in TBI, and the continuing controversy demands further definition of the potential benefit of glutamate receptor antagonism after TBI. As with the study of NO in TBI, some of the controversy may be addressed by systematic assessment of antagonist dosing, delivery, and timing of post-trauma administration. In the future, perhaps the use of a new prospective agent should be successful across many models and several species before advancing to clinical trials. That

being said, a recent trial published by Yurkewicz et al. [58] demonstrated clinical benefit from the use of Traxoprodil (CP-101, 66) an NR2B NMDA subunit–specific receptor antagonist that has been neuroprotective in animal models. They reported improved outcome in 6-month motor function and in mortality, with the most profound effect seen in the most severely injured patients. It is possible that continued investigation of highly subunit-specific agents will bridge the gap between the neuroprotective effect in animals and the neuroprotective effect in human TBI.

Calcium

Several studies have demonstrated significant rise in intracellular calcium within minutes after trauma, which can lead to neuronal damage and death. Normally calcium homeostasis is tightly regulated with extracellular Ca^{2+} 10,000-fold in excess of intracellular levels. Disruption of calcium homeostasis results in activation of many secondary brain injury pathways such as activation of proteases, apoptotic pathways, and free radicals [15,47,51,56]. Increased intracellular calcium can occur through activation of voltage-sensitive Ca^{2+} channels as well as via the glutamate activation of the NMDA receptor channels [47]. Other reports suggest that increased intracellular Ca^{2+} may be the result of massive release from the mitochondrial matrix and/or the endoplasmic reticulum calcium stores [59,60]. Currently, the precise source of this change is not well understood, nor is it certain whether calcium *loading* has the same impact if derived from different mechanisms. Increased intracellular Ca^{2+} via NMDA channels was toxic, whereas that resulting from activation of voltage-sensitive Ca^{2+} channels was not [61]. Ca^{2+} influx through voltage-sensitive channels occurs through membrane depolarization and can regulate contraction, secretion, gene expression, cell signaling pathways, and glutamate release [62]. Cytosolic calcium influx can lead to mitochondrial depolarization, reactive oxygen species (ROS) generation, and decreased ATP synthesis. In addition it can activate the mitochondrial permeability transition pore (mPTP), which permeabilizes mitochondrial membranes to low-molecular-weight solutes—a precursor of cell death [63].

As with many other therapies aimed at mechanisms involved with secondary brain injury, preclinical data with Ca^{2+} channel blockers were very promising after experimental TBI. Unfortunately, the voltage-sensitive Ca^{2+} channel blockers nimodipine (L-type) and ziconotide (N-type) have not consistently demonstrated clinical benefit despite great promise in experimental models showing drug effect when administered several hours post-injury [50,64]. Likewise, riluzole, which blocks presynaptic Na^+ channels and thereby prevents glutamate release into the synapse and Ca^{2+} influx, was promising in the prevention of intracellular calcium accumulation from excess glutamate exposure. To date decreased edema and contusion volume can be seen in animal models, but no hopeful human data exist for the treatment of TBI [65]. It is, however, being used for several neurodegenerative diseases such as ALS with great promise [65]. As for glutamate, a significant increase in cytosolic Ca^{2+} may have several etiologies, including transmembrane influx through NMDA channels or voltage-sensitive channels or release from the mitochondria or the endoplasmic reticulum [60]. In this regard, treatment with voltage-sensitive Ca^{2+} channel or Na^+ channel blockade may only affect one possible mechanism, and it is possible that it may not be the most significant pathway involved. Clearly more work is necessary to fully understand the mechanisms behind TBI-mediated Ca^{2+} influx and its effect on mitochondrial dysfunction as well as on other cell signaling pathways involved in neuronal injury after trauma.

Oxidative Stress

A great deal of data indicate that oxidant stress is an important aspect of neuronal damage after TBI. The pathways known to result in free radical elaboration include Ca^{2+} activation of phospholipases, intracellular Ca^{2+} overload, excitotoxicity, activation of nitric oxide synthase and xanthine oxidase, activation of eicosanoid pathway, and inflammatory responses [66]. High levels of ROS and intracellular Ca^{2+} can lead to structural alterations of the mitochondria and electron transport chain, which then can result in further increases in ROS [11,67,68]. The brain is highly predisposed to free radical–mediated injury because of high oxidative metabolic activity with high production of ROS, poor repair mechanisms, nonreplicating neurons, low antioxidant capacity, and high surface to membrane ratio [15,69]. Reactive nitrogen species (RNS) react with superoxide to form peroxynitrite, leading to oxidation of DNA, proteins, and lipids [56,70]. Reactive oxygen species are also toxic to neurons by reacting with fatty acids leading to lipid peroxidation with cell membrane damage and excess permeability to water and solute [11,56,71]. Byproducts of lipid peroxidation can interfere with glutamate uptake potentially contributing to excitotoxic stimulation, and it can interfere with mitochondrial function at the synaptosome [72]. Free radicals also activate the transcription factors AP-1 and NFκB, thereby altering intracellular signaling pathways [66]. The development of mice deficient in or overexpressing genes such as copper-zinc superoxide dismutase, manganese superoxide dismutase, iNOS, and Bcl-2 (antiapoptotic family of proteins) has contributed significantly to the generation and impact of oxidant stress after TBI [66]. Given the extremely short-lived nature of free radicals, these efforts as well as administration of pharmacologic antioxidants have been necessary to significantly advance the biology of this field. Cerebral microdialysis sampling of extracellular brain fluid has also advanced the analysis of free radicals and oxidant stress in TBI in both animal and human models [11,66,73]. Again, despite many promising preclinical studies, none has been beneficial in clinical use even though the evidence for free radical injury is compelling.

Mitochondrial Failure

Many of the pathways activated after TBI, including excitotoxicity and free radical–induced injury, can alter the structure and function of the mitochondria. Neurons are highly metabolically active and virtually dependent on mitochondrial-derived ATP production [69,74]. When ATP production is compromised, significant cellular dysfunction and/or death can occur [69,74]. Excitotoxicity can result in intracellular Ca^{2+} overload. The mitochondria are part of the intracellular Ca^{2+} buffering mechanism [63,75]. When excess excitotoxicity occurs, Ca^{2+} uptake by the mitochondria leads to formation of ROS in the cytosol and mitochondria, leading to mitochondrial inner membrane lipid peroxidation and destabilization with failure to maintain mitochondrial membrane potentials. Inhibition of ATP production worsens the dysfunction with cell necrosis or apoptosis as a consequence [63,75].

Another consequence of excess Ca^{2+} uptake into the mitochondria is induction of mitochondrial permeability transition (mPT) [63]. The mPT is defined as a sudden increase in mitochondrial membrane permeability to small-molecular-weight solutes through the mPT pore (mPTP), a voltage-dependent anion channel (VDAC) [11,63,76,77]. One hypothesis is that the mPTP provides the mitochondria with a fast Ca^{2+} extrusion mechanism by operating at a low conductance mode. After injury, mitochondrial Ca^{2+} accumulation in response to cytosolic Ca^{2+} overloading may cause the transition of the mPTP to a high-conductance state, allowing permeability to low-molecular-weight solutes [11,63,78]. Solute entry could collapse membrane potential, leading to further ROS production, uncoupling of the electron transport from ATP production, mitochondrial osmotic swelling, release of apoptogenic proteins (soluble cytochrome c, apoptosis inducing factor, and caspases) with activation of apoptotic and/or necrotic cell death pathways [11,63,78].

The mPTP is located between the inner and outer mitochondrial membranes and is associated with the matrix isomerase cyclophilin-D (CyP-D) [76]. Cyclosporine A (CsA) binds and inhibits the activity of CyP-D, thereby inhibiting the mPTP. In a dose-dependent fashion CsA reduces cortical damage in a rat CCI model [79,80]. Reports have shown that CsA administered intraperitoneally postinjury (from 15 minutes to 24 hours) reduced cortical damage by 50% experimentally [80]. At 15 minutes post-injury, CsA significantly attenuated mitochondrial dysfunction as indicated by preservation of the mitochondrial membrane potential, resistance to mPT, and lower Ca^{2+} and ROS levels, indicating that CsA may have a neuroprotective benefit by inhibiting mPT and maintaining mitochondrial homeostasis [80]. In fact, CsA delivered by intraperitoneal bolus or subcutaneous infusion over several days showed protective effects. Interestingly, a post-injury therapeutic window of up to 24 hours was demonstrated, suggesting that tissue destruction persists for several days and is amenable to pharmacologic manipulation beyond the immediate post-trauma interval [79]. Currently, ongoing experiments are exploring NIM811, a more potent, selective, and nonimmunosuppressive CsA derivative capable of inhibiting Ca^{2+}-mediated activation of the mPTP [76]. These agents are being investigated in many disease models, including myocardial ischemia reperfusion, in which NIM811 was shown to prevent both necrotic and apoptotic cell death [81]. Given the prolonged post-injury therapeutic window and development of new, more selective CsA derivatives, it is possible that TBI in humans might be amenable to CyP-D manipulation, leading to inhibition of the mPTP up to several hours after injury.

Both CsA and FK506 inhibit Calcineurin; however, FK506 does not bind CyP-D. Much more data have demonstrated neuroprotective effects from CsA than from FK506, presumably because of the ability of CsA (and its derivatives) to bind CyP-D and inhibit the mPTP rather than via calcineurin inhibition (immunosuppressive effects) [82,83]. The fact that FK506 does not impact on mPTP and the success of NIM811, which does not inhibit Calcineurin, supports this concept. Interestingly, however, calcineurin protein, mRNA, and enzymatic activity are increased and translocated to the postsynaptic region of neurons for several days in the FP TBI model [84–86]. These data support a possible role for calcineurin in the pathophysiology of TBI, although its specific activity in this process is not well defined. Given this, further exploration of neuronal calcineurin function is warranted.

Mitochondrial complexes I, III, and IV transfer protons to the intermembrane space, thereby creating a gradient and establishing the mitochondrial membrane potential. This serves as a driving force for the influx of protons through the ATP synthase channel forming ATP [75]. Mitochondrial uncoupling occurs when electron transport (ETS) is disconnected from the production of ATP. The consequences of uncoupling are decreased mitochondrial membrane potential, decreased calcium influx, and decreased free radical formation [75]. Long-term inhibition of mitochondrial function would be harmful; however, transient uncoupling could have neuroprotective effects [75,87]. *Mild uncoupling* during injury-related excitotoxicity could reduce membrane potentials, thereby decreasing Ca^{2+} uptake and ROS production and leading to neuro-protection [87]. Several studies have demonstrated that mitochondrial Ca^{2+} influx and ROS generation are dependent on the magnitude of the membrane potential [87]. The use of pharmacologic uncoupling agents such as 2,4-dinitrophenol (DNP) or carbonyl cyanide *p*-(trifluoromethoxy) phenyl-hydrazone (FCCP) [75], has further validated the importance of uncoupling of the ETS and ATP production. Both DNP and FCCP were neuroprotective in TBI and stroke models as indicated by reduced lesion volume, improved behavioral outcomes, and reduced mitochondrial dysfunction, oxidative damage, and Ca^{2+} influx [87,88].

Several endogenous uncoupling protein subtypes exist throughout the body; however, the main subtypes in neuronal tissue are uncoupling protein 2 (UCP2) and brain mitochondrial carrier protein-1 (BMCP-1) [89]. Models using UCP2 overexpression support a neuroprotective role of uncoupling with reduced ROS and cell death from oxidant stress [89]. Known inducers of UCP2 include fatty acids, a ketogenic (high-fat) diet, sublethal ischemia, tumor necrosis factor- α (TNF-α), and experimental TBI [87,90]. There are human data demonstrating the presence of ischemic markers (via microdialysis measurement of lactate/pyruvate ratios) from areas of the brain with normal perfusion by CBF imaging [91]. This ischemia unrelated to hypoperfusion may be evidence for mitochondrial metabolic crisis caused by impaired oxidative metabolism [91]. Future studies will need to examine the role of UCPs in impairment of oxidative metabolism after injury. Other tissue injury models including stroke, myocardial infarction, and septic shock have demonstrated a tissue UCP protective effect [87,89,90]. It is possible that uncoupling may be a widespread endogenous protective mechanism and may be a potential target for pharmacologic manipulation in TBI as well as other disease processes.

Apoptosis

Cell death after TBI occurs via multiple pathways. Many have attempted to characterize pathways leading to necrosis in contrast to those leading to apoptosis. One hypothesis is that in the presence cell injury below the threshold required for necrosis, apoptosis may occur [92]. Another aspect of this idea holds that necrotic cell death may be the fate of cells with membrane disruption and irreversible metabolic abnormality early on after injury [92]. Apoptotic cell death is thought to occur later after TBI and to continue longer based on the timing of histopathologic changes and gene activation data consistent with apoptotic patterns [93]. Given the delay in occurrence of apoptotic cell death, it is possible that there is a wider interval between TBI and apoptotic cell death for pharmacologic intervention [93]. Apoptotic pathways can be separated into two pathways differentiated by the role of activation of a family of caspase proteins. One pathway is caspase dependent, and the other pathway is caspase independent and involves mediators such as apoptosis-inducing factor (AIF).

Caspase-dependent apoptosis can occur by extrinsic or intrinsic signaling [93]. The intrinsic type is triggered by cellular metabolic stress involving both the mitochondria and endoplasmic reticulum, resulting in membrane depolarization, Ca^{2+} influx, and

opening of the mPTP with release of cytochrome c into the cytoplasm, leading to activation of caspases and ATP and resulting in apoptotic cell death [92,93]. The extrinsic pathway involves receptors on the cell surface such as the Fas receptor and the TNF receptor, which bind their respective ligands (Fas ligand or TNF). This ligand–receptor complex interacts with TNF receptor-associated death domain (TRADD) and Fas-associated protein with death domain (FADD), respectively. Both of these complexes activate the caspase cascade, ending with cleavage of caspase 3, the *effector caspase* leading to apoptosis [92,93]. Pan-caspase inhibitors and specific caspase inhibitors have been explored as therapies for TBI. Caspase 3 inhibition improved lesion volume without functional outcome changes in rat TBI models, and other studies have not shown consistent improvement post-injury [94,95].

The caspase-independent pathway has been confirmed by its resistance to caspase inhibitors. Poly(ADP-ribose) polymerase-1 (PARP-1) is a DNA binding protein activated by oxidative stress–induced DNA damage [96–98]. Many of the known consequences of overactivation of PARP-1 have been investigated as pathways leading to apoptosis. These include consumption of cellular NAD^+ and ATP in poly(ADP) ribosylation, contributing to energy depletion and AIF translocation to the nucleus where it causes chromatin condensation and significant DNA fragmentation [96–98]. This is a complex pathway and not yet fully understood; however, like the caspase pathway, pharmacologic inhibition of PARP-1 as well as the use of PARP-1 knockout mice has identified PARP-1 as an important apoptotic pathway [93,96–98]. Multiple pharmacologic inhibitors of PARP-1 have been explored. However, no inhibitors of AIF are known. Several PARP-1 inhibitors have demonstrated improvement in neurologic deficits, and some have improved lesion volume after TBI with both pre- and post-trauma intraperitoneal drug administration [96].

Proapoptotic and antiapoptotic proteins are upregulated after TBI in animal models and in humans. The antiapoptotic family Bcl-2 proteins, including Bcl-xL and Mcl-1L, are upregulated in experimental models and are thought to prevent release of mitochondrial cytochrome c, endonuclease G, and AIF, perhaps by inhibiting proteins known to participate in mPTP formation [93,99–101]. The proapoptotic members of the Bcl-2 family, including Bax, truncated Bid, and Bad, are also upregulated in models of TBI and facilitate mitochondrial cytochrome c release [93,99–102]. Bcl-2 overexpression in mouse TBI is neuroprotective. Bcl-2 and Bax have both been found in contusion and pericontusion areas in TBI patients along with evidence of DNA fragmentation, suggesting that apoptosis is ongoing. Evidence of caspase 1, 3, and 8 activation as well as the presence of Bcl-2, Bax, Fas, and Fas ligand in TBI patients in parenchyma and CSF has been reported [93,102–104]. There is some evidence that Bax expression without Bcl-2 was associated with worse outcome than when Bax and Bcl-2 were detected [93,105]. Interestingly, autopsy samples from as long as 12 months post-trauma also showed evidence of DNA fragmentation, suggesting that this process continues beyond the acute and subacute time frames, possibly indicating that a wide therapeutic window for antiapoptotic treatments exists [93,106]. At this point no clinical studies have been published using antiapoptotic strategies despite these promising data.

Cannabinoids

Exogenous (plant-derived) and endogenous cannabinoids have neuroprotective effects through many mechanisms. Endocannabinoids have antiinflammatory, vasomotor, nociceptive, antioxidant, and anti-excitotoxic effects [107]. The best-characterized endocannabinoids are 2-arachidonoyl glycerol (2-AG) and anandamide, which both bind to the cannabinoid receptors CB1 (most prevalent in the central nervous system) and CB2 [108]. By binding to these receptors the effects listed above occur, many of which are important in the pathophysiology of TBI as well as other inflammatory diseases [107,108]. Traumatic brain injury upregulated 2-AG levels in the central nervous system, and, when exogenous 2-AG was administered, decreased edema, infarct volume, and neuronal death with improved clinical recovery were observed. Specific CB1 inhibitor diminished this improvement, demonstrating the role for CB1 in these processes [109]. 2-Arachidonoyl glycerol inhibited glutamate release and Ca influx, which may be the basis of its neuroprotective effect. It also inhibited the release of TNF and ROS from macrophages and the vasoconstrictor ET-1 from endothelial cells—all of which are important contributors in TBI pathophysiology.

The synthetic cannabinoid dexanabinol does not bind to either CB1 or CB2 and is nonpsychotropic; however, it has significant neuroprotective effects in experimental TBI with post-injury administration and therefore is a promising pharmacologic adjunct in the treatment of TBI [110,111]. To date, a phase II randomized, placebo-controlled clinical trial demonstrated some mild benefit; however, very recent results of a phase III study failed to demonstrate significant benefit [110]. Because cannabinoids target several pathophysiologic mechanisms, hopefully further trials with adjusted dosing and/or patient selection or possibly alternative cannabinoid analogs will be performed before this pharmacologic avenue is abandoned.

Microdialysis

In addition to therapeutic agents, another advance that promises to allow for more sophisticated real-time biochemical monitoring for TBI is cerebral microdialysis. The assessment parameters obtainable by microdialysis include biochemical markers of ischemia and cell damage and drug delivery to the brain [18,112]. Many of the markers of brain injury and the understanding of their physiology in TBI as well as in harmful secondary insults have come from the use of this device in animal models. To date, only a few institutions are using this technology to study and to assist in clinical decision making in human TBI. There are currently no clinical management guidelines incorporating this technology into the levels of supportive and surgical care for human TBI [18,112]. As such, these institutions are at the forefront of developing this tool and establishing useful protocols and interpretations of neurochemical variations during the pathophysiology of TBI.

A simplified description of the device is as follows [18,112]. A flexible and sterile dialysis probe (FDA approved for use in the human brain) is inserted into the brain parenchyma. The probe has a dialysis membrane at the distal end, allowing it to function similar to a blood capillary. Small-molecular-weight chemical substances from the interstitial fluid diffuse across the membrane into the perfusion fluid inside the catheter. A long catheter and low perfusate flow allows equilibration of the interstitial concentration with the perfusate providing a high recovery rate for the neurochemicals in question. The currently used volume rate is 0.3 μL/min, and a current device allows for the system to be used continuously for 133 hours. Bedside point of care analysis is performed on glucose, lactate, pyruvate, glutamate, glycerol, and urea [18,112]. These substances and their relationships to each other are particu-

larly useful in the assessment of cerebral energy and metabolic derangements. This is especially helpful in assessment of the impact of known causes of secondary injury and the correlation between alterations of blood flow and metabolic derangements. Researchers are establishing normal ranges and ischemic ranges as well as those seen in fatal conditions [18,112]. Of course pediatric values will need to be established before the use of this technology in children. There are many limitations to the technology, including sampling at only one site, which will require interpretation of utility on a case-by-case basis and will never allow this to be a standalone assessment of pathophysiology [18,112]. Nonetheless, this technology remains an exciting adjuvant to current care and evaluation of future therapies.

Age

Probably no aspect of critical care research requires more careful study than that of TBI in the developing brain—another place in which children are substantially different from adults. Pediatric norms for biochemical markers, CBF alterations, and the impact of secondary insults will need to be established in order to allow proper assessment of new agents in an age-dependent fashion. Many adaptations to TBI models have been designed to scale the magnitude of TBI proportionally to account for growth, size, and age differences between adult, juvenile, and neonatal animals. In addition, models have been adapted to simulate diffuse TBI and shaken baby syndrome [4,113–115]. This is essential for delineation of age differences to avoid misinterpretation based on unequal insults because of size and mechanism. In addition, baseline developmental differences have been demonstrated in the juvenile rat compared with adult [94,102]. For instance, mitochondrial structure is different and activity is higher in young rats [116]. Multiple studies demonstrate significant differences in the pathophysiology and response to experimental therapies on an age-dependent basis. For instance, more pial artery vasoconstriction and diminished regional CBF were seen in newborn than in juvenile pigs after FP [117]. Furthermore, NMDA antagonists had paradoxical results in newborn pigs, showing less early excitotoxic neuronal injury, but more apoptotic cell death was seen later compared with older animals. Similarly, newborn rats developed more apoptotic cell death after weight drop injury than did rats of increasing age [114,118]. Post-trauma behavioral differences have also been reported, with older juvenile rats showing worse cognitive function after FPI than younger rats [119]. Thus, a significant body of literature exists showing age and developmental differences in response to TBI, cell death mechanism, as well as responsiveness to therapeutic agents. For this reason, great pains will need to be taken to adjust therapies to appropriate age groups for which they might be beneficial.

Septic Shock

Research into the biochemical and immunologic mechanisms of septic shock has been massive over the past several decades. Basic science work has greatly advanced the understanding of gene expression, genetic differences, and important mediators as well as intracellular signaling pathways. Unfortunately, little of this work has been incorporated into the clinical care of septic shock. Treatment of adrenal dysfunction with low-dose hydrocortisone and the use of activated protein C (APC) have been the major advances recently. Unfortunately, even the use of APC did not receive FDA approval for use in children, and a recent follow-up trial has been halted because of an unfavorable risk/benefit ratio. Although understanding of the disease process continues and animal and in vitro modeling continue to more closely simulate human septic shock, minimal translation from bench to bedside has occurred to date.

What determines the outcome of the systemic inflammatory response syndrome (SIRS) and septic shock remains quite elusive. The proinflammatory cytokines produced in early SIRS include TNF-α, interferon interferon-γ (IFN-γ), IL-1β, and IL-12 with high-mobility group box 1 (HMGB1) being produced several hours later [120]. Antiinflammatory cytokines are also induced during SIRS/septic shock and include IL-10, IL-4, IL-1 receptor antagonist (IL-1Ra), soluble TNF receptor (sTNFR), IL-6, and TFG-β. Cellular sources of these cytokines include natural killer (NK) cells, monocytes, macrophages, neutrophils, and T cells. A dynamic and evolving balance among these components of the immune system exists. Under physiologic conditions, these mediators provide a communication network throughout the body for activation, amplification, and recruitment of immune cells in order to eradicate pathogens, debride and repair injured tissue, and stimulate T and B cells to differentiate into memory cell types for future defense. The function of antiinflammatory cytokines is postulated to be downregulation of the proinflammatory response and to promote wound healing and memory responses.

The systemic inflammatory response is elicited in a multitude of clinical scenarios, including infection, tissue injury (surgical or traumatic), ischemia-reperfusion, postcardiopulmonary bypass, as well as autoimmune phenomena. There are many factors capable of modulating the magnitude and quality of the immune response during critical illness/injury. Some factors precede critical illness/injury, such as chronic poor nutrition, chronic stress (physiologic and/or psychological), and underlying infectious disease (chronic and acute). Other factors become important modulators during a critical illness/injury, including acute stress, infection, tissue injury, poor nutrition, and pharmacologic agents not usually associated with immunomodulation [121]. Certainly these entities make the risk for developing sepsis higher, but how they can impact on the evolution of the septic inflammatory response is unclear. Is a multitrauma patient who develops *Pseudomonas* pneumonia and septic shock the same as an otherwise healthy, well-nourished victim of meningococcemia or necrotizing fasciitis? Is the inflammatory response mounted in both situations the same? Which patient group is most similar to animal models of sepsis? Will future adjuvant septic shock treatments have the same effect in both types of patients? Did they in past trials? Clearly there is much work to do in terms of optimizing models to investigate these differences as new potential mediators come to the forefront.

The recent failures of antiinflammatory strategies in sepsis and multiple organ failure have raised a myriad of hypotheses for this observation Some focus on timing, suggesting that administration of anti-endotoxin, anti-TNF antibodies, IL-1 receptor antagonists, and antiplatelet activating factor was unsuccessful because of an inability to treat early enough after initiation of the disease process, endpoints in clinical trials were too focused on mortality instead of important morbidities, and the possibility that these efforts were aimed at the antagonism of a physiologic rather than a maladaptive response [1,122]. Other strategies have been aimed at mediators deemed *end effector molecules* such as NO, and these, too, have yet to be successful in reducing morbidity or mortality in critical illness/injury [1]. This section reviews some of the mediators and pathways being currently explored for future use in treating septic shock.

Endothelium/Coagulation

Hemostasis is a finely tuned balance between procoagulant and anticoagulant forces (Figure 15.2 [123,124]. Perturbation of this hemostasis is frequently seen in septic shock as well as in other severe systemic inflammatory conditions, resulting in a shift toward the procoagulant state and, when severe, results in disseminated intravascular coagulation [125]. Activation of the inflammatory response in sepsis results in several key alterations in the coagulation cascade. The production of fibrinogen, an acute phase reactant, is increased, but, most importantly, tissue factor (TF) is

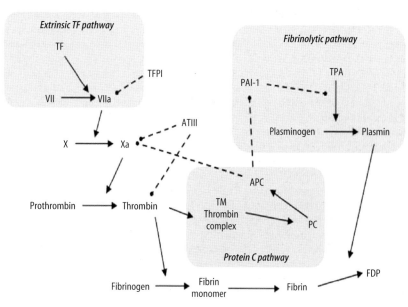

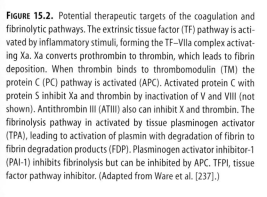

FIGURE 15.2. Potential therapeutic targets of the coagulation and fibrinolytic pathways. The extrinsic tissue factor (TF) pathway is activated by inflammatory stimuli, forming the TF–VIIa complex activating Xa. Xa converts prothrombin to thrombin, which leads to fibrin deposition. When thrombin binds to thrombomodulin (TM) the protein C (PC) pathway is activated (APC). Activated protein C with protein S inhibit Xa and thrombin by inactivation of V and VIII (not shown). Antithrombin III (ATIII) also can inhibit X and thrombin. The fibrinolysis pathway in activated by tissue plasminogen activator (TPA), leading to activation of plasmin with degradation of fibrin to fibrin degradation products (FDP). Plasminogen activator inhibitor-1 (PAI-1) inhibits fibrinolysis but can be inhibited by APC. TFPI, tissue factor pathway inhibitor. (Adapted from Ware et al. [237].)

induced and expressed on leukocyte cell surfaces. Mediators known to induce TF are lipopolysaccharide (LPS), TNF-α, and CD40 ligand (present in activated platelets) [124–126]. Stimulated monocytes release TF and complexes of microparticles containing TF and P selectin glycoprotein ligand (PSGL-1). These particles bind to activated platelets at wound sites, concentrating TF at the endothelium. Tissue factor binds with circulating factor VII, forming TF–VIIa complexes that activate factor Xa. Factor Xa complexes with factor Va to form prothrombin-converting complex, triggering thrombin to cleave fibrinogen thereby leading to fibrin deposition and clot formation [124–126]. The TF–VIIa complexes can *cross-talk* with the initiators of the intrinsic clotting system by activating factor IXa, which together with factor VIIIa can further activate factor Xa and thereby ultimately generating more fibrin clot. In addition, when thrombin is activated it feeds back through factors XI, VIII, and V to amplify factor Xa conversion, further enhancing thrombin formation [124–126].

C reactive protein, another acute phase protein upregulated in septic shock, has a number of procoagulant effects, including enhancement of chemotaxis of monocytes to activated endothelium, inhibition of tissue plasminogen activator activity, activation of complement leading to platelet activation, induction of TF from monocytes, and downregulation of thrombomodulin and the endothelial protein C receptor [127–131]. Activated endothelial cells release ultralarge von Willebrand factor multimers in response to inflammatory cytokines. Under normal circumstances, homeostasis between release and cleavage of these multimers occurs through the action of the metalloprotease called ADAMTS13. Inflammatory cytokines diminish the activity of ADAMTS13, resulting in circulating platelet thrombi and development of microvascular thrombosis [132].

The endogenous anticoagulant pathway is also impacted upon by systemic inflammation. The pathways affected by inflammation include the fibrinolytic tissue factor pathway inhibitor (TFPI), antithrombin III (ATIII) pathway, and the protein C–protein S–thrombomodulin pathway [126]. Fibrinolysis is activated by inflammatory cytokines via conversion of plasminogen to plasmin, which degrades many clotting factors [126]. In septic shock, formation of plasmin is downregulated by the induction of plasminogen activator inhibitors 1 and 2 (PAI-1 and -2) [126,133,134]. Thrombin-activatable fibrinolysis inhibitor (TAFI) is activated by thrombin–thrombomodulin (thrombin receptor) complexes and also results in impaired fibrinolysis [135]. Antithrombin III, an endogenous serine protease inhibitor, can regulate the activity of many of the serine protease types of clotting factors. It is, however, rapidly degraded in sepsis concurrent with activated clotting factors [133]. It is common to find antithrombin inhibitory activity at 50% or less of normal in septic shock [133]. Antithrombin III also has antiinflammatory effects, including induction of prostacyclin, which inhibits platelet aggregation, neutrophil attachment to endothelial cells, production of inflammatory cytokines, and activation of NFκB by endothelial cells and monocytes [126,133]. Despite these promising preclinical data, large randomized controlled trials using antithrombin III or TFPI supplementation failed to show clinical improvement [124,136].

Thrombomodulin has recently been shown to have direct antiinflammatory properties emanating from the N-terminal lectin-like domain, an aspect of the extracellular portion of thrombomodulin that is structurally distinct from the domain responsible for its anticoagulant activity [137]. Interestingly, this N-terminal domain sequesters HMGB1, a very potent late-acting proinflamma-

tory cytokine, discussed in depth below. Thrombomodulin competitively binds HMGB1, thereby reducing binding of HMGB1 to one of its receptors, the receptor for advanced glycation endproducts, thereby diminishing NFκB activation [138]. Administration of recombinant soluble thrombomodulin (rsTM) has been tried in several models of inflammatory disease, including septic shock, and is being currently pursued as an anticoagulant for postoperative hip replacement surgery [139]. Thrombomodulin supplementation has been a potential therapeutic target for septic shock and disseminated intravascular coagulation because of its anticoagulant activity via its interaction with thrombin and activation of APC (see later) [126]. With this new information regarding its potent antiinflammatory activity, thrombomodulin should be explored as a therapeutic agent in septic shock.

The thrombin–thrombomodulin complex formation alters the thrombin enzymatic substrate preference to protein C rather than fibrinogen, resulting in protein C activation rather than fibrin [140]. This is especially efficient when protein C is bound to the endothelial cell protein C receptor (EPCR) [125,141]. In this way, activation of protein C is a negative feedback loop initiated by the clotting cascade [126]. Once activated, protein C binds to protein S and inactivates factors Va and VIIIa, effectively shutting off factors Xa and XIa and thereby inhibiting thrombin and fibrin formation [141]. Some data indicate that APC has further anticoagulant effects via inhibiting the inhibitors of plasmin generation: PAI-1 and TAFI [142].

During septic shock, expression of both thrombomodulin and EPCR is downregulated, resulting in a limited potential for protein C activation [143,144]. Neutrophil elastase cleaves thrombomodulin from the endothelial cell surface, and oxidant stress can significantly diminish the function of thrombomodulin [125,145]. Endothelial cell protein C receptor also is shed and present in serum. If either EPCR or thrombomodulin is not cell surface bound, activation of protein C is much less efficient [145,146]. Because of decreased hepatic synthesis and consumption, protein C and APC levels in septic shock patients are profoundly low as has been seen in multiple trials of APC in septic shock [142,147,148]. Over the past several years the use of APC infusion in adult patients with septic shock has become a commonplace event because of a large clinical trial demonstrating significant survival advantage with a reduction in absolute 28-day mortality from 30% to 24% [147]. Unfortunately, its use for children has not been FDA approved, and there are no published randomized prospective clinical trials with this population, although a recent multicenter trial was recently halted because of an unfavorable risk/benefit ratio.

In addition to the anticoagulant effects of APC, numerous antiinflammatory and antiapoptotic effects have been described that may have contributed to the differences seen between the results of the APC and ATIII trials for septic shock in adults [141,149]. Experimentally, APC has been shown to downregulate proinflammatory cytokine production as well as cytokine-mediated TF induction. In addition, APC can inhibit NFκB, decrease adhesion molecule expression, neutrophil adhesion, and chemotactic responses by binding directly to the EPCR. The EPCR is also expressed on neutrophils and monocytes, and many of these actions are EPCR dependent [142,149,150].

Antiapoptotic actions of APC may also have contributed to its protective benefit in septic shock. Interaction between APC and EPCR can decrease endothelial cell apoptosis and maintain the integrity of an endothelial cell monolayer through the activation of protease activated receptor 1 expressed on endothelial cells [151].

This protective effect is in direct contrast with thrombin signaling through protease activated receptor 1, leading to disruption of endothelial integrity [125,152]. Activated protein C induces antiapoptotic proteins on endothelial cells (Bcl-2 homolog protein and inhibitor of apoptosis protein), making cells more resistant to apoptosis and maintaining the integrity of the endothelial barrier [149,153].

There are numerous points of intersection between the coagulation and inflammatory cascades, some of which have been described earlier. Many mediators appear to be good therapeutic targets; however, the failures of ATIII and TFPI indicate that more understanding and better clinical design will be necessary to flush out the next successful agent [154]. The use of rhAPC for septic shock in the PROWESS trial was successful in decreasing absolute 28-day mortality rate by 6% [147]. A later study showed no benefit and an increased risk of bleeding when adult patients were enrolled who were less severely ill—characterized as severe sepsis with low risk of death (APACHE score <25 or single organ failure only) [155]. Unfortunately, to date, rhAPC has not received FDA approval for use in pediatric septic shock because of a lack of evidence to support a favorable risk/benefit ratio (Eli Lilly communication). With further examination rhAPC may find its place in pediatric critical care for the highest mortality risk groups; however, at this point no clinical trials are in progress.

The complex interplay between the inflammatory cascade and the coagulation cascade may reveal targets capable of acting to improve both systems (as most believe APC does) with less bleeding risk. Strategies might include tailored APC to have higher EPCR affinity and less anticoagulant effect on factors Va and VIIIa. Possibly inhibitors targeting the initiation of the TF cascade might provide partial anticoagulant with antiinflammatory benefits [152]. Another approach, although less clean and linear, is to target attenuation of multiple pathways simultaneously such as inflammation, coagulation, apoptosis, fibrinolysis, as well as endothelial cell and leukocyte activation. In fact, it is possible that rhAPC has actually accomplished that because it is now clear that all of these pathways can be altered by APC, and this may be a factor in its success [124]. Further work will be required to reduce the bleeding risk and to find ideal candidates for APC, especially for children.

Inflammatory Mediators

Countless inflammatory mediators have been identified in septic shock. The importance of many cytokines, chemokines, and biochemical mediators has typically been identified by in vitro or in vivo animal models of severe inflammation, such as endotoxin or systemic bacterial infection. Both antibody neutralization before sepsis resulting in a beneficial effect and administration of recombinant forms resulting in sepsis-like pathology have been used to demonstrate relevance of a new mediator [156]. Many mediators have been investigated in this way, and a few have reached clinical trials. This list includes LPS, TNF-α, IL-1β, platelet activating factor, arachidonic acid metabolites, free radicals, NO, anticoagulation factors, bradykinins, and complement factors. Some mediators have been blocked directly with antibodies or soluble receptors, and the formation of some has been diminished by enzyme inhibition. Unfortunately, none has shown survival benefit in human septic shock [1,122,156].

Eichacker et al. [157] performed a retrospective meta-regression analysis combining data from a multitude of preclinical studies and demonstrated that the higher the risk of mortality for a given patient, the higher the likelihood of benefit from any of the antiinflammatory agents in the trials listed earlier. By combining these data, it was clear that the mortality rate of the animal models was higher than that seen in the large clinical trials (88% median preclinical study mortality vs. 39% median clinical trial mortality). When examining all of the large clinical trials of antiinflammatory agents combined, the same relationship was present in that more benefit occurred for the sicker patients with a higher risk of death. In fact, statistically the antiinflammatory agents as a group were harmful to those patients at low risk of death [157]. These researchers then studied antiinflammatory agents in animal models employing an escalating dose of bacteria aimed at producing a wide range of mortality. Using this framework they demonstrated that, even in an animal model, antiinflammatory agents were most beneficial at the highest mortality rates and that when the mortality rate was less, fewer beneficial effects were seen [157]. These data implore us to develop better means of identification of the highest risk patients in order to select only those for early clinical trials.

High-Mobility Group Box 1

Theoretically, there are many proinflammatory cytokine/chemokine targets; however, some are more promising based on the timing of induction relative to the onset of septic shock. High-mobility group box 1 is dubbed a *late* mediator in septic shock because serum levels of HMGB1 do not begin to rise for several hours after endotoxin injection and persist at elevated levels for 16–36 hours [158]. The delay in the HMGB1 response clearly distinguishes it from TMF-α and other early-acting proinflammatory cytokines [159]. Administration of rHMGB1 can be lethal, and neutralizing anti-HMGB1 antibodies protect against mortality from LPS and cecal ligation and puncture (CLP) even when administered up to 24 hours after CLP or 2 hours after LPS [158]. It is highly conserved and ubiquitously expressed in the nucleus and cytoplasm in all cell types [159]. Intracellularly it functions as a DNA binding protein with several functions, including maintenance of nucleosome structure, regulation of transcription, and modulation of steroid hormone receptors [159].

High-mobility group box 1 also functions as a cytokine and can be released by innate immune cells and by cells undergoing necrosis but not apoptosis [159]. It binds to a number of receptors on the cell surface, such as the receptor for advanced glycation and endproducts (RAGE), toll-like receptors 2 (TLR -2) and 4 (TLR4) [159,160]. In doing so, it activates many intracellular pathways leading to activation of NFκB, mitogen-activated protein kinases, maturation of dendritic cells, and secretion of TNF-α, IL-1β, IL-6, and IL-8 [161]. In addition, HMGB1 induces vascular cell adhesion molecule 1 (VCAM-1), intercellular adhesion molecule 1 (ICAM 1), RAGE, monocyte chemotactic protein 1 (MCP-1), PAI-1, and tissue plasminogen activator [120,122,159,162]. Others have found that HMGB1 can alter gut barrier function via NO production, leading to increased permeability and bacterial translocation [163].

Serum HMGB1 has been reported in animal models of septic shock and hemorrhagic shock [159]. In addition, elevated levels have been reported in humans with septic shock, hemorrhagic shock, and disseminated intravascular coagulopathy. Septic patients demonstrated high serum levels that persisted for at least 1 week. Some reports show an association between high levels and increased disease severity [158,164]. As mentioned before, administration of neutralizing antibodies to HMGB1 was protective in septic animal models. Other substances found to inhibit HMGB1 and to provide a protective effect in septic shock models include recombinant A box (an HMGB1 DNA binding domain with antagonistic activity), ethyl pyruvate, and nicotine [158,165,166]. Ethyl pyruvate and nicotine both block HMGB1 production, and both were protective against lethality when administered 24 hours after CLP and 2 hours after LPS [158,166]. Given the failures of clinical trials aimed at early inflammatory mediators, these data suggest that pursuit of anti-HMGB1 therapies is warranted and very promising. In this case, the preclinical data suggest that a much wider therapeutic window may exist in which to administer this therapy after the onset of sepsis.

Migration Inhibitory Factor

Macrophage migration inhibitory factor (MIF) is an interesting proinflammatory mediator. Primarily it is expressed constitutively by monocytes, macrophages, T cells, anterior pituitary cells, as well as many other cell types, making it unusual for a typical cytokine [167]. When administered concurrent with LPS it enhances lethality. Models using MIF−/− mice and those treated with anti-MIF neutralizing antibodies were hyporesponsive and protected from LPS-induced lethality [168]. Some of the mechanisms involved in MIF enhancement of the response to LPS have been defined. These include the counterregulatory effects seen with regard to glucocorticoid effects. In animal models, MIF production by macrophages is induced by low levels of glucocorticoids. Migration inhibitory factor is upregulated by activation of the hypothalamic–pituitary axis–mediated stress response [122,169]. This also is unique for a typical cytokine. Administration of rMIF was found to override glucocorticoid-mediated antiinflammatory effects [169]. Signaling pathway alterations induced by MIF include regulation of TLR4 expression as demonstrated in MIF−/− mice, which express significantly less TLR4 on macrophages. Specific hyporesponsiveness to TLR4 activators but not to TLR2 activators was reported, identifying a unique role for this cytokine in the response to Gram-negative rods [122,167,170]. A key pathway altered by MIF is suppression of p53-mediated apoptosis of activated macrophages, allowing for increased cytokine production and a sustained proinflammatory response [171]. Apoptosis and removal of activated macrophages is considered to be a critical downregulatory aspect of the inflammatory responses and is dependent on NO, p53, and the caspase cascade [167,171].

Patients with septic shock have high levels of MIF, which correlate with poor outcome. Interestingly, nonseptic, critically ill surgical patients also demonstrate higher levels, suggesting that MIF may be an important mediator of culture-negative SIRS induced by such issues as trauma or hemorrhagic shock [122,172]. Interestingly, red blood cell lysates were extremely potent inducers of MIF, which might suggest a reason for upregulated MIF in culture-negative SIRS from trauma or hemorrhage, especially if associated with disseminated intravascular coagulopathy and hemolysis. In septic patients, MIF serum levels were negatively correlated with the cortisol response to adrenocorticotropic hormone, and MIF levels decreased after administration of stress dose hydrocortisone [172]. These data suggest a counterregulatory effect between MIF and circulating cortisol levels during septic shock. As mentioned earlier, in naïve mice MIF was upregulated by activation of the stress response and important in overcoming glucocorticoid immune suppressive effects. These data are somewhat conflicting; however, it is possible that measuring MIF levels hours into septic shock may not be equivalent to measuring MIF acutely after incit-ing a stress response in the mouse. Nonetheless, higher levels of MIF may be critical to sustaining inflammatory responses by suppressing p53 and upregulating TLR4, thereby contributing to the immune dysregulation seen in septic shock. For this reason MIF remains a promising therapeutic target albeit far from clinical use at this point. Furthermore, these data may provide a clue as to part of the beneficial actions of stress dose glucocorticoid administration in adrenally suppressed septic patients.

Mitochondrial Dysfunction

Tissue hypoxia has long been appreciated to be critical to the pathogenesis of septic shock–related organ failure. An enormous amount of data support this association. The most compelling of which are those reports showing that *very early* fluid resuscitation, inotropic therapy, red cell transfusion, and other strategies targeted at improving oxygen delivery ultimately improved outcome [173–175]. Much clinical work and research has focused on microcirculatory flow problems as the etiology of tissue dysoxia in septic shock. The reasons for flow disturbances are many, including abnormal leukocyte–endothelial interactions, impaired deformability of red blood cells and neutrophils, increased blood viscosity, fibrin deposition and microthrombi in the vasculature, dysfunction of vascular autoregulatory mechanisms, microvascular permeability leading to tissue edema, and secondary enhancement of arteriovenous shunt perfusion [176,177]. Despite this evidence and rationale, two large prospective randomized clinical trials failed to demonstrate outcome benefit (one showed detriment) from efforts designed to optimize tissue oxygenation based on oxygen delivery and consumption parameters [178–180]. In these cohorts, nonsurvivors exhibited impaired ability to increase O_2 consumption despite augmented delivery, which was very different from survivors [181].

Other animal models and human clinical data further support these observations in a more specific fashion. If normal O_2 utilization is present in cells, poor O_2 delivery to tissues (hypoperfusion, anemia) would result in greater extraction of O_2 from red blood cells, resulting in diminished PO_2 in venous blood. Supplementation of O_2 delivery would decrease extraction. If mitochondrial dysfunction is present, cells extract less O_2 from that supplied, resulting in either no change or in increased venous PO_2 compared with normal when O_2 delivery is increased [182]. In several fluid-resuscitated animal septic shock models this idea has been confirmed [183–186]. In addition, these data were replicated in human muscle tissue during septic shock [187–188]. Others have shown depressed adenosine triphosphate and decreased activity of specific elements of the electron transport system in muscle biopsy specimens of septic shock nonsurvivors compared with survivors [189]. This critical work supports the concept of tissue dysoxia unrelated to blood flow. Some refer to this as *impaired cellular oxygen utilization* or as *cytopathic hypoxia* rather than *circulatory hypoxia* [177,180,182,189]. The data mentioned earlier support mitochondrial dysfunction as an etiology. Several possible causes for this dysfunction include depletion of substrate (pyruvate) to the tricarboxylic acid cycle caused by sepsis-induced pyruvate dehydrogenase inhibition as well as increased adenosine triphosphate consumption by enzymes like PARP that consume nicotinamide adenine dinucleotide in efforts to repair damaged DNA as well as mitochondrial injury (see later) [180,189–191].

Inflammatory cytokines can lead to the formation of other mediators (ceramide, caspase 8) that result in activation of the terminal caspase effector molecule caspase 3. This can promote mPT, exaggerated ROS formation, and apoptotic cell death [180,192]. Cytokines also can upregulate the Bcl-2 family proteins. Tumor necrosis factor-α can increase the ratio of proapoptotic to antiapoptotic proteins of this family (Bax to Bcl-2), leading to mPT and subsequent apoptosis [180,193,194]. In addition, Bcl-2 overexpression, which decreases the ratio between Bax and Bcl-2 and prevents mPT, prevents apoptosis and lethality in animal models of sepsis, demonstrating the important relationship between mPT and apoptosis [195,196]. Increased oxidant stress can both cause and result from mitochondrial dysfunction from sepsis-induced mPT, outer membrane damage, and impaired oxidative phosphorylation. This leads to excess ROS and reactive nitrogen species (RNS) formation, which further amplifies mitochondrial dysfunction [180,188]. Another issue that adds to mitochondrial dysfunction is that mitochondrial damage can lead to mitochondrial loss and delayed repair, leaving a state of mitochondrial depletion [180,197,198].

New work is being published at a rapid pace that explores mitochondrial uncoupling proteins (UCPs), which have been shown to protect mitochondrial membranes from ROS. This work is largely being done in the settings of myocardial protection, neuronal injury, and obesity. Uncoupling proteins are activated by free fatty acids and superoxide. Activated UCPs can reduce mitochondrial membrane potentials, leading to decreased ROS production by uncoupling adenosine triphosphate from oxygen consumption. Mild uncoupling is hypothesized to reduce ROS formation and protect mitochondria without completely shutting off adenosine

triphosphate production [87,199]. Data from neuronal injury models and myocardial ischemia reperfusion research demonstrate benefits from exogenous uncoupling agents such as 2,4-dinitrophenol [88]. Several reports have demonstrated increased ROS and RNS in macrophages in UCP2−/− mice. In contrast, LPS treatment of macrophages leads to UCP2 suppression and higher ROS, demonstrating the close relationship between UCPs and ROS [200]. Also, UCP2 overexpression can inhibit monocyte–endothelial adhesion [201]. No studies to date have examined UCPs in septic shock with regard to ROS generation from mitochondrial dysfunction; however, these data suggest that this may be an important phenomenon given the oxidant stress present in septic shock. Furthermore, the above-mentioned important body of literature supports efforts aimed at preventing mPT and ROS formation, such as antiinflammatory, antioxidant, and antiapoptotic strategies or combinations thereof to support mitochondrial performance and counter cytopathic hypoxia.

Lipid Switching

Lipid mediators or eicosanoids, including arachidonic acid metabolites such as prostaglandins (PG), thromboxane, and leukotrienes (LT), have been considered proinflammatory mediators in many systemic inflammatory conditions (Figure 15.3). Prostaglandins and LTs are known to participate in amplification of the inflammatory response to facilitate the influx of leukocytes into wound sites, leukocyte activation, and release of inflammatory effector molecules. This aspect of the inflammatory response is generally thought

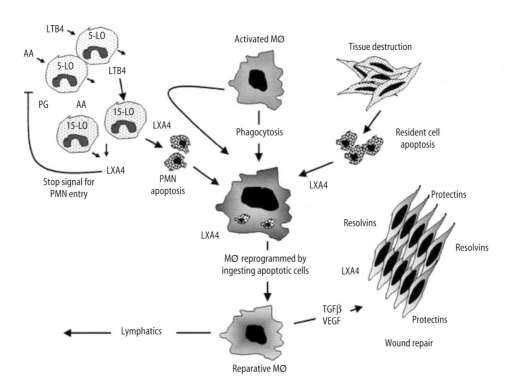

FIGURE 15.3. Lipid switching of wound phenotype. Activated PMNs chemotaxis into wound sites occurs in response to leukotriene B4 (LTB4) and prostaglandins (PG). New polymorphonuclear cells (PMNs) convert arachidonic acid to LTB4 via 5-lipoxygenase (5-LO) and PGs by cyclooxyenase, leading to more PMN influx. Prostaglandins upregulate 15-LO in PMNs, which converts AA to lipoxin A4 (LXA4), which serves as a "stop signal," decreasing PMN influx and accelerating PMN apoptosis leading to phagocytosis by macro-phages (MØ). Exposure to apoptotic cells and LXA4 alters the phenotype of MØ to produce transforming growth factor-β (TGF-β) and vascular endothelial growth factor (VEGF), which promote wound healing. Arachidonic acids are also converted to "resolvins" and "protectins," which are polyunsaturated fatty acid–based and promote wound healing. (Adapted from Serhan and Savill [202]).

to result in microbial eradication and tissue destruction if excessive [202–204]. More recently, an active coordinated program of resolution mediated by lipids has been described that is initiated by and begins after the inflammatory response starts [202]. There are multiple arms of the resolution process, and this section will describe the switch in lipid mediators that occurs at the wound site to dampen the proinflammatory process.

Initially, neutrophil arachidonic acid acts as 5-lipoxygenase (5-LO) substrate, leading to the production of leukotriene B4 (LTB4), which participates in neutrophil chemotaxis [205]. These functions are opposed by lipoxins, which are also derived from a lipoxygenase (15-LO) but serve as a *stop signal* for the amplification and progression of the inflammatory response [202,204]. Neutrophils arriving at a wound site are exposed to LTs and PGs as well as other inflammatory mediators, and at any one time different neutrophils will express different phenotypes (5-LO vs. 15-LO predominance) because of the ambient inflammatory milieu [202,204]. Cell–cell interactions occur at a wound site resulting in arachidonic acid being produced by one cell and metabolized by another (different phenotype) via15-LO to form lipoxins [202,204]. Lipoxins such as LXA4 present in a wound site can serve as a *stop signal* by inhibiting some neutrophil functions, including chemotaxis and enhancing macrophage phagocytosis of apoptotic leukocytes [205,206]. Simultaneously cyclooxygenase 2 (COX2) is induced in macrophages, and prostaglandin E_2 (PGE$_2$) is produced until it negatively feeds back on both COX 2 and 5-LO, resulting in induction of 15-LO in neutrophils. In this setting, PGE$_2$ has *switched* from a pro- to an antiinflammatory participant [202]. Irreversible acetylation of COX2 by aspirin changes COX2 enzymatic activity, resulting in production of a lipoxin moiety called aspirin-triggered 15-epi-LX (ATL) rather than PGE$_2$. Aspirin-triggered 15-epi-LX has similar effects as LXA4, which is important in consideration of the impact of aspirin on inflammatory pathways. Early on, aspirin was thought to simply inhibit COX1 and COX2 based on measurement of PGE$_2$ as a downstream product. Now it is clear that aspirin changes the function of COX2 to produce ATL, resulting in a *stop signal* [202].

The process of inflammatory resolution with a return back to a normal baseline state is referred to as catabasis [207]. Some of the phenomena that contribute to stopping proinflammatory responses are described above. Once stopped, the resolution phase and catabasis occurs. Neutrophil phagocytosis by macrophages signals many events, including an alteration of the macrophage phenotype leading to the production of the antiinflammatory cytokine transforming growth factor and vascular endothelial growth factor, which are both important to tissue repair and regeneration [202]. Several mediators are produced that downregulate neutrophil entry into the tissue, such as IL-12 and IFN-γ. During this phase new lipid mediators appear that have omega 3-polyunsaturated fatty acids as precursors in addition to lipoxins. They include eicosapentaenoic acid (EPA) and docosahexaenoic acid (DHA), which are converted to *resolvins* and *protectins*. These molecules are antiinflammatory and can hasten catabasis [202,207]. The transformation of arachidonic acid to lipoxin, EPA and DHA to resolvins, and DHA to protectins regulates the duration and magnitude of inflammation in part by enhancing uptake of apoptotic neutrophils by macrophages and regulating cellular trafficking into and out of wound sites [202].

This aspect of the inflammatory response is fairly new, and many targets for therapeutic intervention will no doubt emerge focusing on enhancing lipid switching to produce lipoxins as well as resolvins and protectins. One group of targets are the omega 3 fatty acids, which have long been thought to have an important role in healthy organ function; however, a suggested mechanism for this has not been provided until now [202]. Many animal models and human studies have probed the use of these molecules in the critically ill and found that inflammatory cytokines are reduced, but so far clinical trials have not been clearly beneficial [208]. Hopefully, this type of therapy will continue to be investigated perhaps with different study design and/or types of supplements or combination therapies. Aspirin, which can acetylate COX2 to enhance lipoxin formation rather than PGE$_2$ formation, directs COX2 to participate in the resolution phase of inflammation [202]. Timing of the administration of such agents will be important, because the agents may downregulate processes that are important to bacterial containment. It is possible that this type of strategy might be particularly helpful in *culture-negative* septic shock or if administered after cultures have become negative.

Statins

Statins are lipid-lowering drugs with widespread clinical use today for the prevention of atherosclerosis. The mechanism of action involves inhibition of 3-hydroxy 3-methylglutaryl-coenzyme A (HMG-CoA) reductase and the mevalonate pathway to cholesterol formation. Statins have been discovered to have *pleiotropic* effects in addition to cholesterol-lowering effects [209]. Multiple reports demonstrate antiinflammatory, antioxidant, immunomodulatory, and antithrombotic effects. Also, statins protect endothelial function and increase NO bioavailability [209]. Multiple in vitro and in vivo animal studies demonstrate the ability of statins to reduce many LPS-induced proinflammatory cytokines, adhesion molecules, and chemokines [209,210]. Statins also have pleiotropic effects on the coagulation cascade, with reports showing inhibition of TF and thrombin and enhanced fibrinolysis [210,211]. Furthermore, statin treatment up to 6 hours after CLP was associated with prolonged survival [209,212]. There have been no human trials using statins for septic shock; however, human volunteers pretreated with simvastatin produced lower levels of cytokines and procoagulant factors in response to LPS [213]. Retrospectively, clinical data have demonstrated reduced complications such as sepsis, ICU admission, and mortality in hospitalized patients with infection who were taking statins prior to becoming infected [214–216]. Statins are routinely used to lower cholesterol level to prevent atherosclerotic heart disease. A great deal of promising preclinical data support this type of agent as a potential therapy for septic shock. To date, only a mouse model has been used with statins as therapy for septic shock [209]. Further studies using statins after the initiation of sepsis will need to be done to confirm the benefit of statins when given after sepsis has begun. Having multiple sites of interference with septic pathways makes this agent a very exciting prospect to add to current care for septic shock.

Genetics/Genomics/Proteomics

Over the past decade genetic susceptibility for critical illnesses such as septic shock has become recognized in patients other than just those with classic immune deficiency syndromes. Genetic variations in genes crucial for proper functioning and regulation of the inflammatory response have emerged as advancement continues in high-throughput single nucleotide polymorphism (SNP) genotyping [217,218]. Polymorphisms occur through different pathways leading to aberrant gene products, the results of which include altered mRNA stability, altered transcription factor DNA binding with the possibility of either decreasing or increasing gene products, production of truncated proteins, and/or the production of defective proteins [217,218].

To date, many polymorphisms have been identified involving innate immune receptors such as TLR2, TLR4, TLR5, CD14, and heat shock proteins, as well as several others. Cytokine polymorphisms have also been identified for TNF-α, IL-1β, IL-6, IL-8, IL-10, MIF, and IL-1 receptor antagonists [217,218]. Coagulation polymorphisms have also been found, such as Factor V Leiden, PAI-1, and TAFI. Some of these polymorphisms have been associated with septic shock susceptibility to various organisms, risk of developing purpura fulminans (coagulation defects), and mortality [217]. In addition, increased incidences of polymorphic inflammatory genes have also been identified in diseases such as polytrauma with SIRS, arthritis, and atherosclerosis [217,218].

Better characterization of the genetic background of patients with a variety of disorders may lead to individualized and targeted treatments to immunomodulate for loss of the polymorphic protein's function [217]. Immunomodulation may need to be aimed at inhibition or augmentation of inflammatory responses based on the genes affected [219]. Applications of this same concept are utilized in the field of pharmacogenomics aimed at drug development for specific genetic variants. Pharmacogenetics is also important and aimed at genetic variants resulting in alterations in drug metabolism [219].

Genome-wide assessment of gene activation is also being used to gain further understanding of the genes involved in the inflammatory response. For instance, this type of analysis from patients with septic shock can and has revealed activation of genes not ordinarily included in the study of sepsis [220,221]. In addition, patterns of gene activation can be associated with outcome, which may lead to a better understanding of the timing of expression and contribution of a multitude of genes. This work requires careful screening but to date has provided animal data from septic models and is being used in human septic shock using mRNA patterns in peripheral blood mononuclear cells [220]. One recent study examined peripheral blood mononuclear cells from endotoxin-injected human volunteers collected serially over 24 hours [221]. The activity of multiple genes was seen, with some demonstrating reduced and others demonstrating increased activation. The investigators also reported transient modulation of leukocyte bioenergetics, including decreased expression of elements of the mitochondrial respiratory chain complex, ATP synthase, pyruvate dehydrogenase, and VDAC proteins, which are components of the mPT. Coincident with this was upregulated expression of components of the superoxide-producing NADPH-oxidase system. Modulation of translational enzymes and proteins was also seen [221]. Importantly, many of these genes and pathways are critical to the pathophysiology of septic shock as well as other critical illness as discussed earlier, validating these results.

Proteomics studies the expression of proteins in the peripheral blood mononuclear cells in a high-throughput fashion, allowing the examination of differences among gene expression and the production of gene products as well as their isoforms, modifications and protein–protein interactions [222]. Given the changes in translational machinery cited earlier, this is of particular significance in interpretation of gene expression patterns. Hopefully, like genomics, protein expression patterns will be identifiable and useful in correlation with disease severity and disease evolution.

Acute Lung Injury/Acute Respiratory Distress Syndrome

Much of the pathophysiology in the lung during ARDS is similar to that observed throughout the body in septic shock with activation of the inflammatory cascade, production of cytokines and chemokines, influx of neutrophils and monocytes, increased vascular permeability, activation of the coagulation cascade, and liberation of ROS (Figure 15.4). This section will touch on several interesting and hopeful therapeutic candidates for future therapies.

Alveolar Edema

A hallmark of ARDS is increased permeability of the alveolar-capillary barrier, resulting in accumulation of proteinaceous fluid and inflammatory cells into the alveolus with impairment of oxygenation. This edema is, by definition, noncardiogenic and therefore not based on hydrostatic back pressure from the left atrium. The cause of this edema remains ill defined; however, given the influx of neutrophils and the multitude of inflammatory mediators present in bronchoalveolar lavage fluid during ARDS, increased vascular permeability clearly is a factor. Maintenance of an Na^+ gradient between the intracellular and extracellular spaces is an important homeostatic mechanism responsible for alveolar fluid clearance in healthy lungs [223]. This is achieved by epithelial Na channels (ENa^+C), some of which are inhibited by amiloride, Na^+/K^+ ATPase pumps, Cl^- transporters such as the cystic fibrosis transmembrane conductance receptor (CFTR) and water channels (aquaporins). Na^+ and water can both also flow passively through their respective channels; however; it is the Na^+/K^+ ATPase pump that actively maintains the Na^+ gradient [223,224].

Many studies have shown that alveolar fluid clearance can be increased by catecholamines, particularly epinephrine but also β_2-specific agents via cAMP-dependent pathways. Amiloride blocks the effect of catecholamines, indicating that the ENa^+C are altered by catecholamines [224]. In addition, increased synthesis of ENa^+C and Na^+/K^+ ATPase pumps as well as their recruitment to the cell membrane from the cytosol have been demonstrated after stimulation with β-agonists [225,226]. There are conflicting data regarding the status of these mechanisms during lung injury. Data from a septic shock model and an ischemia reperfusion rat model demonstrated 70%–100% increased alveolar fluid clearance [227]. Others report the opposite, and it is thought that this conflict results from differences in model severity [224,228]. In milder injury, an adaptive response may occur with increased fluid clearance that is overcome by increasing lung injury severity [224]. Many mechanisms are thought to decrease fluid clearance, including hypoxia, inflammatory mediators, ROS, RNS, ventilator-induced lung injury (VILI), and atelectasis [223,224].

β-Agonists

A growing body of literature supports the use of β-agonists in ARDS. Animal models as well as human lung models have demonstrated that β-agonists ($\beta_2 > \beta_1$) can accelerate the rate of alveolar fluid clearance by upregulation of Na^+ transporters and channels as well as the CFTR [228–230]. β-Agonists have increased fluid clearance in multiple experimental lung injury models [230]. The use of β_2-receptor –/– mice and β_2-receptor overexpression models

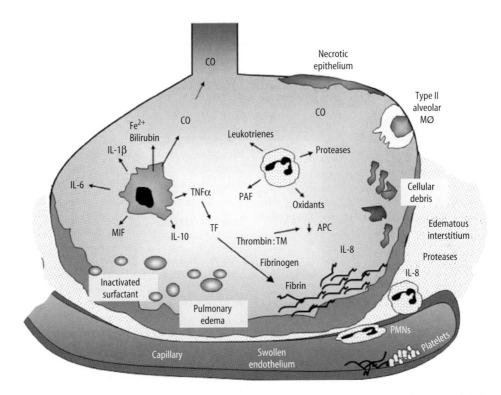

FIGURE 15.4. Acutely injured alveolus. Early acute respiratory distress syndrome has intraalveolar evidence of activation of both the inflammatory and coagulation cascades with cytokine/chemokine production, fibrin deposition, vascular permeability with pulmonary edema, cellular infiltrates, reactive oxygen species production, inactivated surfactant, epithelial damage, interstitial edema, capillary endothelial activation, and activation of the hemoxygenase pathway with carbon monoxide (CO) production. APC, activated protein C; IL, interleukin; MIF, migration inhibitory factor; PAF, platelet activating factor; TF, tissue factor; TNF-α, tissue necrosis factor-α. (Adapted from Matthay and Zimmerman [224].)

has validated the role of the β2-receptor in resolution of pulmonary edema and recovery from ARDS [231]. Interestingly, β2-agonists also reduced the incidence of high-altitude pulmonary edema in at-risk volunteers [229,232]. In a rat model of acid-induced lung injury, treatment with aerosolized β-agonists increased alveolar fluid clearance and decreased lung endothelial permeability, supporting previous observations. The results from a randomized placebo-controlled trial, the β-Agonist Lung Injury Trial (BALTI) were recently reported. The objective was to study the use of intravenous salbutamol (albuterol) in patients with ARDS [229]. Less extravascular lung water and lower plateau ventilatory pressures on day 7 were seen in the salbutamol-treated patients. No differences in mortality were noted, however, although the trial was not powered for mortality assessment because it included only 40 patients [229].

In addition to impacting on alveolar fluid clearance, β-agonists also have many antiinflammatory effects, which are important to consider in the setting of ARDS [reviewed in 230]. Some of the antiinflammatory effects of β-agonists on neutrophils include reductions in the following: pulmonary neutrophil sequestration, CD11b/18 adhesion molecule expression, chemotaxis, ROS and RNS production, lipid peroxidation, and proinflammatory cytokine production; with an increase in antiinflammatory cytokines [reviewed in 230]. Furthermore, β-agonist treatment can augment secretion of surfactant proteins and in particular SP-B and SP-C [233]. Finally, β-agonists have been shown to induce apoptosis of several cell types, including human neutrophils [230]. All of these actions support larger randomized controlled trials to further evaluate the use of β-agonists in the setting of ARDS.

Pulmonary Coagulopathy

Systemic inflammation and the coagulation cascade are intimately associated and capable of having reciprocal amplifying effects [234]. Similar to the evidence supporting activation of the inflammatory response in bronchoalveolar lavage fluid during pneumonia or ARDS, evidence of activation of the coagulation cascade can also be seen. These findings indicate the presence of what some authors refer to as a local *pulmonary coagulopathy* [234]. Resident cells in the lung, including epithelial cells, fibroblasts, and alveolar macrophages, can secrete TF, tissue plasminogen activator, and PAI-1. Endothelial cells can express TF when inflammatory stimuli are present [235]. Hence, the coagulation balance can be shifted when the inflammatory response begins, and both are amplified by the influx of neutrophils and macrophages into the lung. Activated coagulation factors present in bronchoalveolar lavage fluid from ARDS/pneumonia include increased TF, thrombin–antithrombin complexes, factor VII, factor X, fibrin, and thrombomodulin. Disease severity correlated with bronchoalveolar lavage fluid thrombomodulin levels and experimental blockade of the TF–VIIa pathway attenuated lung injury and cytokine release induced by intratracheal LPS [234,236,237]. Fibrin deposition in the lung can inhibit surfactant function, disrupt endothelial cells, alter neutrophil and macrophage migration, and increase vascular permeability [235,238]. In addition, bronchoalveolar lavage APC levels are suppressed in ARDS as well as nonseptic patients with ventilator-associated pneumonia. *Escherichia coli* were instilled into the lung of human volunteers by bronchoscopy after receiving systemic rhAPC or placebo. Treatment with rhAPC decreased

E. coli–induced TF, TAT, and PAI-1 in bronchoalveolar lavage fluid [234,239,240].

Fibrinolytic activity was also suppressed in pneumonia and ARDS and associated with increased alveolar PAI-1 as well as decreased fibrin degradation products [241–243]. One study showed that patients at risk for ventilator-associated pneumonia demonstrated diminished fibrinolysis during ventilator-associated pneumonia and several days before its onset [234,244]. Mechanical ventilation with larger tidal volumes can activate coagulation factors as it does cytokines in the lung [234]. These data clearly demonstrate local coagulation cascade activation in models of lung disease as well as in human lung disease. Clinical trials are being organized currently to focus on the use of APC in lung injury specifically rather than septic shock in adults.

Heme Oxygenase-1

Heme oxygenase is an enzyme involved in the breakdown of heme. There are three isoforms: HO-1, which is inducible; and HO-2 and HO-3, which are constitutively activated and expressed in a wide variety of cells. Over the past several years, it has become evident that HO-1 can provide cytoprotection against cellular stress and is largely expressed in inflammatory cells [245]. Heme oxygenase-1 is a stress-induced protein (formerly named *heat shock protein 32* [HSP32]) and as such can be induced by a wide variety of stimuli, such as hyperthermia, LPS, hyperoxia, oxidant stress, and oleic acid in an ARDS model [245]. Once induced, stress proteins are cytoprotective for further insults [246]. Heme oxygenase catalyzes oxidative cleavage of heme to release equimolar amounts of carbon monoxide (CO), Fe^{2+}, and biliverdin, which is converted to bilirubin by bilirubin reductase. Fe^{2+} then induces ferritin synthesis [246].

At low concentrations CO can have many biologic roles, including acting as a neurotransmitter. In addition, it has antiapoptotic, antiinflammatory, antioxidant, antiproliferative, and tolerogenic effects [reviewed in 246]. In addition, it can cause smooth muscle relaxation and prevent platelet aggregation, much like NO via a cGMP-dependent mechanism [246]. Antiinflammatory and antiapoptotic effects are mediated through the mitogen-activated protein kinase (MAPK) pathways, including p38 and the c-Jun N-terminal kinase. Carbon monoxide downregulates proinflammatory cytokines and upregulates IL-10, providing a net antiinflammatory benefit [246]. The pathway for this has been defined as CO-mediated activation of MAPK (process unknown), leading to upregulation of heat shock factor 1, which induces another stress protein, heat shock protein 70. Heat shock protein 70 induces many antiinflammatory and antiapoptotic effects [247]. In a pig LPS acute lung injury model, pretreatment with inhaled CO diminished pathologic changes in lung resistance and compliance as well as gas exchange. Carbon monoxide also protected against disseminated intravascular coagulopathy and renal and hepatic dysfunction in this model, as well as suppressing inflammatory cytokine production. In addition, ICAM expression on lung endothelium and leukocyte marginalization in lung parenchyma was blocked by CO [248]. In a nebulized LPS model for ARDS, HO-1-/- mice exhibited significantly reduced surfactant protein B expression. This was reversed when mice were reconstituted with HO-1 WT cells. Maintaining SP-B in the alveoli may have contributed to the beneficial role of HO-1 in ARDS [249]. There are some conflicting animal data, and at this time it is unclear whether the conflict derives from differences in animal models or techniques [250,251]. More work

will be needed to resolve these differences; however, most of the available work points to HO-1 being protective.

The other byproducts of heme metabolism also provide cytoprotective effects that may contribute to those provided by CO. Bilirubin has powerful antioxidant effects, and the implications of this are being widely examined. Normal human serum is thought to have enough bilirubin to provide a good part of the total antioxidant capacity of serum [246,252]. Fe^{2+} from HO-1 conversion of heme induces ferritin, which also has cytoprotective effects, and its induction may provide some of the HO-1–mediated protection.

In vivo studies have confirmed that HO-1 is very active in producing CO in the lung by demonstrating higher carboxyhemoglobin levels in arterial blood than in venous blood drawn from a central vein [253]. Made in the lung, CO can be analyzed in exhaled gas. The concentration of CO in exhaled gas is being studied for the possibility of using it as a diagnostic or monitoring strategy for lung disease with the assumption that higher CO indicates higher HO-1 function and expression. Theoretically, this may provide a marker of the degree of inflammation and oxidative stress in the lung [246]. In terms of using CO as a therapeutic gas, much work will be needed to establish unequivocally its benefit at below-toxic levels of administration to examine the brain and neurologic function in animal models to confirm no evidence of toxicity and to evaluate dose–response information and pharmacokinetics in various disease entities [245,246]. One exciting new strategy has been put forth that involves the use of CO releasing molecules to produce the vasodilating effect of inhaled CO in animal models [254]. Work is ongoing to examine the HO system and CO-mediated protective effects in ARDS and sepsis models.

Conclusion

As is evident in the this chapter, there is a great deal of overlap in the pathophysiology of TBI, septic shock, and ARDS with respect to activation of the inflammatory response, the coagulation cascade, the production of ROS and RNS with oxidant stress, and, as a consequence of these issues, mitochondrial dysfunction leading to bioenergetic failure and cell death by apoptosis and necrosis. It is possible that future antioxidant or mitochondrial protection strategies will benefit all three disease categories because there is involvement of each process in all. Although it is unlikely that we will see the use of anticoagulants such as APC or soluble thrombomodulin in TBI, both agents may prove to be beneficial in septic shock and ARDS.

Of course all of these models must be validated in young (juvenile and/or newborn) animals in order to confirm shared pathophysiology regardless of age. Models must also be developed to simulate septic shock and ARDS in chronically ill and/or stressed patients because they are frequently the ones who develop these severe complications. In order to bring promising agents to the bedside, we may always trail the early adult studies in order for there to be unequivocal safety testing in adults before use in children. However, because the mortality rate of pediatric septic shock is lower than that of adults, we must anticipate this and select only those patients at extremely high mortality risk for testing. Because pediatric outcomes are so favorable, most children will survive with no need for unconventional therapies. To separate these children from those at extremely high risk of mortality, we need more reliable severity markers, and we may need to wait a bit longer before enrollment. The window of opportunity may be smaller at that point; however, if the overall mortality of the cohort studied is higher, the risk/benefit ratio may be favorable to allow further use and exploration of an agent. There is much to be done, and, hopefully, as our community-wide research efforts, skills, and manpower continue to grow, the pace of the translation from the bench to the bedside will improve.

References

1. Vincent JL, Abraham E. The last 100 years of sepsis. Am J Respir Crit Care Med 2006;173(3):256–263.
2. Watson RS, Carcillo JA, Linde-Zwirble WT, Clermont G, Lidicker J, Angus DC. The epidemiology of severe sepsis in children in the United States. Am J Respir Crit Care Med 2003;167(5):695–701.
3. Statler KD, Jenkins LW, Dixon CE, Clark RS, Marion DW, Kochanek P. The simple model versus the super model: translating experimental traumatic brain injury research to the bedside. J Neurotrauma 2001; 18:1195–1206.
4. Prins ML, Hovda DA. Developing experimental models to address traumatic brain injury in children. J Neurotrauma 2003;20:123–137.
5. Kochanek P, Clark RSB, Ruppel RA, Adelson PD, Bell MJ, Whalen MJ, et al. Biochemical, cellular and molecular mechanisms in the evolution of secondary damage after severe TBI in infants and children. Lessons learned from the bedside. Pediatr Crit Care 2000;1: 4–19.
6. Ito J, Marmarou A, Barzo P, Fatouros P, Corwin F. Characterization of edema by diffusion-weighted imaging in experimental traumatic brain injury. J Neurosurg 1996;84(1):97–103.
7. Graham DI, Adams JH, Doyle D. Ischaemic brain damage in fatal non-missile head injuries. J Neurol Sci 1978;39(2–3):213–234.
8. Bouma GJ, Muizelaar JP, Stringer WA, Choi SC, Fatouros P, Young HF. Ultra-early evaluation of regional cerebral blood flow in severely head-injured patients using xenon-enhanced computerized tomography. J Neurosurg 1992;77:360–368.
9. Obrist WD, Langfitt TW, Jaggi JL, Cruz J, Gennarelli TA. Cerebral blood flow and metabolism in comatose patients with acute head injury. Relationship to intracranial hypertension. J Neurosurg 1984; 61:241–253.
10. Schroder ML, Muizelaar JP, Bullock MR, Salvant JB, Povlishock JT. Focal ischemia due to traumatic contusions documented by stable xenon–CT and ultrastructural studies. J Neurosurg 1995;82:966–971.
11. Enriquez P, Bullock R. Molecular and cellular mechanisms in the pathophysiology of severe head injury. Curr Pharm Design 2004; 10:2131–2143.
12. Bullock R, Zauner A, Woodward JJ, Myseros J, Choi SC, Ward JD. Factors affecting excitatory amino acid release following severe human head injury. J Neurosurg 1998;89:507–518.
13. Adelson PD, Dixon CE, Robichaud P, Kochanek P. Motor and cognitive functional deficits following diffuse traumatic brain injury in the immature rat. J Neurotrauma 1997;14:99–108.
14. Thomale UW, Schaser K, Kroppenstedt SN, Unterberg AW, Stover JF. Cortical hypoperfusion precedes hyperperfusion following controlled cortical impact injury. Acta Neurochir Suppl 2002;81:229–231.
15. Leker RR, Shohami E. Cerebral ischemia and trauma-different etiologies yet similar mechanisms: neuroprotective opportunities. Brain Res Brain Res Rev 2002;39:55–73.
16. Cherian L, Hlatky R, Robertson CS. Nitric oxide in traumatic brain injury. Brain Pathol 2004;14(2):195–201.
17. Andresen J, Shafi NI, Bryan RM. Endothelial influences on cerebrovascular tone. J Appl Physiol 2006;100:318–327.
18. Hillered L, Vespa PM, Hovda DA. Translational neurochemical research in acute human brain injury: the current status and potential future for cerebral microdialysis. J Neurotrauma 2005;22:3–41.
19. Cherian L, Goodman JC, Robertson CS. Brain nitric oxide changes after controlled cortical impact injury in rats. J Neurophysiol 2000; 83:2171–2178.
20. Ahn MJ, Sherwood ER, Prough DS, Lin CY, DeWitt DS. The effects of traumatic brain injury on cerebral blood flow and brain tissue nitric oxide levels and cytokine expression. J Neurotrauma 2004;21: 1431–1442.
21. Cherian L, Chacko G, Goodman C, Robertson CS. Neuroprotective effects of L-arginine administration after cortical impact injury in rats: dose–response and time window. J Pharmacol Exp Ther 2003; 304:617–623.
22. Cherian L, Robertson CS. L-arginine and free radical scavengers increase cerebral blood flow and brain tissue nitric oxide concentrations after controlled cortical impact injury in rats. J Neurotrauma 2003;20:77–85.
23. Dewitt DS, Smith TG, Deyo DJ. L-arginine and superoxide dismutase prevent or reverse cerebral hypoperfusion after fluid-percussion TBI. J Neurotrauma 1997;14:223–233.
24. Mendez DR, Cherian L, Robertson CS. Laser Doppler flow and brain tissue PO_2 after cortical impact injury complicated by secondary ischemia in rats treated with arginine. J Trauma 2004;57: 244–250.
25. Bayir H, Kagan VE, Tyurina YY, Tyurin V, Ruppel RA, Adelson PD. Assessment of antioxidant reserves and oxidative stress in cerebrospinal fluid after severe traumatic brain injury in infants and children. Pediatr Res 2002;51:571–578.
26. Bayir V, Kagan V, Borisenko GG, Tyurina YY, Janesko KL, Vagni VA, et al. Enhanced oxidative stress in iNOS-deficient mice after traumatic brain injury: support for a neuroprotective role of iNOS. J Cereb Blood Flow Metab 2005;25:673–684.
27. Wada K, Chatzipanteli K, Kraydieh S, Busto R, Dietrich WD. Inducible nitric oxide synthase expression after traumatic brain injury and neuroprotection with aminoguanidine treatment in rats. Neurosurgery 1998;43(6):1427–1436.
28. Orihara Y, Ikematsu K, Tsuda R, Nakasono I. Induction of nitric oxide synthase by traumatic brain injury. Forensic Sci Int 2001;123(2–3): 142–149.
29. Louin G, Marchand-Verreccia C, Palmier B, Plotkine M, Jafarian-Tehrani M. Selective inhibition of inducible nitric oxide synthase reduces neurological deficit but not cerebral edema following traumatic brain injury. Neuropharmacology 2006;50(2):182–190.
30. Jafarian-Tehrni M, Louin G, Royo NC, Besson VC, Bohme GA, Plotkine M, et al. 1400W, a potent selective inducible NOS inhibitor, improves histopathological outcome following traumatic brain injury in rats. Nitric Oxide 2005;12:61–69.
31. Jones NC, Constantin D, Gibson CL, Prior MJ, Morris PG, Marsden CA, et al. A detrimental role for nitric oxide synthase-2 in the pathology resulting from acute cerebral injury. J Neuropathol Exp Neurol 2004;63:708–720.
32. Sinz EH, P K, Dixon CE, Clark RS, Carcillo JA, Schiding JK, et al. Inducible nitric oxide synthase is an endogenous neuroprotectant after traumatic brain injury in rats and mice. J Clin Invest 1999; 104:647–656.
33. Clark RS, P K, Obrist WD, Wong HR, Billiar TR, Wisniewski SR, et al. Cerebrospinal fluid and plasma nitrite and nitrate concentrations after head injury in humans. Crit Care Med 1996;24: 1243–1251.
34. Bayir H, Kochanek P, Liu SX, Arroyo A, Osipov A, Jiang J, et al. Increased S-nitrosothiols and S-nitrosoalbumin in cerebrospinal fluid after severe traumatic brain injury in infants and children: indirect association with intracranial pressure. J Cereb Blood Flow Metab 2003;23:51–61.
35. Armstead WM. Endothelins and the role of endothelin antagonists in the management of posttraumatic vasospasm. Curr Pharm Design 2004;10:2185–2192.
36. Provencio JJ, Vora N. Subarachnoid hemorrhage and inflammation: bench to bedside and back. Semin Neurol 2005;25(4):435–444.
37. Petrov T, Rafols JA. Acute alterations of endothelin-1 and iNOS expression and control of the brain microcirculation after head trauma. Neurol Res 2001;23:139–143.

38. Kasemri T, Armstead WM. Endothelin impairs ATP-sensitive K⁺ channel function after brain injury. Am J Physiol 1997;273:H2639–H2647.

39. Zubkov A, Miao L, Zhang J. Signal transduction of ET-1 in contraction of cerebral arteries. J Cardiovasc Pharmacol 2004;44:24–26.

40. Barone FC, Ohlstein EH, Hunter AJ, Campbell CA, Hadingham SH, Parsons AA. Selective antagonism of endothelin A receptors improves outcome in both head trauma and focal stroke in rat. J Cardiovasc Pharmacol 2000;36:S357–S361.

41. Armstead WM. Role of endothelin in pial artery vasoconstriction and altered responses to vasopressin following brain injury. J Neurosurg 1996;85:901–907.

42. Armstead WM. Hypotension dilates pial arteries by KATP and KCa channel activation. Brain Res. 1999;815:158–164.

43. Steiner J, Rafols D, Park HK, Katar MS, Rafols JA, Petrov T. Attenuation of iNOS mRNA exacerbates hypoperfusion and upregulates endothelin-1 expression in hippocampus and cortex after brain trauma. Nitric Oxide 2004;10:162–169.

44. Motte S, McEntee K, Naeije R. Endothelin receptor antagonists. Pharmacol Ther 2006;110(3):386–414.

45. Ros J, Jones D, Pecinska N, Alessandri B, Boutelle M, Landolt H. Glutamate infusion coupled with hypoxia has a neuroprotective effect in the rat. J Neurosci Methods 2002;119:129–233.

46. Ros J, Pecinska N, Alessandri B, Landolt H, Fillenz M. Lactate reduces glutamate-induced neurotoxicity in rat cortex. J Neurosci Res 2001;66:790–794.

47. Choi DW. Ionic dependence of glutamate neurotoxicity. J Neurosci 1987;7(2):369–379.

48. Morris GF, Bullock R, Marshall SB, Marmarou A, Maas A, Marshall LF. Failure of the competitive N-methyl-D-aspartate antagonist Selfotel (CGS 19755) in the treatment of severe head injury: results of two phase III clinical trials. The Selfotel Investigators. J Neurosurg 1999;91(5):737–743.

49. Farin A, Marshall LF. Lessons from epidemiologic studies in clinical trials of traumatic brain injury. Acta Neurochir Suppl 2004;89:101–107.

50. Muir KW. Glutamate-based therapeutic approaches: clinical trials with NMDA antagonists. Curr Opin Pharmacol 2006;6(1):53–60.

51. Zipfel GJ, Babcock DJ, Lee JM, Choi DW. Neuronal apoptosis after CNS injury: the roles of glutamate and calcium. J Neurotrauma 2000;17(10):857–869.

52. Hardingham GE, Fukunaga Y, Bading H. Extrasynaptic NMDARs oppose synaptic NMDARs by triggering CREB shut-off and cell death pathways. Nat Neurosci 2002;5(5):405–414.

53. Royo NC, Shimizu S, Schouten JW, Stover JF, McIntosh TK. Pharmacology of traumatic brain injury. Curr Opin 2003;3:27–32.

54. Maas AI, Steyerberg EW, Murray GD, Bullock R, Baethmann A, Marshall LF. Why have recent trials of neuroprotective agents in head injury failed to show convincing efficacy? A pragmatic analysis and theoretical considerations. Neurosurgery 1999;44:1286–1298.

55. Narayan RK, Michel ME, Ansell B, Baethmann A, Biegon A, Bracken MB. Clinical trials in head injury. J Neurotrauma 2002;19:503–557.

56. Bayir H, Kochanek P, Clark RS. Traumatic brain injury in infants and children. Mechanisms of secondary damage and treatment in the intensive care unit. Crit Care Clin 2003;19:529–549.

57. Doppenberg EM, Choi SC, Bullock R. Clinical trials in traumatic brain injury: lessons for the future. J Neurosurg Anesthesiol 2004;16(1):87–94.

58. Yurkewicz L, Weaver J, Bullock MR, Marshall LF. The effect of the selective NMDA receptor antagonist traxoprodil in the treatment of traumatic brain injury. J Neurotrauma 2005;22:1428–1443.

59. Paschen W. Calcium neurotoxicity. J Neurochem 1999;72(6):2625–2626.

60. Paschen W, Frandsen A. Endoplasmic reticulum dysfunction–a common denominator for cell injury in acute and degenerative diseases of the brain? J Neurochem 2001;79(4):719–725.

61. Sattler R, Tymianski M. Molecular mechanisms of calcium-dependent excitotoxicity. J Mol Med 2000;78(1):3–13.

62. Lee LL, Galo E, Lyeth BG, Muizelaar JP, Berman RF. Neuroprotection in the rat lateral fluid percussion model of traumatic brain injury by SNX-185, an N-type voltage-gated calcium channel blocker. Exp Neurol 2004;190(1):70–78.

63. Sullivan PG, Rabchevsky AG, Waldmeier PC, Springer JE. Mitochondrial permeability transition in CNS trauma: cause or effect of neuronal cell death? J Neurosci Res 2005;79:231–239.

64. Verweij BH, Muizelaar JP, Vinas FC, Peterson PL, Xiong Y, Lee CP. Improvement in mitochondrial dysfunction as a new surrogate efficiency measure for preclinical trials: dose–response and time-window profiles for administration of the calcium channel blocker ziconotide in experimental brain injury. J Neurosurg 2000;93(5):829–834.

65. Stover JF, Beyer TF, Unterberg AW. Riluzole reduces brain swelling and contusion volume in rats following controlled cortical impact injury. J Neurotrauma 2000;17(12):1171–1178.

66. Lewen A, Matz P, Chan PH. Free radical pathways in CNS injury. J Neurotrauma 2000;17:871–890.

67. Pellegrini-Giampietro DE, Cherici G, Alesiani M, Carla V, Moroni F. Excitatory amino acid release and free radical formation may cooperate in the genesis of ischemia-induced neuronal damage. J Neurosci 1990;10:1035–1041.

68. Dykens JA. Isolated cerebral and cerebellar mitochondria produce free radicals when exposed to elevated CA^{2+} and Na^+: implications for neurodegeneration. J Neurochem 1994;63:584–591.

69. Evans PH. Free radicals in brain metabolism and pathology. Br Med Bull 1993;49:577–587.

70. Mohanakumar KP, Thomas B, Sharma SM, Muralikrishnan D, Chowdhury R, Chiueh C. Nitric oxide: an antioxidant and neuroprotector. Ann NY Acad Sci 2002;962:389–401.

71. Lewen A, Fujimura M, Sugawara T, Matz P, Copin JC, Chan PH. Oxidative stress-dependent release of mitochondrial cytochrome c after traumatic brain injury. J Cereb Blood Flow Metab 2001;21:914–920.

72. Keller JN, Mark RJ, Bruce AJ, Blanc E, Rothstein JD, Uchida K. 4-Hydroxynonenal, an aldehydic product of membrane lipid peroxidation, impairs glutamate transport and mitochondrial function in synaptosomes. Neuroscience 1997;80:685–696.

73. Marklund N, Clausen F, Lewander T, Hillered L. Monitoring of reactive oxygen species production after traumatic brain injury in rats with microdialysis and the 4-hydroxybenzoic acid trapping method. J Neurotrauma 2001;18(11):1217–1227.

74. Reiter RJ. Oxidative processes and antioxidative defense mechanisms in the aging brain. FASEB J 1995;9:526–533.

75. Maragos WF, Korde AS. Mitochondrial uncoupling as a potential therapeutic target in acute central nervous system injury. J Neurochem 2004;91:257–262.

76. Hansson MJ, Persson T, Friberg H, Keep MF, Rees A, Wieloch T, et al. Powerful cyclosporin inhibition of calcium-induced permeability transition in brain mitochondria. Brain Res 2003;960:99–111.

77. Ichas F, Mazat JP. From calcium signaling to cell death: two conformations for the mitochondrial permeability transition pore. Switching from low- to high-conductance state. Biochem Biophys Acta 1998;1366:33–50.

78. Lifshitz J, Sullivan PG, Hovda DA, Wieloch T, McIntosh TK. Mitochondrial damage and dysfunction in traumatic brain injury. Mitochondrion 2004;4:705–713.

79. Sullivan PG, Thompson M, Scheff SW. Continuous infusion of cyclosporin A postinjury significantly ameliorates cortical damage following traumatic brain injury. Exp Neurol 2000;161:631–637.

80. Scheff SW, Sullivan PG. Cyclosporin A significantly ameliorates cortical damage following experimental traumatic brain injury in rodents. J Neurotrauma 1999;16:783–792.

81. Arguad L, Gateau-Roesch O, Muntean D, Chalabreysse L, Loufouat J, Robert D, et al. Specific inhibition of the mitochondrial permeability transition prevents lethal reperfusion injury. J Mol Cell Cardiol 2004;38:367–374.

82. Singleton RH, Stone JR, Okonkwo DO, Pellicane AJ, Povlishock JT. The immunophilin ligand FK506 attenuates axonal injury in an impact-acceleration model of traumatic brain injury. J Neurotrauma 2001;18:607–614.

83. Suehiro E, Singleton RH, Stone JR, Povlishock JT. The immunophilin ligand FK506 attenuates the axonal damage associated with rapid rewarming following posttraumatic hypothermia. Exp Neurol 2001; 172:199–210.

84. Price M, Lang MG, Frank AT, Goetting-Minesky MP, Patel SP, Silviera ML, et al. Seven cDNAs enriched following hippocampal lesion: possible roles in neuronal responses to injury. Brain Res Mol Brain Res 2003;117:58–67.

85. Kurz JE, Hamm RJ, Singleton RH, Povlishock JT, Churt SB. A persistent change in subcellular distribution of calcineurin following fluid percussion injury in the rat. Brain Res 2005;1048:153–160.

86. Kurz JE, Parsons JT, Rana A, Gibson CJ, Hamm RJ, Churn SB. A significant increase in both basal and maximal calcineurin activity following fluid percussion injury in the rat. J Neurotrauma 2005;22: 476–490.

87. Sullivan PG. Mitochondrial uncoupling as a therapeutic target following neuronal injury. J Bioenergeics Biomembranes 2004;36:353–356.

88. Korde AS, Pettigrew LC, Craddock SD, Maragos WF. The mitochondrial uncoupler 2,4-dinitrophenol attenuates tissue damage and improves mitochondrial homeostasis following transient focal cerebral ischemia. J Neurochem 2005;94(6):1676–1684.

89. Mattiasson G, Shamloo M, Gido G, Mathi K, Tomasevic G, Yi S, et al. Uncoupling protein-2 prevents neuronal death and diminishes brain dysfunction after stroke and brain trauma. Nat Med 2003;9: 1062–1068.

90. Roshon MJ, Kline JA, Thornton LR, Watts JA. Cardiac UCP2 expression and myocardial oxidative metabolism during acute septic shock in the rat. Shock 2003;19(6):570–576.

91. Vespa P, Bergsneider M, Hattori N, Wu HM, Huang SC, Martin NA, et al. Metabolic crisis without brain ischemia is common after traumatic brain injury: a combined microdialysis and positron emission tomography study. J Cereb Blood Flow Metab 2005;25:763–774.

92. Wong J, Hoe MW, Zhiwei F, Ng I. Apoptosis and Traumatic Brain Injury. Neurocrit Care 2005;3:177–182.

93. Zhang X, Chen Y, Jenkins LW, Kochanek P, Clark RS. Bench-to-bedside review: apoptosis/programmed cell death triggered by traumatic brain injury. Critical Care 2005;9:66–75.

94. Clark RS, Kochanek P, Watkins SC. Caspase-3 mediated neuronal death after traumatic brain injury in rats. J Neurochem 2000;74: 740–753.

95. Yakovlev AG, Ota K, Wang G, Movsesyan V, Bao WL, Yoshihara K, et al. Differential expression of apoptotic protease-activating factor-1 and caspase-3 genes and susceptibility to apoptosis during brain development and after traumatic brain injury. J Neurosci 2001;21(19): 7439–7446.

96. Besson VC, Zsengeller Z, Plotkine M, Szabo C, Marchand-Verrecchia C. Beneficial effects of PJ34 and INO-1001, two novel water-soluble poly(ADP-ribose) polymerase inhibitors, on the consequences of traumatic brain injury in rat. Brain Res 2005;1041:149–156.

97. Hong SJ, Dawson TM, Dawson VL. Nuclear and mitochondrial conversations in cell death: PARP-1 and AIF signaling. Trends Pharmacol Sci 2004;25:259–264.

98. Koh DW, Dawson TM, Dawson VL. Mediation of cell death by poly (ADP-ribose) polymerase-1. Pharmacol Res 2005;52:5–14.

99. Li LY, Luo X, Wang X. Endonuclease G is an apoptotic DNase when released from mitochondria. Nature 2001;412:95–99.

100. Graham SH, Chen J, Clark RS. Bcl-2 family gene products in cerebral ischemia and traumatic brain injury. J Neurotrauma 2000;17: 831–841.

101. Concha NO, Abdel-Meguid SS. Controlling apoptosis by inhibition of caspases. Curr Medicinal Chem 2002;9:713–726.

102. Clark RS, Kochanek PM, Schwartz MA, Schiding JK, Turner DS, Chen M, et al. Inducible nitric oxide synthase expression in cerebrovascular smooth muscle and neutrophils after traumatic brain injury in immature rats. Pediatr Res 1996;39:784–790.

103. Ang BT, Yap E, Lim J, Tan WL, Ng PY, Ng I, et al. Poly(adenosine diphosphate-ribose) polymerase expression in human traumatic brain injury. J Neurosurg 2003;99(1):125–130.

104. Lenzlinger PM, Marx A, Trentz O, Kossman T, Morganti-Kossman MC. Prolonged intrathecal release of soluble Fas following severe traumatic brain injury in humans. J Neuroimmunol 2002;122:167–174.

105. Ng I, Yeo TT, Tang WY, Soong R, Ng PY, Smith DR. Apoptosis occurs after cerebral contusions in humans. Neurosurgery 2000;46(4):949–956.

106. Williams S, Raghupathi R, MacKinnon MA, McIntosh TK, Saatman KE, Graham DI. In situ DNA fragmentation occurs in white matter up to 12 months after head injury in man. Acta Neuropathol (Berl) 2001;102(6):581–590.

107. Biegon A. Cannabinoids as neuroprotective agents in traumatic brain injury. Curr Pharm Design 2004;10:2177–2183.

108. Mechoulam R, Spatz M, Shohami E. Endocannabinoids and neuroprotection. Science 2002;129:1–6.

109. Panikashvill D, Simeonidou C, Ben-Shabat S, Hanus L, Breuer A, Mechoulam R, et al. An endogenous cannabinoid (2-AG) is neuroprotective after brain injury. Nature 2001;413:527–531.

110. Knoller N, Levi L, Shoshan I, Reichenthal E, Razon N, Rappaport ZH, et al. Dexanabinol (HU-211) in the treatment of severe closed head injury: a randomized, placebo-controlled, phase II clinical trial. Crit Care Med 2002;30:548–554.

111. Shohami E, Mechoulam R. Dexanabinol (HU-211): A nonpsychotropic cannabinoid with neuroprotective properties. Drug Dev Res 2000; 50:211–215.

112. Ungerstedt U, Rostami E. Microdialysis in neurointensive care. Curr Pharm Design 2004;10:2145–2152.

113. Grate LL, Golden JA, Hoopes PJ, Hunter JV, Duhaime AC. Traumatic brain injury in piglets of different ages: techniques for lesion analysis using histology and magnetic resonance imaging. J Neurosci Methods 2003;123:201–206.

114. Armstead WM. Age dependent NMDA contribution to impaired hypotensive cerebral hemodynamics following brain injury. Dev Brain Res 2002;139:19–28.

115. Smith SL, Andous PK, Gleason DG, Hall ED. Infant rat model of the shaken baby syndrome: preliminary characterization and evidence for the role of free radicals in cortical hemorrhaging and progressive neuronal degeneration. J Neurotrauma 1998;15:693–705.

116. Robertson CL. Mitochondrial dysfunction contributes to cell death following traumatic brain injury in adult and immature animals. J Bioenergeics Biomembranes 2004;36:363–368.

117. Armstead WM, Kurth CD. Different cerebral hemodynamic responses following fluid percussion brain injury in the newborn and juvenile pig. J Neurotrauma 1994;11:487–497.

118. Bittigau P, Sifringer M, Pohl D. Apoptotic neurodegeneration following trauma is markedly enhanced in the immature brain. Ann Neurol 1999;45:724–735.

119. Prins ML, Hovda DA. Fluid percussion brain injury in the developing rat: effects of the maturation on Morris water maze acquisition. J Neurotrauma 1998;15:799–811.

120. Dumitriu IE, Baruah P, Manfredi AA, Bianchi ME, Rovere-Querini P. HMGB1: guiding immunity from within. Trends Immunol 2005; 26(7):381–387.

121. Doughty L. Modulation of the immune response in critical illness/injury. In: Doughty LA, Linden P, eds. Immunology and Infectious Disease. Norwell, MA: Kluwer Academic Publishers; 2003:115–154.

122. Riedemann NC, Guo RF, Ward PA. Novel strategies for the treatment of sepsis. Nat Med 2003;9:517–524.

123. Aird WC. The role of the endothelium in severe sepsis and multiple organ dysfunction syndrome. Blood 2003;101:3765–3777.

124. Aird WC. Coagulation. Crit Care Med 2005;33:S485.

125. Esmon CT. The interactions between inflammation and coagulation. Br J Haematol 2005;131:417–430.

126. Opal SM, Esmon CT. Bench-to-bedside review: functional relationships between coagulation and the innate immune response and their respective roles in the pathogenesis of sepsis. Crit Care 2003;7: 23–38.

127. Han KH, Hong KH, Park JH, Ko J, Kang DH, Choi KJ, et al. C-reactive protein promotes monocyte chemoattractant protein-1–mediated chemotaxis through upregulating CC chemokine receptor 2 expression in human monocytes. Circulation 2004;109:2566–2571.

128. Han KH, Tangirala RK, Green SR. Chemokine receptor CCR2 expression and monocyte chemoattractant protein-1 mediated chemotaxis in human monocytes: a regulatory role for plasma low-density lipoprotein. Arterioscler Thromb Vasc Biol 1998;17:1983–1991.

129. Wolbink GJ, Bossink AW, Groeneveld AB, DeGroot MC, Thijs LG, Hack CE. Complement activation in patients with sepsis is in part mediated by C-reactive protein. J Infect Dis 1998;177:81–87.

130. Singh U, Devaraj S, Jialal I. C-reactive protein decreases tissue plasminogen activator activity in human aortic endothelial cells: evidence that C-reactive protein is a procoagulant. Arterioscler Thromb Vasc Biol 2005;25:2216–2221.

131. Nan B, Yang H, Yan S, Lin PH, Lumsden AB, Yao Q, et al. C-reactive protein decreases expression of thrombomodulin and endothelial protein C receptor in human endothelial cells. Surgery 2005;138: 212–222.

132. Bernardo A, Ball C, Nolasco L, Moake JF, Dpmg J. Effects of inflammatory cytokines on the release and cleavage of the endothelial cell-derived ultralarge von Willebrand factor multimers under flow. Blood 2004;104:100–106.

133. Opal SM. Therapeutic rationale for antithrombin III in sepsis. Crit Care Med 2000;28:S34–S37.

134. Voss R, Matthias FR, Borkowski G, Reitz D. Activation and inhibition of fibrinolysis in septic patients in an internal intensive care unit. Br J Haematol 1990;75(1):99–105.

135. Zeerleder S, Schroeder V, Hack CE, Kohler HP, Wuillemin WA. TAFI and PAI-1 levels in human sepsis. Thromb Res 2006;118(2):205–212.

136. Warren BL, Eid A, Singer P, Pillay SS, Carl P, Novak I, et al. Caring for the critically ill patient. High-dose antithrombin III in severe sepsis: a randomized controlled trial. JAMA 2001;286(15):1869–1878.

137. Conway EM. The lectin-like domain of thrombomodulin confers protection from neutrophil-mediated tissue damage by suppressing adhesion molecule expression via nuclear factor kB and mitogen-activated protein kinase pathways. J Exp Med 2002;196:565–577.

138. Abeyama K, Stern DM, Ito Y, Kawahara KI, Yoshimoto Y, Tanaka M, et al. The N-terminal domain of thrombomodulin sequesters high-mobility group-B1 protein, a novel antiinflammatory mechanism. J Clinical Invest 2005;115:1267–1274.

139. Kearon C, Comp C, Douketis D, Royds R, Yamada K, Gent M. A dose-response study of a recombinant human soluble thrombomodulin (ART-123) for prevention of venous thromboembolism after unilateral total hip replacement. J Thromb Haemost 2003;Abstract 0C330.

140. Esmon CT. The roles of protein C and thrombomodulin in the regulation of blood coagulation. J Biol Chem 1989;264:4743–4746.

141. Esmon CT. The protein C pathway. Chest 2003;124:26–32.

142. Macias WL, Yan SB, Williams MD, Um SL, Sandusky GE, Ballard DW, et al. New insights into the protein C pathway: potential implications for the biological activities of drotrecogin alfa (activated). Crit Care 2005;9:S38–S45.

143. Faust SN, Levin M, Harrison OB, Goldin RD, Lockhart MS. Dysfunction of endothelial protein C activation in severe meningococcal sepsis. N Engl J Med 2001;345:408–416.

144. Conway EM, Rosenberg RD. Tumor necrosis factor suppresses transcription of the thrombomodulin gene in endothelial cells. Mol Cell Biol 1988;8:5588–5592.

145. Takano S, Kimura S, Ohdama S, Aoki N. Plasma thrombomodulin in health and diseases. Blood 1990;76:2024–2029.

146. Glaser CB, Morser J, Clarke JH, Blasko E, McLean K, Kuhn I, et al. Oxidation of a specific methionine in thrombomodulin by activated neutrophil products blocks cofactor activity. A potential rapid mechanism for modulation of coagulation. J Clin Invest 1992;90(6): 2565–2573.

147. Bernard GR, Ely EW, Wright TJ, Fraiz J, Stasek JE, Russell JA, et al. Safety and dose relationship of recombinant human activated protein C for coagulopathy in severe sepsis. Crit Care Med 2001;29:2051–2059.

148. Macias WL, Khainaut JF, Yan SC, Helterbrand JD, Seger M, Johnson G, et al. Pharmacokinetic–pharmacodynamic analysis of drotrecogin alfa (activated) in patients with severe sepsis. Clin Pharmacol Ther 2002;72:391–402.

149. Joyce DE, Gelbert L, Ciaccia A, DeHoff B, Grinnell BW. Gene expression profile of antithrombotic protein C defines new mechanisms modulating inflammation and apoptosis. J Biol Chem 2001;276: 11199–11203.

150. Sturn DH, Kaneider NC, Feistritzer C, Djanani A, Fukudome K, Wiedermann CJ. Expression and function of the endothelial protein C receptor in human neutrophils. Blood 2003;102:1499–1505.

151. Feistritzer C, Lenta R, Riewald M. Protease-activated receptors-1 and -2 can mediate endothelial barrier protection: role in factor Xa signaling. J Thromb Haemost 2005;3:2798–2805.

152. Riewald M, Ruf W. Science review: role of coagulation protease cascades in sepsis. Crit Care 2003;7:123–129.

153. Bannerman DD, Tupper JC, Ricketts WA, Bennett CF, Winn RK, Harlan JM. A constitutive cytoprotective pathway protects endothelial cells from lipopolysaccharide-induced apoptosis. J Biol Chem 2001; 276(18):14924–1432.

154. Abraham E, Reinhart K, Opal S, Demeyer I, Doig C, Rodriguez AL, et al. Efficacy and safety of tifacogin (recombinant tissue factor pathway inhibitor) in severe sepsis: a randomized controlled trial. JAMA 2003;290:238–247.

155. Abraham E, Laterre PF, Garg R, Levy H, Talwar D, Trzaskoma BL, et al. Drotrecogin alfa (activated) for adults with severe sepsis and a low risk of death. N Engl J Med 2005;353:1332–1341.

156. Deans KJ, Haley M, Natanson C, Eichacker PQ, Minneci PC. Novel therapies for sepsis: a review. J Trauma 2005;58:867–874.

157. Eichacker PQ, Parent C, Kalil A, Esposito C, Cui X, Banks SM, et al. Risk and the efficacy of antiinflammatory agents. Am J Respir Crit Care Med 2002;166:1197–1205.

158. Wang H. Cholinergic agonists inhibit HMGB1 release and improve survival in experimental sepsis. Nat Med 2004;10:1216–1221.

159. Yang H, Wang H, Czura CJ, Tracey KJ. The cytokine activity of HMGB1. J Leukocyte Biol 2005;78:1–8.

160. Park JS, Gamboni-Robertson F, He Q, Svetkauskaite D, Kim JY, Strassheim D, et al. High mobility group box 1 protein (HMGB1) interacts with multiple toll like receptors. Am J Physiol Cell Physiol 2006;290(3):C917–C924.

161. Andersson U, Erlandsson-Harris H, Yang H, Tracey KJ. HMGB1 as a DNA-binding cytokine. J Leukocyte Biol 2002;72:1084–1091.

162. Fluza C. Inflammatory promoting activity of HMGB1 on human microvascular endothelial cells. Blood 2002;101:2652–2660.

163. Sappington PL. HMGB1 B box increases the permeability of Caco-2 enterocytic monolayers and impairs intestinal barrier function in mice. Gastroenterology 2002;123:790–802.

164. Sunden-Cullberg J, Norrby-Teglund A, Rouhiainen A, Rauvala H, Herman G, Tracey KJ, et al. Persistent elevation of high mobility group box-1 protein (HMGB1) in patients with severe sepsis and septic shock. Crit Care Med 2005;34:564–573.

165. Li J. Structural basis for the proinflammatory cytokine activity of high mobility group box 1. Mol Med 2003;9:37–45.

166. Ulloa L. Ethyl pyruvate prevents lethality in mice with established lethal sepsis and systemic inflammation. Proc Natl Acad Sci USA 2002;99:12351–12356.

167. Roger T, David J, Glauser MP, Calandra T. MF regulates innate immune responses through modulation of Toll-like receptor 4. Nature 2001; 414:920–923.

168. Bernhagen J, Calandra T, Mitchell RA, Martin SB, Tracey KJ, Voelter W, et al. MIF is a pituitary-derived cytokine that potentiates lethal endotoxaemia. Nature 1993;365(6448):756–759.

169. Calandra T, Bernhagen J, Metz CN, Spiegel LA, Macher M, Donnelly T, et al. MIF as a glucocorticoid-induced modulator of cytokine production. Nature 1995;365:756–759.

170. Leng L, Bucala R. Macrophage migration inhibitory factor. Crit Care Med 2005;33(12 Suppl):S475–S477.

171. Mitchell RA, Liao H, Chesney J, Fingerle-Rowson G, Baugh J, David J, et al. Macrophage migration inhibitory factor (MIF) sustains macrophage proinflammatory function by inhibiting p53: regulatory role in the innage immune response. Proc Natl Acad Sci USA 2002;99: 345–350.

172. Maxime V, Fitting C, Annane D, Cavaillon JM. Corticoids normalize leukocyte production of macrophage migration inhibitory factor in septic shock. J Infect Dis 2005;191:138–144.

173. Carcillo JA, Davis AL, Zaritsky A. Role of early fluid resuscitation in pediatric septic shock. JAMA 1991;266:1242–1245.

174. Han YY, Carcillo JA, Dragotta MA, Bills DM, Watson RS, Westerman ME, et al. Early reversal of pediatric-neonatal septic shock by community physicians is associated with improved outcome. Pediatrics 2003;112:793–799.

175. Rivers E, Nguyen B, Havstad S, Ressler J, Muzzin A, Knoblich B, et al. Early goal-directed therapy in the treatment of severe sepsis and septic shock. N Eng J Med 2001;345:1368–1377.

176. Spronk PE, Zandstra DF, Ince C. Bench-to-bedside review: sepsis is a disease of the microcirculation. Crit Care 2004;8:462–468.

177. Sibbald WJ. Shockingly complex: the difficult road to introducing new ideas to critical care. Crit Care 2004;8:419–421.

178. Hayes MA, Timmins AC, Yau EHS, Palazzo M, Hinds CJ, Watson D. Elevation of systemic oxygen delivery in the treatment of critically patients. N Engl J Med 1994;330:1717–1722.

179. Gattinoni L, Brazzi L, Pelosi P, Latini R, Tagnoni G, Pesenti A, et al. A trial of goal-oriented hemodynamic therapy in critically ill patients. N Engl J Med. 1995;333:1025–1032.

180. Crouser ED. Mitochondrial dysfunction in septic shock and multiple organ dysfunction syndrome. Mitochondrion 2004;4:729–741.

181. Hayes MA, Timmins AC, Yau EH, Palazzo M, Watson D, Hinds CJ. Oxygen transport patterns in patients with sepsis syndrome or septic shock: influence of treatment and relationship to outcome. Crit Care Med 1997;25:926–936.

182. Fink MP. Bench-to-bedside review: cytopathic hypoxia. Crit Care 2002;6:491–499.

183. Hotchkiss RS, Song SK, Neil JJ, Chen RD, Manchester JK, Karl IE, et al. Sepsis does not impair tricarboxylic acid cycle in the heart. Am J Physiol 1991;260(1 Pt 1):C50–C57.

184. Astiz M, Rackow EC, Weil MH, Schumer W. Early impairment of oxidative metabolism and energy production in severe sepsis. Circ Shock 1988;26(3):311–320.

185. Rosser DM, Stidwill RP, Jacobson D, Singer M. Oxygen tension in the bladder epithelium rises in both high and low cardiac output endotoxemic sepsis. J Appl Physiol 1995;79(6):1878–1882.

186. Boekstegers P, Weidenhofer S, Pilz G, Werdan K. Peripheral oxygen availability within skeletal muscle in sepsis and septic shock: comparison to limited infection and cardiogenic shock. Infection 1991; 19(5):317–323.

187. Sair M, Etherington PJ, Peter Winlove C, Evans TW. Tissue oxygenation and perfusion in patients with systemic sepsis. Crit Care Med 2001;29(7):1343–1349.

188. Brealey D, Brand M, Hargreaves I, Heales S, Land J, Smolenski R, et al. Association between mitochondrial dysfunction and severity and outcome of septic shock. Lancet 2002;360:219–223.

189. Fink MP. Cytopathic hypoxia: mitochondrial dysfunction as mechanism contribution to organ dysfunction in sepsis. Crit Care Clin 2001;17:219–237.

190. Cuzzocrea S. Shock, inflammation and PARP. Pharmacol Res 2005; 52:72–82.

191. Vary TC, Siegel JH, Nakatani T, Sato T, Aoyama H. Effect of sepsis on activity of pyruvate dehydrogenase complex in skeletal muscle and liver. Am J Physiol 1986;250:E634–E640.

192. von Haefen C, Wieder T, Gillissen B, Starck L, Graupner V, Dorken B, et al. Ceramide induces mitochondrial activation and apoptosis via a Bax-dependent pathway in human carcinoma cells. Oncogene 2002;21(25):4009–4019.

193. Kim BC, Kim HT, Mamura M, Ambudkar IS, Choi KS, Kim SJ. Tumor necrosis factor induces apoptosis in hepatoma cells by increasing C12+release from the endoplasmic reticulum and suppressing Bcl–2 expression. J Biol Chem 2002;277:31381–31389.

194. Tsujimoto Y. Bcl-2 family of proteins: life-or-death switch in mitochondria. Biosci Rep 2002;22(1):47–58.

195. Coopersmith CM, Stromberg PE, Dunne WM, Davis CG, Amiot DM, Buchman TG, et al. Inhibition of intestinal epithelial apoptosis and survival in a murine model of pneumonia-induced sepsis. JAMA 2002;287:1716–1721.

196. Coopersmith CM, Chang KC, Swanson PE, Tinsley KW, Stromberg PE, Buchman TG, et al. Overexpression of Bcl–2 in the intestinal epithelium improves survival in septic mice. Crit Care Med 2002;30:195–201.

197. Tavakoli H, Mela L. Alterations of mitochondrial metabolism and protein concentrations in subacute septicemia. Infect Immun 1982;38(2):536–541.

198. Prins JB, Ledgerwood EC, Ameloot P, Vandenabeele P, Faraco PR, Bright NA, et al. Tumor necrosis factor–induced cytotoxicity is not related to rates of mitochondrial morphological abnormalities or autophagy-changes that can be mediated TNFR-I or TNFR-II. Biosci Rep 1998;18:329–340.

199. Jezek P, Hlavata L. Mitochondria in homeostasis of reactive oxygen species in cell, tissues, and organism. International J Biochem Cell Biol 2005;37:2478–2503.

200. Kizaki T, Suzuki K, Hitomi Y, Taniguchi N, Saitoh D, Watanabe K, et al. Uncoupling protein 2 plays an important role in nitric oxide production of lipopolysaccharide-stimulated macrophages. Proc Natl Acad Sci USA 2002;99(14):9392–9397.

201. Ryu JW, Hong KH, Maeng JH, Kim JB, Ko J, Park JY, et al. Overexpression of uncoupling protein 2 in THP1 monocytes inhibits b2, integrin-mediated firm adhesion and transendothelial migration. Arterioscler Thromb Vasc Biol 2004;24:864–870.

202. Serhan CN, Savill J. Resolution of inflammation: the beginning programs the end. Nat Immunol 2005;6:1191–1197.

203. Serhan CN. Novel w—3–derived local mediators in anti-inflammation and resolution. Pharmacol Ther 2005;105:7–21.

204. Nathan C. Points of control in inflammation. Nature 2002;420: 846–852.

205. Levy BD, Clish CB, Schmidt B, Gronert K, Serhan CN. Lipid mediator class switching during acute inflammation: signals in resolution. Nat Immunol 2001;2:612–619.

206. Godson C. Cutting edge: lipoxins rapidly stimulate nonphlogistic phagocytosis of apoptotic neutrophils by monocyte-derived macrophages. J Immunol 2000;164:1663–1667.

207. Bannenberg GL, Chiang N, Ariel A, Arita M, Tjonahen E, Gotlinger KH, et al. Molecular circuits of resolution: formation and actions of resolvins and protectins[1]. J Immunol 2005;174:4345–4355.

208. Calder PC. n-3 fatty acids, inflammation, and immunity—relevance to postsurgical and critically ill patients. Lipids 2004;39(12):1147–1161.

209. Mekontso-Dessap A, Brun-Buisson C. Statins: the next step in adjuvant therapy for sepsis? Intensive Care Med 2006;32:11–14.

210. Schonbeck U, Libby P. Inflammation, immunity, and HMG-CoA reductase inhibitors. Statins as antiinflammatory agents? Circulation 2004;109:II-18–II-26.

211. Krysiak R, Okopien B, Herman Z. Effects of HMG-CoA reductase inhibitors on coagulation and fibrinolysis processes. Drugs 2003; 63:1821–1854.

212. Merx MW, Liehn EA, Graf J, van de Sandt A, Schaltenbrand M, Schrader J, et al. Statin treatment after onset of sepsis in a murine model improves survival. Circulation 2005;112(1):117–124.

213. Steiner S, Speidl WS, Pleiner J, Seidinger D, Zorn G, Kaun C, et al. Simvastatin blunts endotoxin-induced tissue factor in vivo. Circulation 2005;111:1841–1846.

214. Almog Y, Shefer A, Novack V, Maimon N, Barski L, Eizinger M, et al. Prior statin therapy is associated with a decreased rate of severe sepsis. Circulation 2004;110:880–885.

215. Kruger P, Fitzsimmons K, Cook D, Jones M, Nimmo G. Statin therapy is associated with fewer deaths in patients with bacteraemia. Intensive Care Med 2006;32:75–79.

216. Liappis AP, Kan VL, Rochester CG, Simon GL. The effect of statins on mortality in patients with bacteremia. Clin Infect Dis 2001;33:1352–1357.

217. Arcaroli J, Fessler MB, Abraham E. Genetic polymorphisms and sepsis. Shock 2005;24:300–312.

218. Schroder NWJ, Schumann RR. Single nucleotide polymorphisms of toll-like receptors and susceptibility to infections disease. Lancet Infect Dis 2005;5:156–164.

219. Wheeler DS, Wong HR. The impact of molecular biology on the practice of pediatric critical care medicine. Pediatr Crit Care Med 2001;2:299–310.

220. Feezor RJ, Cheng A, Paddock HN, Baker HV, Moldawer LL. Functional genomics and gene expression profiling in sepsis: beyond class prediction. Clin Infect Dis 2005;41:S427–S435.

221. Calvano SE, Xiao W, Richards DR, Felciano RM, Baker HV, Cho RJ, et al. A network-based analysis of systemic inflammation in humans. Nature 2005;437:1032–1037.

222. Hoehn GT, Suffredini AF. Proteomics. Crit Care Med 2005;33(12 Suppl):S444–S448.

223. Zemans RL, Matthay MA. Bench-to-bedside review: the role of the alveolar epithelium in the resolution of pulmonary edema in acute lung injury. Critical Care 2004;8:469–477.

224. Matthay MA, Zimmerman GA. Acute lung injury and the acute respiratory distress syndrome. Am J Respir Cell Mol Biol 2005;33:319–327.

225. Minakata Y, Suzuki S, Grygorczyk C, Dagenais A, Berthiaume Y. Impact of β-adrenergic agonists on Na channel and Na/K ATPase expression in alveolar type II cells. Am J Physiol 1998;275:L414–L422.

226. Saldias FJ, Comellas A, Ridge KM, Lecuona E, Sznajder JI. Isoproterenol improves ability of lung to clear edema in rats exposed to hyperoxia. J Appl Physiol 1999;87:30–35.

227. Borjesson A, Norlin A, Wang X, Anderson R, Folkesson HG. TNF-alpha stimulates alveolar liquid clearance during intestinal ischemia-reperfusion in rats. Am J Physiol Lung Cell Mol Physiol 2000;278:L3–L12.

228. Matthay MA, Folkesson HG, Clerici C. Lung epithelial fluid transport and the resolution of pulmonary edema. Physiol Res 2002;82:569–600.

229. Perkins GD, McAuley DF, Thickett DR, Gao F. The β-agonists lung injury trial (BALTI). A randomized placebo-controlled clinical trial. Am J Respir Crit Care Med 2006;173:281–287.

230. Perkins GD, McAuley DF, Richter A, Thickett DR, Gao F. Bench-to-bedside review: β2-Agonists and the acute respiratory distress syndrome. Crit Care 2004;8:25–32.

231. Mutlu GM, Dumasius V, Burhop J, McShane PJ, Meng FJ, Welch L, et al. Upregulation of alveolar epithelial active Na+ transport is dependent on β2-adrenergic receptor signaling. Circ Res 2004;94:1091–1100.

232. Sartori C, Allemann Y, Duplain H, Lepori M, Egli M, Lipp E, et al. Salmeterol for the prevention of high-altitude pulmonary edema. N Engl J Med 2002;346:1631–1636.

233. Gobran LI, Rooney SA. Regulation of SP-B and SP-C secretion in rat type II cells in primary culture. Am J Physiol Lung Cell Mol Physiol 2001;281(6):L1413–L1419.

234. Schultz MJ, Haitsma JJ, Zhang H, Slutsky AS. Pulmonary coagulopathy as a new target in therapeutic studies of acute lung injury or pneumonia—a review. Crit Care Med 2006;34:1–7.

235. Idell S. Coagulation, fibrinolysis, and fibrin deposition in acute lung injury. Crit Care Med 2003;31:S213–S220.

236. Miller DL, Welty-Wolf K, Carraway MS. Extrinsic coagulation blockade attenuates lung injury and proinflammatory cytokine release after intratracheal lipopolysaccharide. Am J Respir Cell Mol Biol 2002;26:650–658.

237. Ware LB, Bastarache JA, Wang L. Coagulation and fibrinolysis in human acute lung injury—new therapeutic targets? Keio J Med 2005;54:142–149.

238. Laterre PF, Wittebole X, Dhainaut JF. Anticoagulant therapy in acute lung injury. Crit Care Med 2003;31:S329–S336.

239. Yasui H, Gabazza EC, Tamaki S. Intratracheal administration of activated protein C inhibits bleomycin-induced lung fibrosis in the mouse. Am J Respir Crit Care Med 2001;163:1660–1668.

240. VanderPoll T, Levi M, Nick JA, Abraham E. Activated protein C inhibits local coagulation after intrapulmonary delivery of endotoxin in humans. Am J Respir Crit Care Med 2005;171:1125–1128.

241. Idell S, Koenig KB, Fair DS. Serial abnormalities of fibrin turnover in evolving adult respiratory distress syndrome. Am J Physiol 1991;261:L240–L248.

242. Gunther M, Mosavi P, Heinemann S. Alveolar fibrin formation caused by enhanced procoagulant and depressed fibrinolytic capacities in severe pneumonia. Comparison with the acute respiratory distress syndrome. Am J Respir Crit Care Med 2000;161:454–462.

243. Prabhakaran P, Ware LB, White KE. Elevated levels of plasminogen activator inhibitor-1 in pulmonary edema fluid are associated with mortality in acute lung injury. Am J Physiol Lung Cell Mol Physiol 2003;285:L20–L28.

244. Schultz MJ, Millo J, Levi M. Local activation of coagulation and inhibition of fibrinolysis in the lung during ventilator associated pneumonia. Thorax 2004;59:130–135.

245. Jin Y, Choi AM. Cytoprotection of heme oxygenase-1/carbon monoxide in lung injury. Proc Am Thorac Soc 2005;2:232–235.

246. Morse D, Choi AM. Heme oxygenase-1. From bench-to-bedside. Am J Respir Crit Care Med 2005;172:660–670.

247. Kim HP, Wang X, Zhang J, Suh GY, Benjamin IJ, Ryter SW, et al. Heat shock protein-70 mediates the cytoprotective effect of carbon monoxide: involvement of P38b MAPK and heat shock factor-1[1]. J Immunol 2005;175:2622–2629.

248. Mazzola S, Forni M, Albertini M, Bacci ML, Zannoni A, Gentilini F, et al. Carbon monoxide pretreatment prevents respiratory derangement and ameliorates hyperacute endotoxic shock in pigs. FASEB J 2005;19(4):2045–2047.

249. Fredenburgh LE, Baron RM, Carvajal IM, Mouded M, Macias AA, Ith B, et al. Absence of oxygenase-1 expression in the lung parenchyma exacerbates endotoxin-induced acute lung injury and decreases surfactant protein-B levels. Cell Mol Biol 2005;51:513–520.

250. Dennery PA, Spitz DR, Yang G, Tatarov A, Lee CS, Shegog ML, et al. Oxygen toxicity and iron accumulation in the lungs of mice lacking heme oxygenase-2. J Clin Invest 1998;101:1001–1011.

251. Dennery PA, Visner G, Weng YH, Nguyen X, Lu F, Zander D, et al. Resistance to hyperoxia with heme oxygenase-1 disruption: role of iron. Free Radic Biol Med 2003;34:124–133.

252. Gopinathan V, Miller NJ, Milner AD, Rice-Evans CA. Bilirubin and ascorbate antioxidant activity in neonatal plasma. FEBS Lett 1994;349:197–200.

253. Meyer J, Prien T, Aken HV, Bone HG, Waurick R, Theilmeier G, et al. Arterio-venous carboxyhemoglobin difference suggests carbon monoxide production by human lungs. Biochem Biophys Res Commun 1998;244:230–232.

254. Motterlini R, Clark JE, Foresti R, Sarathchandra P, Mann BE, Green CJ. Carbon monoxide-releasing molecules. Characterization of biochemical and vascular activities. Circ Res 2002;90:e17–e24.

16
Genetic Polymorphisms in Critical Care and Illness

Mary K. Dahmer and Michael W. Quasney

Introduction

Although the vast majority of nuclear DNA is identical from one person to the next, there is a small fraction of DNA sequence (~0.1%) that varies among individuals. The variations in DNA sequence found within regions that make up genes are responsible for the genetically determined variation in our physical characteristics, our physiology, and our personality traits. Genetic variability also appears to be involved in susceptibility to some diseases, as well as therapeutic responses to treatment. Recent data have also suggested that genetic variations may affect the severity of some illnesses, thereby impacting the final outcome of these illnesses. In this chapter, we explore the evidence for whether genetic variation has an impact on critical illness and response to injury. We discuss how genetic variations may influence susceptibility to, severity of, and outcome from critical illness and injury and how they may help to identify risk factors for complications in children in the pediatric intensive care unit (PICU).

Genetic Polymorphisms

The sequencing of the human genome has revealed that many genes are polymorphic, that is, there are small differences in DNA sequences among individuals. Polymorphic genes are genes in which variation at a specific site is found in greater than 1% of the general population. The sites that are variable within the genes are referred to as *polymorphic sites*. The polymorphisms in DNA sequences may exist in several forms, with the most frequent form being a single nucleotide polymorphism (SNP) caused by a base pair substitution. In addition, polymorphisms within genes may also be caused by insertions or deletions of fragments of DNA or to the presence of a variable number of tandem repeats (VNTR) of short, repetitive DNA sequences.

Polymorphic sites can exist in coding and noncoding regions of the gene. They can have no effect, or they can influence the activity and/or level of the resulting protein, thereby affecting cell function. When present in the coding sequences of the gene, these variations can result in an alteration in the amino acid sequence of the protein that can affect the structure and function of the protein. When the polymorphic site exists in a noncoding region of the gene, it can affect the regulation of gene transcription, resulting in altered levels of protein product in the cell.

Genotyping of Polymorphic Sites

Although biochemical analyses of proteins have indicated that protein products are polymorphic, the first demonstration of the extent of polymorphism in the human genome was demonstrated using restriction enzymes that recognize and cut DNA at specific nucleotide sequences. Analyses of the DNA fragments generated by the action of a specific restriction enzyme on human DNA demonstrated that the size of the cleavage products differed among individuals. These restriction fragment length polymorphisms (RFLPs) are generally caused by an SNP within restriction enzyme recognition sites. After the realization that many SNPs were present in the human genome, a number of other methods were used to identify SNPs within genes [1,2].

Once a polymorphic site within a gene is identified, there are a number of methods that can be used to determine the genotype of individuals at that polymorphic site. As individuals have two copies of each gene, at any given polymorphic site an individual can be homozygous for one or the other polymorphism found at that site; or the individual may be heterozygous. Almost all genotyping techniques require amplification of the fragment of DNA containing the site of interest by the polymerase chain reaction (PCR) technique. This technique allows for the amplification of a specific region of the genome (in this case a region containing the polymorphic site) using small fragments of DNA that flank the polymorphic site as primers for the PCR. For insertions or deletions and most VNTRs, the genotype can be determined by examining the size of the PCR products by gel electrophoresis. In the case of SNPs, there are a

D.S. Wheeler et al. (eds.), *Science and Practice of Pediatric Critical Care Medicine*,
DOI 10.1007/978-1-84800-921-9_16, © Springer-Verlag London Limited 2009

number of different techniques that have been used for genotyping. Until recently most of these techniques were labor intensive, required experienced personnel, and were not conducive to genotyping many SNPs rapidly. More recently, with the increased interest in SNPs as tools for mapping genes and for candidate gene association studies, techniques for high-throughput SNP genotyping have begun to be developed. As the underlying strategies for the newer high-throughput techniques and the older, more labor intensive techniques are both based first on a reaction that discriminates which nucleotide is present at the polymorphic site and second on a technique that allows the identification of the product of the reaction, we discuss in detail several of the older techniques that are found in much of the literature published thus far to illustrate the general concepts. A brief discussion of high-throughput techniques is included at the end of this section.

Generally when genotyping an SNP, the two possible nucleotides found at the site are known from sequencing, and a technique is used to distinguish one nucleotide from the other. When the polymorphic site is within a recognition site for a restriction enzyme, the ability of the restriction enzyme to cleave the PCR product can be used to determine which nucleotide is present at the polymorphic site (Figure 16.1A). Whether the PCR product is cleaved is demonstrated by the size of the DNA as determined by electrophoresis.

Another way to determine whether a specific nucleotide is present at a polymorphic site is by performing allele-specific PCR (copies of DNA with different nucleotides at a specific polymorphic site are considered to be different alleles of the gene; Figure 16.1B). Allele-specific primers that are identical except for the last nucleotide are used in the PCR reaction. Polymerase chain reactions generate new pieces of DNA by the addition of nucleotides to the 3′ end of the primer that has hybridized to the DNA of interest, which acts as a template. If there is no match at the 3′ end of the primer, the polymerase extends the primer at a 100- to 10,000-fold lower efficiency, and no PCR product is detected. If the last nucleotide of the primer hybridizes to the specific allele it is designed to detect, a PCR product is formed if the individual has a copy of that allele. Presence or absence of the PCR product is determined by electrophoresis. To genotype an individual using the allele-specific PCR technique, two different PCR reactions are performed with one or the other allele-specific primer and a second primer common to both reactions.

Another technique that is often used to genotype SNPs is based on hybridization with allele-specific oligonucleotide (ASO) probes that are labeled so they can be detected (Figure 16.1C). Such probes differ only by a single nucleotide (the polymorphic site, which is generally in the middle of the ASO). In the simplest of these types of assays, hybridization conditions are chosen such that each ASO hybridizes only to its specific allele. The presence of one mismatched nucleotide is enough to prevent annealing under the hybridization conditions used. The DNA sequence surrounding the polymorphic site determines whether conditions can be identified in which the ASO probe hybridizes only to its matching allele and not to the other allele. If this is not possible, the less stable DNA duplex (that containing the mismatched nucleotide) can be distinguished from the perfect match by its melting temperature (Tm), which is an indicator of the stability of the duplex. The mismatched duplex is less stable and consequently has a lower Tm. This technique, however, is more complicated and time consuming.

In the past several years, new high-throughput techniques have been developed for SNP genotyping, some of which are beginning to be used in studies of critically ill patients [3,4]. These techniques

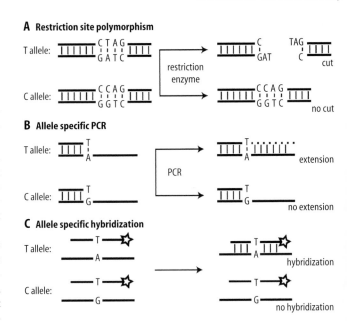

FIGURE 16.1. Genotyping of polymorphic sites. (A) Genotyping by restriction site polymorphism. The polymorphic site has either a T or a C. When the T is present, a restriction enzyme recognition site is formed that is cleaved in the presence of the restriction enzyme as determined by gel electrophoresis. If C is present at the site, the restriction enzyme does not cut. **(B)** Genotyping by allele-specific polymerase chain reaction (PCR). Reactions contain a common primer and an allele-specific primer ending with one of the nucleotides found at the polymorphic site. In this example, the allele-specific primer shown is for the T allele and only extension from the allele-specific primer, not the common primer. If the patient has the T allele, the last nucleotide will hybridize and extension will occur, allowing a productive PCR reaction. If the patient contains the C allele, the last nucleotide of the primer cannot hybridize and extension does not occur, resulting in no PCR product. With this technique two PCR reactions have to be performed with each patient sample. Each reaction contains a common primer and one of the two allele-specific primers. The presence of a PCR product is determined by gel electrophoresis. **(C)** Genotyping by allele-specific hybridization. Two allele-specific oligonucleotide (ASO) probes are made that are identical except for the polymorphic site. The probes are tagged for visualization as indicated by the stars. Only the allele-specific probe for the T allele is shown. The ASO will hybridize only to the DNA that contains a perfectly matched complementary sequence, in this case the T allele. Although only one reaction is shown (that containing the ASO with the T), two reactions containing the two different ASOs are performed for each patient sample. When unhybridized probe is washed away the hybridization can be visualized in a variety of ways.

include some that are performed in solution and others that are solid-phase reactions performed on supports such as beads or microarray chips. Most of these techniques use hybridization, single base pair extension or "mini-sequencing," or allele-specific PCR to distinguish one allele from another. Some of the detection techniques used include fluorescence, fluorescence polarization, and mass spectrometry. The different techniques available and their advantages and disadvantages have been reviewed by others elsewhere [1,2,5–8]. Which of these techniques will prove the most reliable and cost effective is not yet known. Certainly care will have to be used in applying these techniques, and appropriate controls will be required to illustrate reproducibility and reliability.

Genetic Polymorphisms and Sepsis

Individuals respond to infections and antimicrobial therapies in a highly variable fashion. Most patients will recover and do well, while a small but significant portion will develop severe sepsis and may develop multiple organ system failure, refractory hypotension, and die. This variability in the susceptibility to and outcome from sepsis, which is considered to be the most common cause of death in children in the world, has been attributed to a number of factors. These include the virulence of the etiologic agent and the length of time between onset of symptoms and initiation of treatment. However, the genetic makeup of the host also appears to play an important role in the susceptibility to and the development of sepsis, as well as its severity and outcome. For example, familial studies in which there were deaths due to severe infections demonstrated a strong genetic influence [9].

The body's inflammatory response to bacterial infection first requires recognition of pathogen-associated bacterial products. The initial recognition and the resultant response require dozens of cellular proteins, many of which are polymorphic. Genetic variation within these polymorphic genes may influence the overall response to the infection. In this section we discuss the evidence that genetic variability in specific genes plays a role in development of sepsis and its outcome [for review, see 10].

Recognition

Thus far, studies demonstrating associations between genetic polymorphisms in some of the genes coding for proteins involved in recognition and response to bacterial infection, and susceptibility to and outcome from sepsis, have implicated several genes involved with pathogen recognition as possibly being involved in the variability observed in individuals. Such genes include the toll-like receptor 4 (TLR4) gene, the mannose binding lectin (MBL) gene, and the Fcγ receptor (FcγR) genes (Table 16.1).

Lipopolysaccharide (LPS), one of the major components of the cell wall of Gram-negative bacteria, binds to a cell surface receptor composed of at least three proteins: TLR4, CD14, and MD-2 [11–15]. A number of studies suggest that variations in the TLR4 gene can generate variability in susceptibility and/or response to infection. In mice, TLR4 is required for response to LPS [16], and a single amino acid change can significantly reduce response to LPS [14,17] and enhance susceptibility to infection. In the human TLR4 gene, two SNPs have been identified that result in the replacement of an aspartic acid at amino acid position 299 with glycine and a threonine at amino acid position 399 with an isoleucine. The Gly299Ile399 variant appears to be expressed at lower levels in human airway epithelia [18], and a number of studies have demonstrated association of this variant with a reduced response to LPS as determined by examining airway reactivity or systemic cytokine response to inhaled LPS [18–20]. This variant is also associated with a diminished response to LPS in a transfected cell system using primary human epithelial cells [18]. An association of the TLR4 Gly299Ile399 variant with Gram-negative bacterial infections and septic shock [21,22] and mortality in systemic inflammatory response syndrome [23] has also been demonstrated in humans. However, the Gly299Ile399 variant showed no association with susceptibility to, or severity of, meningococcal disease [24], although other rare TLR4 mutations have been implicated in meningococcal susceptibility [25]. The lack of any association of the Gly299Ile399 variant with meningococcal disease may be explained by the observation that *Neisseria meningitides* is capable of eliciting an inflammatory response via the TLR2 receptor in the absence of LPS [26,27].

Another component of the host immune system involved in recognition of bacterial invasion is the group of leukocyte Fcγ receptors (see Table 16.1). These receptors bind to the constant region of

TABLE 16.1. Genetic polymorphisms and risk of infection and sepsis.

Gene	Polymorphism*	Consequence of polymorphism
TLR4	Asp299Gly/Thr399Ile	Gly/Ile associated with decreased expression; associated with increased risk of sepsis and mortality
FcγRIIa	H131R	R associated with decreased affinity to IgG$_2$ and opsonization; associated with increased risk of infection and septic shock
MBL	Variants B, C, D	Variants associated with decreased levels and activity; associated with increased risk of infection
TNF-α	−308 G/A, others	A associated with increased levels; associated with increased mortality in sepsis and meningococcal disease
LT-α or TNF-β	LT-α+250 G/A	A associated with increased levels; associated with increased mortality in sepsis and bacteremia
IL-1RA	Variable 86-bp repeat	A2 associated with increased levels of IL-1RA; variable results of association studies examining risk of sepsis and mortality
IL-6	−174 G/C	G associated with increased IL-6 levels in patients, but C associated with increased levels in monocytes from neonates; associated with sepsis in neonates but not adults
IL-10	−1082 G/A, −819 C/T, −592 C/A	GCC haplotype associated with increased levels; associated with sepsis but not mortality
HSP70-2	+1267 G/A	G associated with lower mRNA levels; A associated with septic shock in adults with CAP
ACE	I/D	DD associated with increased serum and tissue levels; associated with more severe meningococcal disease
PAI-1	4G/5G	4G associated with increased levels; associated with septic shock in meningococcal disease

*The terms used for the various polymorphisms are the ones most commonly used in the literature and may refer to the nucleotide position, amino acid position, or name of the allele. This table is representative of polymorphisms examined in sepsis but does not include all such polymorphisms.
Note: TLR, toll-like receptor; Ig, immunoglobulin; MBL, mannose binding lectin; TNF, tumor necrosis factor; LT, lymphotoxin; IL-1RA, interleukin-1 receptor antagonist (GCC haplotype of the IL-10 promoter is defined by three single-site polymorphisms at −1082, −819, and −592); HSP, heat shock protein; CAP, community-acquired pneumonia; ACE, angiotensin-converting enzyme; PAI, plasminogen activator inhibitor.

IgG and are primarily responsible for the phagocytosis of immunoglobulin G (IgG)–coated bacteria and induction of the inflammatory response [28,29]. The human Fcγ receptors are grouped into three classes, which vary in their affinity for the various IgG subclasses. The FcγRI class consists of the FcγRIa receptor; the FcγRII class consists of FcγRIIa, FcγRIIb, and FcγRIIc; and the FcγRIII class consists of FcγRIIIa and FcγRIIIb. Genetic polymorphisms affecting function have been described in three of the Fcγ receptors [29]. The FcγRIIIa has a polymorphism at amino acid 158 resulting in either a valine (V) or phenylalanine (F) at this position, which in turn affects its affinity for IgG$_1$, IgG$_3$, and IgG$_4$ [30,31]. The FcγRIIIb has a polymorphism that is a four amino acid substitution (allotypes FcγRIIIb-NA1 or -NA2), resulting in differences in glycosylation [32]. This substitution alters the opsonization efficiency required for phagocytosis of IgG$_1$- and IgG$_3$-opsonized particles [33,34]. Individuals homozygous for the FcγRIIIb-NA1 allotype appear to have more efficient phagocytosis. The FcγRIIa gene has a polymorphic site at amino acid position 131 [35,36] that results in either a histidine (FcγRIIa-H131) or an arginine (FcγRIIa-R131) at amino acid position 131. This amino acid is in the extracellular domain of the receptor, and the FcγRIIa-R131 allotype binds the Fc portion of IgG$_2$ with lower affinity than the more common FcγRIIa-H131 allotype [36]. In vitro studies have demonstrated reduced phagocytosis of IgG$_2$-opsonized particles in cells from individuals homozygous for FcγRIIa-R131 compared with cells from individuals homozygous for FcγRIIa-H131 [37,38]. Immunoglobulin G$_2$ is the main antibody subtype directed against encapsulated bacteria such as *Streptococcus pneumoniae*, *Haemophilus influenzae* type b, and *N. meningitides* and plays an important role in their phagocytosis [36,39,40]. Studies have examined the association between the presence of the FcγRIIa-R131 and/or the FcγRIIIb-NA2 polymorphisms in individuals and an increased susceptibility to infections, particularly meningococcal disease. Although the vast majority of reports have shown an association between infection and/or sepsis and the FcγRIIa and FcγRIIIb polymorphisms, there are two reports where no association was seen [41,42]. However, in most studies higher frequencies of the FcγRIIa-R131/R131 or FcγRIIIb-Na2/Na2 genotypes have been found in patients with meningococcal disease [43–48], particularly in patients with severe meningococcal disease [45,46] or fulminant meningococcal septic shock [43,44] when compared with a healthy control population. An association between the FcγRIIa polymorphism and infection with other encapsulated bacteria has also been reported [49,50]. Thus, genetic variation in the gene coding for at least two of the Fcγ receptors appears to influence the susceptibility to and outcome from infection with encapsulated bacteria.

Mannose binding lectin is also involved with the opsonization [51] of bacteria and binds to bacterial surface oligosaccharides N-acetyl glucosamine and mannose [52]. The heterotrimeric MBL protein contains a carbohydrate binding domain and a helical tail domain that is important in polymerization of the three peptides [53]. Polymerization of the heterotrimer is crucial for the stability of MBL. Three genetic polymorphisms have been described in MBL in the amino acids at the positions 52, 54, and 57 (referred to as variants D, C, and B, respectively). These polymorphic sites result in amino acid changes that diminish the ability of the helical tails to polymerize, resulting in an increased degradation of MBL [51,54,55] and reduced serum levels of MBL [55]. Studies have demonstrated associations among these MBL genetic polymorphisms and increased susceptibility to infections [56], hospitalizations because of infections in children [57], number of acute respiratory infections in children [58], increased risk for meningococcal infections [59], susceptibility to infections in patients with systemic lupus erythematosus [60], increased risk for recurrent respiratory infections [61], and increased susceptibility to invasive pneumococcal disease even in individuals with at least one copy of the variant polymorphism [62]. Thus, as with the genetic polymorphisms in the genes coding for the FcγRIIa and FcγRIIIb receptors, there appears to be an association between the MBL genetic variants and susceptibility to bacterial infections.

Response

Proinflammatory cytokines, such as tumor necrosis factor- α (TNF-α), interleukin-1 (IL-1), and IL-6, are produced and secreted within minutes of a pathogenic stimulus and result in the secretion of many other cytokines and chemokines. This is balanced by the subsequent release of antiinflammatory cytokines such as IL-10 and a return to baseline of cytokines and chemokines [63,64]. It is now generally accepted that an overexaggerated proinflammatory response resulting in an imbalance between the proinflammatory and antiinflammatory cytokines results in the clinical manifestation of severe sepsis and septic shock. The mechanism by which this imbalance occurs leading to exaggerated response is an area of intense research. Genetic variability within genes coding for the proinflammatory and antiinflammatory cytokines might influence this balance and could potentially influence the overall susceptibility to and outcome from the sepsis.

Tumor necrosis factor-α and the genetic polymorphisms within the regulatory regions of the gene coding for TNF-α are perhaps the most extensively studied of all sepsis-induced cytokines. We will discuss the genetic polymorphisms found in the TNF-α locus in more detail here and briefly mention other polymorphisms and association studies. As a proinflammatory cytokine, TNF-α plays a key role in the pathogenesis of the acute inflammatory response and is responsible for the activation of the inflammatory response. Tumor necrosis factor-α is also responsible for the development of the harmful effects of the systemic inflammatory response such as capillary leak, hypotension, acute respiratory distress syndrome (ARDS), and multiple organ system failure [65–69]. Several SNPs within the regulatory region of the gene coding for TNF-α have been identified that impact TNF-α production [70–77]. The most studied are the G to A transitions 308 and 238 base pairs upstream from the transcriptional start site for the TNF-α gene. In vitro studies have demonstrated that the rarer TNF-α–308A allele is associated with increased transcription [77] and increased secretion of TNF-α from LPS-stimulated macrophages [72] compared with the more common TNF-α–308G allele. In contrast, the more common TNF-α–238G allele is associated with higher TNF-α production in vitro compared with the rarer TNF-α–238A allele [78]. These polymorphisms lie near putative DNA binding sites for several transcription factors, and in vitro studies have demonstrated differential binding of nuclear proteins to DNA fragments containing either an A or a G at the TNF-α–308 position [79].

Another polymorphism associated with higher levels of TNF-α is approximately 250 base pairs downstream from the transcriptional start site for the gene coding for lymphotoxin-α (LT-α, also known as TNF-β). This site (also referred to as the TNFB allele, LT-α+250, and TNF-β+252 site; for this chapter, LT-α+250 site will be used) is approximately 3.2 kb upstream from the TNF-α gene. Higher serum levels of TNF-α have been demonstrated in septic patients with the LT-α+250A allele [73–75]. Consequently, either this region acts as an enhancer for the TNF-α gene, or it is linked to a regulatory region further downstream. In any case, the data from studies of the TNF-α–308, TNF-α–238, and LT-α+250 alleles provide convincing evidence that genetic variation within regulatory regions of the gene coding for TNF-α influences the amount of TNF-α produced.

Most association studies have suggested that the TNF-α polymorphisms influence the clinical presentation and/or outcome in children with meningococcal infections [80] or bacteremia [73] and in adults with septic shock [70,75,81,82], or community-acquired pneumonia [83]. Specifically, the frequency of the TNF-α–308A allele is higher in adults who died with septic shock [82] and in children who died from meningococcal disease than in controls [80]. Even those children who were heterozygous at this position

(TNF-α–308 G/A) were at increased risk for more fulminant meningococcal disease and death compared with those children who were homozygous for the wild-type genotype (TNF-α–308 G/G). At the LT-α+250 site, analysis of a cohort of adults with community-acquired pneumonia demonstrated that those with the A/A genotype were at greater risk for presenting with the clinical symptoms of sepsis [83]. Patients in postoperative and trauma intensive care units who developed sepsis and were homozygous for the LT-α+250 A allele have higher levels of TNF-α and a higher mortality rate [75,84,85]. Similarly, an association among the LT-α+250 A allele, higher serum levels of TNF-α, and higher mortality rate in bacteremic children has been observed [73]. Children who were heterozygous at this position (LT-α+250 GA) had an intermediate mortality rate. Thus, most evidence appears to support an association among certain genotypes in the regulatory region of the gene coding for TNF-α, levels of TNF-α production, and mortality rate of patients with sepsis.

Genetic polymorphisms in many other proinflammatory and antiinflammatory cytokines that influence the levels or function of the cytokines have also been examined to determine whether these genetic variations are associated with susceptibility to or outcome from sepsis (see Table 16.1). These include IL-1α, IL-1β, IL-1$_{RA}$ [86–88], IL-6 [89–91], IL-8 [92–95], and IL-10 [96–99], and the list continues to grow rapidly as more polymorphisms in cytokine genes are discovered. Several of the above-mentioned cytokines contain polymorphisms that appear to be associated with sepsis. The reader is referred to a recent review for more detail [10].

Genetic polymorphisms within noncytokine genes have also been examined for the influence of genetic variations on critically ill patients. Heat shock proteins (HSPs) are a family of stress-inducible proteins expressed in response to heat as well as a number of other noxious stimuli, including endotoxin and other mediators of severe sepsis [100]. These proteins play an important role in cell survival during stress [101] and are involved in a number of important cellular functions, including the folding, assembly, and translocation of proteins across membranes [102,103]. Polymorphisms within the genes coding for HSPs that influence HSP production [104] have been shown to be associated with more organ system failure in trauma patients [105] and the development of septic shock but not mortality in adults with community-acquired pneumonia [106].

Angiotensin I–converting enzyme (ACE) is present in all tissues, particularly the pulmonary endothelium. Angiotensin I–converting enzyme is primarily responsible for converting angiotensin I to angiotensin II but is also involved in the metabolism of chemotactic peptides, suggesting that it may play a role in the inflammatory response. Individuals have been shown to have variable plasma and tissue levels of ACE, and evidence suggests that these variable levels are caused in part by genetic factors [107]. Specifically, an insertion (I)/deletion (D) of a 287 base repair repeat sequence in the noncoding intron 16 of the gene coding for ACE [108,109] is associated with variable plasma levels; individuals with the DD genotype have higher plasma and tissue levels of ACE than individuals who are heterozygous or are homozygous for the insertion sequence [110,111]. Association studies have suggested that the D/D polymorphism is associated with more severe meningococcal disease in children as measured by a higher predicted risk of mortality, greater prevalence of inotropic support and mechanical ventilation, and longer intensive care unit stay [112].

The pathogenesis of multiple organ system failure in sepsis is believed to involve in part endothelial dysfunction and intravascular fibrin deposition [113]. Diminished activity of anticoagulants, or elevated levels of inhibitors of fibrinolysis, can lead to fibrin deposition and may contribute to multiple organ system failure. Plasminogen activator inhibitor 1 (PAI-1) is an inhibitor of fibrinolysis because of its ability to inhibit the potent fibrinolytic, plasminogen activator. High plasma concentrations of PAI-1 have been observed in sepsis [114] and severe meningococcal disease [115], and high concentrations are correlated with worse outcome. A single nucleotide I/D polymorphism exists within the promoter region of the gene coding for PAI-1 that appears to influence the amount of PAI-1 production, with individuals homozygous for the 4G/4G genotype producing more PAI-1 than either individuals heterozygous (4G/5G) or homozygous for five guanines (5G/5G) [116]. Children with the 4G/4G genotype who had meningococcal disease had higher plasma levels of PAI-1 [117] and an increased risk of death from sepsis than did children with either the 4G/5G or the 5G/5G genotype [117–119]. This polymorphism is not only associated with outcome from meningococcal disease but appears to be a marker for poor outcome after severe trauma [120]. Thus, there appears to be a strong association between the 4G/4G genotype in the PAI-1 gene, high plasma concentrations of PAI-1, and worse outcome in critical illness.

In summary, there are a number of polymorphisms within genes involved in recognition of bacterial pathogens and response to bacterial pathogens that appear to be associated with the development of sepsis and its outcome (see Table 16.1). In a number of cases, changes in the level or the function of the gene's protein product has been documented.

Genetic Polymorphisms in Acute Respiratory Failure and Lung Injury

Respiratory failure is one of the major reasons for admission to both adult ICUs and PICUs. The causes of respiratory failure in children are too numerous to list here but include pulmonary causes such as ARDS, asthma, and bronchopulmonary dysplasia; infectious causes such as pneumonia and bronchiolitis; and neurologic causes such as central hypoventilation and ingestions. Thus, the list of potential genetic polymorphisms that may influence respiratory failure is likely to be very diverse. We discuss two examples of genes that play a role in respiratory physiology and inflammation for which data suggest that polymorphisms may influence the degree of respiratory failure and lung injury in critically ill patients.

Community-acquired pneumonia is a primary cause of respiratory failure in both children and adults. Although most individuals with community-acquired pneumonia have minimal lung injury, a small but significant number develop respiratory failure and severe lung injury. The most severe form of lung injury is ARDS and results in high morbidity and mortality in both children and adults. This variability in the degree of lung injury in patients with community-acquired pneumonia raises the possibility that genetic variation influences the susceptibility to and outcome from lung injury.

Genes coding for proteins involved in normal lung physiology, such as pulmonary surfactant, are ideal candidate genes in which genetic variation might influence the degree of lung injury and respiratory failure. Indeed, it has been suggested that alterations in surfactant may play important roles in these processes [121,122].

Surfactant contains four major proteins, A, B, C, and D, which exhibit a variety of functions, including a role in host defenses in the lung [123–128] and the reduction of surface tension at the air–liquid interface. The surfactant protein-A (SP-A) genes as well as SP-B, -C, and –D genes are polymorphic, and polymorphisms in these genes have been associated with lung disease [129–132]. The polymorphisms in the SP-A genes (A1 and A2) and SP-B gene are the best characterized, and many reports have shown association of these genes with lung disease [130,131,133–136]. We will discuss SP-B and how a common genetic polymorphism in the gene coding for SP-B may influence respiratory failure and lung injury in critically ill children.

Deficiency in, or impaired activity of, SP-B is implicated in a variety of interstitial pulmonary diseases, including acute respiratory failure and death in newborns and mice [137–139], increased sensitivity to hyperoxia [140], human congenital proteinosis [141,142], respiratory distress syndrome in premature infants [143,144], and ARDS [130,145,146]. Indeed, in patients with ARDS, both a lower level of surfactant proteins in bronchoalveolar lavage fluid [146,147] and a diminished ability of surfactant to lower surface tension have been found [148]. In addition, calfactant, a natural lung surfactant containing high levels of SP-B, improved oxygenation and decreased mortality in children with acute lung injury [149]. Genetic variations in the regulatory or functional regions of the gene encoding for SP-B may, therefore, influence susceptibility to, and outcome from, severe lung injury and respiratory failure.

The gene coding for SP-B is located on chromosome 2 and consists of 11 exons, including a 3′-untranslated sequence [150]. Surfactant protein-B is synthesized as a 381-amino acid precursor protein that is proteolytically cleaved to the active 79-amino acid form. Several SNPs within intron 2, exon 4, and the 5′ and 3′ flanking regions of the gene coding for SP-B have been identified. A C/T nucleotide variation at position 1580 in exon 4 changes amino acid 131 from threonine to isoleucine [141], altering a site for N-linked glycosylation [151,152]. Glycosylation of this site may impact the processing and/or function of SP-B [152,153] resulting in decreased functional SP-B. We have examined the genetic polymorphism in the SP-B+1580 site in adults with community-acquired pneumonia and demonstrated that a higher percentage of those individuals with the less common C/C genotype developed respiratory failure requiring mechanical ventilation and met the criteria for ARDS compared with those individuals with the T/C or T/T genotypes [154]. Whether or not this polymorphism is associated with more severe lung injury in children with community-acquired pneumonia is currently being investigated.

Another candidate gene in which polymorphisms might be associated with more severe lung injury is the gene coding for ACE. As mentioned earlier, ACE is present in the pulmonary endothelium and is responsible for converting angiotensin I to angiotensin II (ATII). In adults with ARDS, ACE concentrations in bronchoalveolar lavage fluid are elevated [155] as are the transpulmonary gradient and circulating concentrations of ATII [156]. An association between the D allele, which is associated with higher plasma tissue levels of ACE as described earlier, and ARDS has been observed in adults [157]. A higher percentage of adults with ARDS had the D/D genotype than did adults who were at risk for the development of ARDS, including those who underwent coronary artery bypass graft surgery or were in the ICU for other reasons. Thus, the genetic variation in the ACE gene may be associated with more severe lung injury.

Genetic Polymorphisms in Cardiovascular Surgery

Children who have undergone cardiovascular surgery represent a significant number of patients in pediatric and/or cardiovascular intensive care units. Whether genetic polymorphisms are associated with various complications in the post-operative period in this population is another area of intense research. One of the potential sources of many of the complications observed in the post-operative period may be the release of inflammatory mediators, including TNF-α, IL-6, IL-8, and ATII [158]. Studies of adults and children undergoing cardiovascular surgery involving the use of cardiopulmonary bypass have demonstrated a release of proinflammatory and antiinflammatory cytokines after surgery [159]. Various stimuli have been suggested to initiate cytokine release after cardiopulmonary bypass, including exposure of blood to the foreign surface of the bypass machine, complement activation [160,161], ischemia–reperfusion injury [162], and endotoxin released because of gastrointestinal tract hypoperfusion [163]. Whatever the inciting event, this inflammatory cascade may result in postoperative complications such as cardiovascular instability, systemic inflammatory response syndrome, and multiple organ dysfunction [164–166]. As discussed previously, genetic variation influences the levels of many of the proinflammatory and antiinflammatory cytokines. It is plausible, therefore, that the complications observed in patients after exposure to cardiopulmonary bypass may be, in part, influenced by genetic variation.

Few studies have examined the association between polymorphisms in genes involved in inflammation and complications in children who have undergone cardiac surgery, and, therefore, we will discuss studies examining these associations in adults who have undergone coronary artery bypass graft (CABG) surgery. Mechanical ventilation greater than 24 hours after CABG is considered prolonged and is a well-known complication of CABG observed in adults. Approximately 6% of patients undergoing their first CABG surgery and 11% of those undergoing repeated CABG surgery are unable to be tracheally extubated by 24 hours [167]. The etiologies for prolonged mechanical ventilation include both pulmonary-related (atelectasis, bronchospasm, congestive heart failure [CHF], ARDS, and acute lung injury) and nonpulmonary-related (cerebrovascular accident, cardiogenic shock, and excess postoperative bleeding) events. Understanding the underlying mechanisms resulting in prolonged mechanical ventilation might allow both identification of those patients at increased risk and development of therapies and strategies specific for such patients.

The associations between genetic polymorphisms located in genes coding for TNF-α, LT-α, IL-10, IL-6, and ATII and various complications after cardiopulmonary bypass have been studied [168–172]. We have examined the association between some of these polymorphisms and prolonged mechanical ventilation in adults who have undergone CABG surgery [173]. Adults with the A/A "TNF-α hypersecretor" genotype at either the TNF-α–308 or the LT-α+250 sites demonstrated overall shorter times to extubation and lower risk of prolonged mechanical ventilation. This appears to be contrary to the idea that hypersecretion of proinflammatory mediators may be detrimental to patients in the postoperative period [174,175]. Possible explanations for the apparent beneficial effect of TNF-α are that TNF-α appears to protect the myocardium from hypoxic insults [176,177] and that TNF-α stimulates protective HSPs [178–180]. Further studies are needed to better define the role of proinflammatory mediators in prolonged mechanical ventilation in this population.

Another potential mediator that could play a role in postoperative complications is ATII. Animal studies have demonstrated that ATII plays a role in myocardial ischemia–reperfusion injury [181] and contributes to depression of myocardial function [182]. Elevation of ATII may contribute to various causes of prolonged mechanical ventilation discussed earlier; for instance, its role in ischemia–reperfusion injury may contribute to postoperative ARDS/acute lung injury, whereas cardiac effects may increase postoperative CHF. As mentioned previously, ACE is present in the pulmonary endothelium and converts ATI to ATII. Concentrations of ACE are elevated after CABG surgery [183], and these elevated concentrations appear to be influenced in part by genetic polymorphisms. Other studies have demonstrated that adults with the D allele had higher mortality and restenosis rates after CABG surgery compared with patients with the I allele [184]. Also, as mentioned previously, the D allele appears to be associated with susceptibility to and prognosis of ARDS [157], an important cause of prolonged mechanical ventilation in the postoperative period for adults who have undergone CABG surgery. The ACE D allele is also associated with prolonged mechanical ventilation in this population except for patients who had their CABG procedure off-pump [185]. This observation suggests that the off-pump approach for those patients with the D/D genotype who are at higher risk for prolonged mechanical ventilation may decrease the incidence of this complication.

The risk for prolonged mechanical ventilation in the CABG population (like many of the conditions treated in the ICU) may be influenced by multiple proteins and their genetic polymorphisms. Currently there are an increasing number of studies examining the association of genetic polymorphisms in multiple genes with certain clinical conditions. The associations of the I/D polymorphism in the ACE gene and the TNF-α–308 and LT-α+250 polymorphisms with the risk of prolonged mechanical ventilation in the CABG population have been analyzed. Individuals with the G/G haplotype at TNF-α–308 and LT-α+250 loci and the D/D polymorphism of the ACE gene had a significantly higher adjusted hazards ratio than did individuals who did not have the G/G haplotype at TNF-α–308 and LT-α+250 loci and had the I/I polymorphism of the ACE gene [185]. Thus, data are beginning to suggest that some of the postoperative complications observed after cardiopulmonary bypass may be influenced by genetic variation in the host. In addition, the possible influences of genetic variation in receptors and/or components of the signal transduction pathways of the various inotropic agents, vasoconstrictors, and vasodilators used in the care of children who have undergone cardiovascular surgery are also beginning to be analyzed.

Genetic Polymorphisms in Thrombosis

Thromboses in both arteries and veins are significant problems in children in PICUs [186–192]. These children are exposed to multiple risk factors for thrombosis, including sepsis and central venous catheters, with reports of deep venous thrombosis in 7.5% to 50% of children with central venous catheters [193–196]. A number of inherited defects in the coagulation and thrombolytic systems also predispose children to thrombosis [197–199]. These defects can result in hyperactive coagulation, hypoactive anticoagulation, or hypoactive fibrinolysis. Several genetic variations (Table 16.2) have been identified in genes coding for components of the coagulation system that influence the quantity or function of these proteins and

TABLE 16.2. Genetic polymorphisms examined for associations with risk of thrombosis.

Gene	Polymorphism*	Consequence of polymorphism
Factor V	G1691A; Arg506Gln; (factor V Leiden)	Resists activated protein C
Prothrombin	G20210A (in 3'-UTR)	Increased levels; associated with risk of deep venous thrombosis
Antithrombin	Multiple sites	Decreased levels and activity
Protein C	Multiple sites in promoter	Decreased levels; associated with risk of venous thrombosis
Protein S	Multiple sites	Decreased levels; increased thrombosis
Fibrinogen	Thr312Ala	Affects structure/function and FXIII cross-linking; associated with pulmonary embolism
Methylentetrahydrofolate reductase	C677T; Val/Ala	Decreased enzymatic activity; increased levels of homocysteine; associated with arteriovenous fistula
Endothelial nitric oxide synthase	G894T; Glu298Asp	Less stable enzyme; associated with restenosis of stents; associated with myocardial infarcts
Factor XIII A	Val34Leu	Increased cleavage and activation; associated with deep venous thrombosis

*The terms used for the various polymorphisms are the ones most commonly used in the literature and may refer to the nucleotide position, amino acid position, or name of the allele. This table is representative of polymorphisms examined in thrombosis but does not include all such polymorphisms.

have been shown to be significant risk factors for thrombosis [198,200]. These include variations in genes coding for factor V [201], prothrombin [202–205], antithrombin [206–210], protein C [211–215], protein S [216–221], methylentetrahydrofolate reductase [222], endothelial nitric oxide synthase [223–225], α-fibrinogen [226–229], and factor XIII [228,230–235]. However, no researchers have reported the relative risks of these various genetic polymorphisms in the development of thrombosis in children in PICUs. The Arg506Gln polymorphism in the factor V gene (factor V Leiden) has been reported in 13%–45% of pediatric patients with thromboembolism [236–239], but this population may not necessarily reflect the population of PICU patients who also have the other nonhereditary risk factors mentioned earlier. Because the development of thrombosis can be deterred with anticoagulants, knowledge of a child's genetic polymorphisms in the genes coding for components of the coagulation system might identify children who could benefit most by anticoagulant therapies.

Pharmacogenomics

Another area of pediatric critical care in which genetic polymorphisms influence critical illness is pharmacology. Pharmacogenomics attempts to determine the genetic factors that affect the various aspects of drug action, including drug transport, binding to receptors and signal transduction, and metabolism. That genetics can influence some drug responses was first suggested by associations between inheritance or ethnicity and abnormal drug responses and further defined through biochemistry and molecular genetics [for review, see refs. 240–243]. While the list of genetic polymorphisms in genes coding for drug transporters, receptors, and enzymes involved in drug metabolism is growing rapidly [244], there are very few examples of genetic polymorphisms that influence the action of drugs commonly used in PICUs.

The best-described examples of genetic polymorphisms that influence drug response are those that are found in genes coding for enzymes involved in drug metabolism (Table 16.3). One example is briefly described here in order to demonstrate the clinical relevance of such genetic variations. Thiopurine S-methyltransferase (TPMT) is an enzyme primarily responsible for inactivation of the thiopurines mercaptopurine and azathioprine used as immunosuppressants and chemotherapeutic drugs. Genetic polymorphisms in the gene coding for TPMT result in a nonfunctioning enzyme; thus, patients receiving mercaptopurine or azathioprine who inherit the nonfunctional allele accumulate high concentrations of the active metabolites and are at risk for developing life-threatening hematopoietic toxicities [245–247]. Clinical diagnostic tests are available for detecting the SNPs in the TPMT gene that result in TPMT deficiency, thereby allowing for the identification of patients at high risk for thiopurine toxicities. Patients receiving mercaptopurine or azathioprine who are genetically predisposed to be TPMT deficient have been treated successfully for their oncologic diseases using approximately 5%–10% of the conventional dose of the thiopurines [245,246] without the toxicities. This represents a good example of modifying drug therapies based on an individual's genetic makeup.

A second example of a genetic variability that may influence drug action involves the β_2-adrenergic receptor (β_2-AR). β_2-Adrenergic receptor agonists are the most potent bronchodilators and continue to be the mainstay treatment for exacerbations of asthma [248]. β_2-Agonists activate the β_2-AR, resulting in coupling of the receptor–agonist complex to G_s, which in turn activates adenylate cyclase and increases the intracellular production of cyclic AMP (cAMP), resulting in the dilation of the smooth muscle lining the small bronchiolar airways [249]. Substantial variation in β_2-AR response between individuals has been observed [250]. Over the past several years many studies have examined the possibility that alterations in β_2-AR function might be associated with asthma, severity of asthma, or asthma phenotypes.

A number of SNPs within the gene coding for the β_2-AR have been identified [251]. An SNP upstream of the coding region (−47 C/T) appears to be associated with the regulation of β_2-AR expression in the cell [252,253]. In addition, the two most common SNPs, glycine or arginine at position 16 (Gly16 or Arg16) and glutamic acid or glutamine at position 27 (Glu27 or Gln27), alter the amino acid sequence of the β_2-AR, which in turn alters properties of the receptor [251]. More recently, Drysdale et al. [254] genotyped 13 SNPs in ~80 individuals and identified 12 different combinations of these individual SNPS in the β_2-AR gene, meaning that there are 12 β_2-AR haplotypes (and hence alleles). Only one haplotype has Glu at amino acid 27; this is also the only haplotype with C at the −47 polymorphic site [254]. The β_2-AR variant with C at −47 has been shown to express lower levels of the receptor than variants with T at that site [252,253].

Studies have investigated the association of β_2-AR SNPs with asthma, asthma phenotype, or treatment modalities. Such studies have been performed primarily with single SNPs in the adult Caucasian population. Although there is no strong evidence linking a specific β_2-AR genotype to asthma, there are a number of studies linking specific genotypes to asthma phenotypes [255–260]. In children there is an association between the homozygous Gly16 genotype and bronchodilator desensitization [261], and we have recently reported an association of the Gln27Glu genotype with the need for aminophylline treatment in African-American children with status asthmaticus [262]. Aminophylline inhibits phosphodiesterase, the enzyme responsible for degradation of cAMP, and consequently the level of β_2-AR–stimulated cAMP is greater and its degradation is delayed, prolonging the elevated cAMP levels in the cell. These results suggest that African-American children with this genotype may have diminished response to β_2-agonist therapy and may respond more effectively to treatment with a phosphodiesterase inhibitor in addition to the β_2-agonist therapy. One possible explanation for the association of the Gln27Glu genotype with aminophylline treatment is that these patients may have a lower β_2-agonist–stimulated cAMP response than patients with the Gln27Gln genotype, and aminophylline addition may be required to increase cAMP to levels that are clinically efficacious. Presumably the Glu27 variant is responsible, as the need for aminophylline treatment is seen only in patients who have this variant of the receptor. A lower cAMP response could be caused by lower expression of the Glu27 variant, which has been reported in in vitro studies [252,253], or by increased desensitization of the β_2-AR Glu27 variant, which is still controversial as different studies have concluded that the Glu27 variant undergoes greater [263] or lesser [264] desensitization than the Gln27 variant.

Limitations

Association studies attempting to examine the influence of genetic polymorphisms in specific diseases have several limitations that are important to keep in mind when reading the literature. A few of these limitations are briefly discussed here, and the reader is referred to a more comprehensive review of these limitations [265]. First, it is important that the correct control population is used in

TABLE 16.3. Genes in which polymorphisms alter drug effects.

Gene*	Specific drug or drug class	Consequence of polymorphism
β_2-Adrenergic receptor	Albuterol, terbutaline	Decreased bronchodilation
α_1-Adrenergic receptor	α_1-Agonists	Decreased cardiovascular response to α_1-agonsts
G_s protein β	β-Blockers	Decreased antihypertensive effect
ALOX5	Leukotriene receptor antagonists	Decreased effect on FEV_1
Serotonin transporter	Antidepressants	Decreased clozapine effects, decreased antidepressant response
CYP2C9	Warfarin, phenytoin, nonsteroidal antiinflammatories	Increased anticoagulant effects of warfarin
CYP2D6	Antidepressants, codeine, β-blockers	Decreased codeine analgesia, increased antidepressant toxicity
CYP3A4/3A5/3A7	Midazolam, steroids, calcium channel blockers	Altered clearance of midazolam and steroids
CYP2C19	Omeprazole	Altered peptic ulcer response to omeprazole

*This table is representative of genes in which genetic polymorphisms have been shown to alter drug effects but does not include all such genes and their polymorphisms.

the study. For example, in some sepsis studies the frequency of a polymorphism in the group of patients with sepsis is compared with the frequency of the polymorphism in a healthy control population. However, healthy individuals are not the appropriate control population, as they may not have been exposed to the same pathogens to which the patients with sepsis were exposed. A more appropriate control group for comparison would be a group of patients with a similar infection who did not develop sepsis.

A second limitation is that in many studies subjects within the study and control groups are from various ethnic groups. It is now well known that the frequency of many of these polymorphisms varies between ethnic groups and so comparisons should only be made within ethnic groups. Finally, the specific nucleotide variation being investigated may in fact not be directly involved but rather closely linked to the actual gene responsible for the effect.

Conclusion

In summary, there is little doubt that host genetic variation is responsible for some of the variable disease presentation, response to therapy, and final outcome observed in critically ill children. Identification of genetic polymorphisms that will ultimately be useful in identifying critically ill children at increased risk will allow for a more individualized approach to therapy. Carefully controlled studies examining candidate genes alone and in combination with other genes will be required to determine whether patient treatment can be tailored more specifically to an individual patient's genetic makeup.

References

1. Kirk BW, Feinsod M, Favis R, Kliman RM, Barany F. Single nucleotide polymorphism seeking long term association with complex disease. Nucleic Acids Res 2002;30(15):3295–3311.
2. Shi MM. Enabling large-scale pharmacogenetic studies by high-throughput mutation detection and genotyping technologies. Clin Chem 2001;47(2):164–172.
3. Freeman BD, Buchman TG, McGrath S, Tabrizi AR, Zehnbauer BA. Template-directed dye-terminator incorporation with fluorescence polarization detection for analysis of single nucleotide polymorphisms implicated in sepsis. J Mol Diagn 2002;4(4):209–215.
4. Freeman BD, Buchman TG, Zehnbauer BA. Template-directed dye-terminator incorporation with fluorescence polarization detection for analysis of single nucleotide polymorphisms associated with cardiovascular and thromboembolic disease. Thromb Res 2003;111(6):373–379.
5. Chen X, Sullivan PF. Single nucleotide polymorphism genotyping: biochemistry, protocol, cost and throughput. Pharmacogenomics J 2003;3(2):77–96.
6. Kwok PY. Methods for genotyping single nucleotide polymorphisms. Annu Rev Genomics Hum Genet 2001;2:235–258.
7. Syvanen AC. From gels to chips: "minisequencing" primer extension for analysis of point mutations and single nucleotide polymorphisms. Hum Mutat 1999;13(1):1–10.
8. Syvanen AC. Accessing genetic variation: genotyping single nucleotide polymorphisms. Nat Rev Genet 2001;2(12):930–942.
9. Sorensen TI, Nielsen GG, Andersen PK, Teasdale TW. Genetic and environmental influences on premature death in adult adoptees. N Engl J Med 1988;318(12):727–732.
10. Dahmer MK, Randolph A, Vitali S, Quasney MW. Genetic polymorphisms in sepsis. Pediatr Crit Care Med 2005;6(3 Suppl):S61–S73.
11. Aderem A, Ulevitch RJ. Toll-like receptors in the induction of the innate immune response. Nature 2000;406(6797):782–787.
12. Beutler B, Poltorak A. Sepsis and evolution of the innate immune response. Crit Care Med 2001;29(7 Suppl):S2–S7.
13. Chow JC, Young DW, Golenbock DT, Christ WJ, Gusovsky F. Toll-like receptor-4 mediates lipopolysaccharide-induced signal transduction. J Biol Chem 1999;274(16):10689–10692.
14. Poltorak A, He X, Smirnova I, Liu MY, Van Huffel C, Du X, et al. Defective LPS signaling in C3H/HeJ and C57BL/10ScCr mice: mutations in Tlr4 gene. Science 1998;282(5396):2085–2088.
15. Ulevitch RJ. Regulation of receptor-dependent activation of the innate immune response. J Infect Dis 2003;187(Suppl 2):S351–S355.
16. Hoshino K, Takeuchi O, Kawai T, Sanjo H, Ogawa T, Takeda Y, et al. Cutting edge: toll-like receptor 4 (TLR4)–deficient mice are hyporesponsive to lipopolysaccharide: evidence for TLR4 as the LPS gene product. J Immunol 1999;162(7):3749–3752.
17. Qureshi ST, Lariviere L, Leveque G, Clermont S, Moore KJ, Gros P, et al. Endotoxin-tolerant mice have mutations in Toll-like receptor 4 (Tlr4). J Exp Med 1999;189(4):615–625.
18. Arbour NC, Lorenz E, Schutte BC, Zabner J, Kline JN, Jones M, et al. TLR4 mutations are associated with endotoxin hyporesponsiveness in humans. Nat Genet 2000;25(2):187–191.
19. Michel O, LeVan TD, Stern D, Dentener M, Thorn J, Gnat D, et al. Systemic responsiveness to lipopolysaccharide and polymorphisms in the toll-like receptor 4 gene in human beings. J Allergy Clin Immunol 2003;112(5):923–929.
20. Werner M, Topp R, Wimmer K, Richter K, Bischof W, Wjst M, et al. TLR4 gene variants modify endotoxin effects on asthma. J Allergy Clin Immunol 2003;112(2):323–330.
21. Agnese DM, Calvano JE, Hahm SJ, Coyle SM, Corbett SA, Calvano SE, et al. Human toll-like receptor 4 mutations but not CD14 polymorphisms are associated with an increased risk of Gram-negative infections. J Infect Dis 2002;186(10):1522–1525.
22. Lorenz E, Mira JP, Frees KL, Schwartz DA. Relevance of mutations in the TLR4 receptor in patients with Gram-negative septic shock. Arch Intern Med 2002;162(9):1028–1032.
23. Child NJ, Yang IA, Pulletz MC, de Courcy-Golder K, Andrews AL, Pappachan VJ, et al. Polymorphisms in toll-like receptor 4 and the systemic inflammatory response syndrome. Biochem Soc Trans 2003;31(Pt 3):652–653.
24. Read RC, Pullin J, Gregory S, Borrow R, Kaczmarski EB, di Giovine FS, et al. A functional polymorphism of toll-like receptor 4 is not associated with likelihood or severity of meningococcal disease. J Infect Dis 2001;184(5):640–642.
25. Smirnova I, Mann N, Dols A, Derkx HH, Hibberd ML, Levin M, et al. Assay of locus-specific genetic load implicates rare Toll-like receptor 4 mutations in meningococcal susceptibility. Proc Natl Acad Sci USA 2003;100(10):6075–6080.
26. Ingalls RR, Lien E, Golenbock DT. Membrane-associated proteins of a lipopolysaccharide-deficient mutant of Neisseria meningitidis activate the inflammatory response through toll-like receptor 2. Infect Immun 2001;69(4):2230–2236.
27. Pridmore AC, Wyllie DH, Abdillahi F, Steeghs L, van der Ley P, Dower SK, et al. A lipopolysaccharide-deficient mutant of Neisseria meningitidis elicits attenuated cytokine release by human macrophages and signals via toll-like receptor (TLR) 2 but not via TLR4/MD2. J Infect Dis 2001;183(1):89–96.
28. van der Pol W, van de Winkel JG. IgG receptor polymorphisms: risk factors for disease. Immunogenetics 1998;48(3):222–232.
29. van Sorge NM, van der Pol WL, van de Winkel JG. FcγR polymorphisms: implications for function, disease susceptibility and immunotherapy. Tissue Antigens 2003;61(3):189–202.
30. Koene HR, Kleijer M, Algra J, Roos D, von dem Borne AE, de Haas M. FcγRIIIa-158V/F polymorphism influences the binding of IgG by natural killer cell FcγRIIIa, independently of the FcγRIIIa–48L/R/H phenotype. Blood 1997;90(3):1109–1114.
31. Wu J, Edberg JC, Redecha PB, Bansal V, Guyre PM, Coleman K, et al. A novel polymorphism of FcγRIIIa (CD16) alters receptor function

and predisposes to autoimmune disease. J Clin Invest 1997;100(5): 1059–1070.

32. Huizinga TW, Kleijer M, Tetteroo PA, Roos D, von dem Borne AE. Biallelic neutrophil Na-antigen system is associated with a polymorphism on the phospho-inositol–linked Fcγ receptor III (CD16). Blood 1990;75(1):213–217.

33. Salmon JE, Millard SS, Brogle NL, Kimberly RP. Fcγ receptor IIIb enhances Fcγ receptor IIa function in an oxidant-dependent and allele-sensitive manner. J Clin Invest 1995;95(6):2877–2885.

34. Salmon JE, Edberg JC, Kimberly RP. Fcγ receptor III on human neutrophils: allelic variants have functionally distinct capacities. J Clin Invest 1990;85:1287–1295.

35. Warmerdam PA, van de Winkel JG, Gosselin EJ, Capel PJ. Molecular basis for a polymorphism of human Fcγ receptor II (CD32). J Exp Med 1990;172(1):19–25.

36. Warmerdam PA, van de Winkel JG, Vlug A, Westerdaal NA, Capel PJ. A single amino acid in the second Ig-like domain of the human Fcγ receptor II is critical for human IgG2 binding. J Immunol 1991; 147(4):1338–1343.

37. Salmon JE, Edberg JC, Brogle NL, Kimberly RP. Allelic polymorphisms of human Fcγ receptor IIA and Fcγ receptor IIIB. Independent mechanisms for differences in human phagocyte function. J Clin Inves. 1992;89(4):1274–1281.

38. Sanders LA, Feldman RG, Voorhorst-Ogink MM, de Haas M, Rijkers GT, Capel PJ, et al. Human immunoglobulin G (IgG) Fc receptor IIA (CD32) polymorphism and IgG2-mediated bacterial phagocytosis by neutrophils. Infect Immun 1995;63(1):73–81.

39. Herrmann DJ, Hamilton RG, Barington T, Frasch CE, Arakere G, Makela O, et al. Quantitation of human IgG subclass antibodies to *Haemophilus influenzae* type b capsular polysaccharide. Results of an international collaborative study using enzyme immunoassay methodology. J Immunol Methods 1992;148(1–2):101–114.

40. Siber GR, Schur PH, Aisenberg AC, Weitzman SA, Schiffman G. Correlation between serum IgG-2 concentrations and the antibody response to bacterial polysaccharide antigens. N Engl J Med 1980; 303(4):178–182.

41. Smith I, Vedeler C, Halstensen A. FcγRIIa and FcγRIIIb polymorphisms were not associated with meningococcal disease in Western Norway. Epidemiol Infect 2003;130(2):193–199.

42. Tezcan I, Berkel AI, Ersoy F, Sanal O, Kanra G. Fcγ receptor allotypes in children with bacterial meningitis. A preliminary study. Turk J Pediatr 1998;40(4):533–538.

43. Bredius RG, Derkx BH, Fijen CA, de Wit TP, de Haas M, Weening RS, et al. Fcγ receptor IIa (CD32) polymorphism in fulminant meningococcal septic shock in children. J Infect Dis 1994;170(4):848–853.

44. Domingo P, Muniz-Diaz E, Baraldes MA, Arilla M, Barquet N, Pericas R, et al. Associations between Fcγ receptor IIA polymorphisms and the risk and prognosis of meningococcal disease. Am J Med 2002; 112(1):19–25.

45. Platonov AE, Kuijper EJ, Vershinina IV, Shipulin GA, Westerdaal N, Fijen CA, et al. Meningococcal disease and polymorphism of FcγRIIa (CD32) in late complement component–deficient individuals. Clin Exp Immunol 1998;111(1):97–101.

46. Platonov AE, Shipulin GA, Vershinina IV, Dankert J, van de Winkel JG, Kuijper EJ. Association of human Fcγ RIIa (CD32) polymorphism with susceptibility to and severity of meningococcal disease. Clin Infect Dis 1998;27(4):746–750.

47. van der Pol WL, Huizinga TW, Vidarsson G, van der Linden MW, Jansen MD, Keijsers V, et al. Relevance of Fcγ receptor and interleukin-10 polymorphisms for meningococcal disease. J Infect Dis 2001;184(12):1548–1555.

48. Fijen CA, Bredius RG, Kuijper EJ. Polymorphism of IgG Fc receptors in meningococcal disease. Ann Intern Med 1993;119(7 Pt 1):636.

49. Yee AM, Phan HM, Zuniga R, Salmon JE, Musher DM. Association between FcγRIIa-R131 allotype and bacteremic pneumococcal pneumonia. Clin Infect Dis 2000;30(1):25–28.

50. Lieke A, Sanders M, J.G.J. vdW. Fcγ receptor IIa (CD32) heterogeneity in patients with recurrent bacterial respiratory tract infections. J Infect Dis 1994;170:854–861.

51. Turner MW. Mannose-binding lectin (MBL) in health and disease. Immunobiology 1998;199(2):327–339.

52. Kuhlman M, Joiner K, Ezekowitz RA. The human mannose-binding protein functions as an opsonin. J Exp Med 1989;169(5):1733–1745.

53. Sastry K, Herman GA, Day L, Deignan E, Bruns G, Morton CC, et al. The human mannose-binding protein gene. Exon structure reveals its evolutionary relationship to a human pulmonary surfactant gene and localization to chromosome 10. J Exp Med 1989;170(4):1175–1189.

54. Lipscombe RJ, Sumiya M, Hill AV, Lau YL, Levinsky RJ, Summerfield JA, et al. High frequencies in African and non-African populations of independent mutations in the mannose binding protein gene. Hum Mol Genet 1992;1(9):709–715.

55. Sumiya M, Super M, Tabona P, Levinsky RJ, Arai T, Turner MW, et al. Molecular basis of opsonic defect in immunodeficient children. Lancet 1991;337(8757):1569–1570.

56. Summerfield JA, Ryder S, Sumiya M, Thursz M, Gorchein A, Monteil MA, et al. Mannose binding protein gene mutations associated with unusual and severe infections in adults. Lancet 1995;345(8954): 886–889.

57. Summerfield JA, Sumiya M, Levin M, Turner MW. Association of mutations in mannose binding protein gene with childhood infection in consecutive hospital series. BMJ 1997;314(7089):1229–1232.

58. Koch A, Melbye M, Sorensen P, Homoe P, Madsen HO, Molbak K, et al. Acute respiratory tract infections and mannose-binding lectin insufficiency during early childhood. JAMA 2001;285(10):1316–1321.

59. Hibberd ML, Sumiya M, Summerfield JA, Booy R, Levin M. Association of variants of the gene for mannose-binding lectin with susceptibility to meningococcal disease. Meningococcal Research Group. Lancet 1999;353(9158):1049–1053.

60. Garred P, Madsen HO, Halberg P, Petersen J, Kronborg G, Svejgaard A, et al. Mannose-binding lectin polymorphisms and susceptibility to infection in systemic lupus erythematosus. Arthritis Rheum 1999;42(10):2145–2152.

61. Gomi K, Tokue Y, Kobayashi T, Takahashi H, Watanabe A, Fujita T, et al. Mannose-binding lectin gene polymorphism is a modulating factor in repeated respiratory infections. Chest 2004;126(1):95–99.

62. Roy S, Knox K, Segal S, Griffiths D, Moore CE, Welsh KI, et al. MBL genotype and risk of invasive pneumococcal disease: a case–control study. Lancet 2002;359(9317):1569–1573.

63. Nathan C. Points of control in inflammation. Nature 2002;420(6917): 846–852.

64. Cohen J. The immunopathogenesis of sepsis. Nature. 2002;420(6917): 885–891.

65. Furman WL, Strother D, McClain K, Bell B, Leventhal B, Pratt CB. Phase I clinical trial of recombinant human tumor necrosis factor in children with refractory solid tumors: a Pediatric Oncology Group study. J Clin Oncol 1993;11(11):2205–2210.

66. Selleri C, Sato T, Anderson S, Young NS, Maciejewski JP. Interferon-γ and tumor necrosis factor-α suppress both early and late stages of hematopoiesis and induce programmed cell death. J Cell Physiol 1995;165(3):538–546.

67. Tracey KJ, Beutler B, Lowry SF, Merryweather J, Wolpe S, Milsark IW, et al. Shock and tissue injury induced by recombinant human cachectin. Science 1986;234(4775):470–474.

68. van Hinsbergh VW, Bauer KA, Kooistra T, Kluft C, Dooijewaard G, Sherman ML, et al. Progress of fibrinolysis during tumor necrosis factor infusions in humans. Concomitant increase in tissue-type plasminogen activator, plasminogen activator inhibitor type-1, and fibrin(ogen) degradation products. Blood 1990;76(11):2284–2289.

69. Wheeler AP, Jesmok G, Brigham KL. Tumor necrosis factor's effects on lung mechanics, gas exchange, and airway reactivity in sheep. J Appl Physiol 1990;68(6):2542–2549.

70. Appoloni O, Dupont E, Vandercruys M, Andriens M, Duchateau J, Vincent JL. Association of tumor necrosis factor-2 allele with plasma

tumor necrosis factor-α levels and mortality from septic shock. Am J Med 2001;110(6):486–488.

71. Higuchi T, Seki N, Kamizono S, Yamada A, Kimura A, Kato H, et al. Polymorphism of the 5'-flanking region of the human tumor necrosis factor (TNF)-α gene in Japanese. Tissue Antigens 1998;51(6):605–612.

72. Louis E, Franchimont D, Piron A, Gevaert Y, Schaaf-Lafontaine N, Roland S, et al. Tumour necrosis factor (TNF) gene polymorphism influences TNF-α production in lipopolysaccharide (LPS)–stimulated whole blood cell culture in healthy humans. Clin Exp Immunol 1998;113(3):401–406.

73. McArthur JA, Zhang Q, Quasney MW. Association between the A/A genotype at the lymphotoxin-α+250 site and increased mortality in children with positive blood cultures. Pediatr Crit Care Med 2002;3(4):341–344.

74. Pociot F, Briant L, Jongeneel CV, Molvig J, Worsaae H, Abbal M, et al. Association of tumor necrosis factor (TNF) and class II major histocompatibility complex alleles with the secretion of TNF-α and TNF-β by human mononuclear cells: a possible link to insulin-dependent diabetes mellitus. Eur J Immunol 1993;23(1):224–231.

75. Stuber F, Petersen M, Bokelmann F, Schade U. A genomic polymorphism within the tumor necrosis factor locus influences plasma tumor necrosis factor-α concentrations and outcome of patients with severe sepsis. Crit Care Med 1996;24(3):381–384.

76. Wilson AG, di Giovine FS, Blakemore AI, Duff GW. Single base polymorphism in the human tumour necrosis factor α (TNF α) gene detectable by NcoI restriction of PCR product. Hum Mol Genet 1992;1(5):353.

77. Wilson AG, Symons JA, McDowell TL, McDevitt HO, Duff GW. Effects of a polymorphism in the human tumor necrosis factor α promoter on transcriptional activation. Proc Natl Acad Sci USA 1997;94(7):3195–3199.

78. Huizinga TW, Westendorp RG, Bollen EL, Keijsers V, Brinkman BM, Langermans JA, et al. TNF-α promoter polymorphisms, production and susceptibility to multiple sclerosis in different groups of patients. J Neuroimmunol 1997;72(2):149–153.

79. Kroeger KM, Carville KS, Abraham LJ. The -308 tumor necrosis factor-α promoter polymorphism effects transcription. Mol Immunol 1997;34(5):391–399.

80. Nadel S, Newport MJ, Booy R, Levin M. Variation in the tumor necrosis factor-α gene promoter region may be associated with death from meningococcal disease. J Infect Dis 1996;174(4):878–880.

81. Majetschak M, Obertacke U, Schade FU, Bardenheuer M, Voggenreiter G, Bloemeke B, et al. Tumor necrosis factor gene polymorphisms, leukocyte function, and sepsis susceptibility in blunt trauma patients. Clin Diagn Lab Immunol 2002;9(6):1205–1211.

82. Mira JP, Cariou A, Grall F, Delclaux C, Losser MR, Heshmati F, et al. Association of TNF2, a TNF-α promoter polymorphism, with septic shock susceptibility and mortality: a multicenter study. JAMA 1999;282(6):561–568.

83. Waterer GW, Quasney MW, Cantor RM, Wunderink RG. Septic shock and respiratory failure in community-acquired pneumonia have different TNF polymorphism associations. Am J Respir Crit Care Med 2001;163(7):1599–1604.

84. Majetschak M, Flohe S, Obertacke U, Schroder J, Staubach K, Nast-Kolb D, et al. Relation of a TNF gene polymorphism to severe sepsis in trauma patients. Ann Surg 1999;230(2):207–214.

85. Stuber F, Udalova IA, Book M, Drutskaya LN, Kuprash DV, Turetskaya RL, et al. −308 Tumor necrosis factor (TNF) polymorphism is not associated with survival in severe sepsis and is unrelated to lipopolysaccharide inducibility of the human TNF promoter. J Inflamm 1995;46(1):42–50.

86. Fang XM, Schroder S, Hoeft A, Stuber F. Comparison of two polymorphisms of the interleukin-1 gene family: interleukin-1 receptor antagonist polymorphism contributes to susceptibility to severe sepsis. Crit Care Med 1999;27(7):1330–1334.

87. Arnalich F, Lopez-Maderuelo D, Codoceo R, Lopez J, Solis-Garrido LM, Capiscol C, et al. Interleukin-1 receptor antagonist gene polymorphism and mortality in patients with severe sepsis. Clin Exp Immunol 2002;127(2):331–336.

88. Read RC, Cannings C, Naylor SC, Timms JM, Maheswaran R, Borrow R, et al. Variation within genes encoding interleukin-1 and the interleukin-1 receptor antagonist influence the severity of meningococcal disease. Ann Intern Med 2003;138(7):534–541.

89. Harding D, Dhamrait S, Millar A, Humphries S, Marlow N, Whitelaw A, et al. Is interleukin-6 −174 genotype associated with the development of septicemia in preterm infants? Pediatrics 2003;112(4):800–803.

90. Schluter B, Raufhake C, Erren M, Schotte H, Kipp F, Rust S, et al. Effect of the interleukin-6 promoter polymorphism (−174 G/C) on the incidence and outcome of sepsis. Crit Care Med 2002;30(1):32–37.

91. Sutherland AM, Walley KR, Manocha S, Russell JA. The association of interleukin 6 haplotype clades with mortality in critically ill adults. Arch Intern Med 2005;165(1):75–82.

92. Hull J, Ackerman H, Isles K, Usen S, Pinder M, Thomson A, et al. Unusual haplotypic structure of IL8, a susceptibility locus for a common respiratory virus. Am J Hum Genet 2001;69(2):413–419.

93. Hull J, Rowlands K, Lockhart E, Sharland M, Moore C, Hanchard N, et al. Haplotype mapping of the bronchiolitis susceptibility locus near IL8. Hum Genet 2004;114(3):272–279.

94. Hacking D, Knight JC, Rockett K, Brown H, Frampton J, Kwiatkowski DP, et al. Increased in vivo transcription of an IL-8 haplotype associated with respiratory syncytial virus disease-susceptibility. Genes Immun 2004;5(4):274–282.

95. Hull J, Thomson A, Kwiatkowski D. Association of respiratory syncytial virus bronchiolitis with the interleukin 8 gene region in UK families. Thorax 2000;55(12):1023–1027.

96. Wilson J, Rowlands K, Rockett K, Moore C, Lockhart E, Sharland M, et al. Genetic variation at the IL10 gene locus is associated with severity of respiratory syncytial virus bronchiolitis. J Infect Dis 2005;191(10):1705–1709.

97. Gallagher PM, Lowe G, Fitzgerald T, Bella A, Greene CM, McElvaney NG, et al. Association of IL-10 polymorphism with severity of illness in community acquired pneumonia. Thorax 2003;58(2):154–156.

98. Schaaf BM, Boehmke F, Esnaashari H, Seitzer U, Kothe H, Maass M, et al. Pneumococcal septic shock is associated with the interleukin-10-1082 gene promoter polymorphism. Am J Respir Crit Care Med 2003;168(4):476–480.

99. Lowe PR, Galley HF, Abdel-Fattah A, Webster NR. Influence of interleukin-10 polymorphisms on interleukin-10 expression and survival in critically ill patients. Crit Care Med 2003;31(1):34–38.

100. Deitch EA, Beck SC, Cruz NC, De Maio A. Induction of heat shock gene expression in colonic epithelial cells after incubation with *Escherichia coli* or endotoxin. Crit Care Med 1995;23(8):1371–1376.

101. Hightower LE. Heat shock, stress proteins, chaperones, and proteotoxicity. Cell 1991;66(2):191–197.

102. Hendrick JP, Hartl FU. Molecular chaperone functions of heat-shock proteins. Annu Rev Biochem 1993;62:349–384.

103. Parsell DA, Lindquist S. The function of heat-shock proteins in stress tolerance: degradation and reactivation of damaged proteins. Annu Rev Genet 1993;27:437–496.

104. Temple SE, Cheong KY, Ardlie KG, Sayer D, Waterer GW. The septic shock associated HSPA1B1267 polymorphism influences production of HSPA1A and HSPA1B. Intensive Care Med 2004;30(9):1761–1767.

105. Schroder O, Schulte KM, Ostermann P, Roher HD, Ekkernkamp A, Laun RA. Heat shock protein 70 genotypes HSPA1B and HSPA1L influence cytokine concentrations and interfere with outcome after major injury. Crit Care Med 2003;31(1):73–79.

106. Waterer GW, El Bahlawan L, Quasney MW, Zhang Q, Kessler LA, Wunderink RG. Heat shock protein 70-2+1267 AA homozygotes have an increased risk of septic shock in adults with community-acquired pneumonia. Crit Care Med 2003;31(5):1367–1372.

107. Cambien F, Alhenc-Gelas F, Herbeth B, Andre JL, Rakotovao R, Gonzales MF, et al. Familial resemblance of plasma angiotensin-converting enzyme level: the Nancy Study. Am J Hum Genet 1988;43(5):774–780.

108. Rigat B, Hubert C, Alhenc-Gelas F, Cambien F, Corvol P, Soubrier F. An insertion/deletion polymorphism in the angiotensin I–converting enzyme gene accounting for half the variance of serum enzyme levels. J Clin Invest 1990;86(4):1343–1346.

109. Rigat B, Hubert C, Corvol P, Soubrier F. PCR detection of the insertion/deletion polymorphism of the human angiotensin converting enzyme gene (DCP1) (dipeptidyl carboxypeptidase 1). Nucleic Acids Res 1992;20(6):1433.

110. Costerousse O, Allegrini J, Lopez M, Alhenc-Gelas F. Angiotensin I–converting enzyme in human circulating mononuclear cells: genetic polymorphism of expression in T-lymphocytes. Biochem J 1993;290 (Pt 1):33–40.

111. Tiret L, Rigat B, Visvikis S, Breda C, Corvol P, Cambien F, et al. Evidence, from combined segregation and linkage analysis, that a variant of the angiotensin I–converting enzyme (ACE) gene controls plasma ACE levels. Am J Hum Genet 1992;51(1):197–205.

112. Harding D, Baines PB, Brull D, Vassiliou V, Ellis I, Hart A, et al. Severity of meningococcal disease in children and the angiotensin-converting enzyme insertion/deletion polymorphism. Am J Respir Crit Care Med 2002;165(8):1103–1106.

113. Aird WC. Vascular bed–specific hemostasis: role of endothelium in sepsis pathogenesis. Crit Care Med 2001;29(7 Suppl):S28–S35.

114. Paramo JA, Perez JL, Serrano M, Rocha E. Types 1 and 2 plasminogen activator inhibitor and tumor necrosis factor α in patients with sepsis. Thromb Haemost 1990;64(1):3–6.

115. Brandtzaeg P, Joo GB, Brusletto B, Kierulf P. Plasminogen activator inhibitor 1 and 2, α-2-antiplasmin, plasminogen, and endotoxin levels in systemic meningococcal disease. Thromb Res 1990;57(2): 271–278.

116. Eriksson P, Kallin B, van 't Hooft FM, Bavenholm P, Hamsten A. Allele-specific increase in basal transcription of the plasminogen-activator inhibitor 1 gene is associated with myocardial infarction. Proc Natl Acad Sci USA 1995;92(6):1851–1855.

117. Hermans PW, Hibberd ML, Booy R, Daramola O, Hazelzet JA, de Groot R, et al. 4G/5G promoter polymorphism in the plasminogen-activator-inhibitor-1 gene and outcome of meningococcal disease. Meningococcal Research Group. Lancet 1999;354(9178):556–560.

118. Haralambous E, Hibberd ML, Hermans PW, Ninis N, Nadel S, Levin M. Role of functional plasminogen-activator-inhibitor-1 4G/5G promoter polymorphism in susceptibility, severity, and outcome of meningococcal disease in Caucasian children. Crit Care Med 2003;31(12):2788–2793.

119. Geishofer G, Binder A, Muller M, Zohrer B, Resch B, Muller W, et al. 4G/5G promoter polymorphism in the plasminogen-activator-inhibitor-1 gene in children with systemic meningococcaemia. Eur J Pediatr 2005;164(8):486–490.

120. Menges T, Hermans PW, Little SG, Langefeld T, Boning O, Engel J, et al. Plasminogen-activator-inhibitor-1 4G/5G promoter polymorphism and prognosis of severely injured patients. Lancet 2001;357(9262): 1096–1097.

121. Lewis JF, Jobe AH. Surfactant and the adult respiratory distress syndrome. Am Rev Respir Dis 1993;147(1):218–233.

122. Seeger W, Gunther A, Walmrath HD, Grimminger F, Lasch HG. Alveolar surfactant and adult respiratory distress syndrome. Pathogenetic role and therapeutic prospects. Clin Invest 1993;71(3):177–190.

123. Chiba H, Pattanajitvilai S, Mitsuzawa H, Kuroki Y, Evans A, Voelker DR. Pulmonary surfactant proteins A and D recognize lipid ligands on *Mycoplasma pneumoniae* and markedly augment the innate immune response to the organism. Chest 2003;123(3 Suppl):426S.

124. Floros J, Karinch AM. Human SP-A: then and now. Am J Physiol 1995;268(2 Pt 1):L162–L165.

125. LeVine AM, Kurak KE, Bruno MD, Stark JM, Whitsett JA, Korfhagen TR. Surfactant protein-A–deficient mice are susceptible to

126. *Pseudomonas aeruginosa* infection. Am J Respir Cell Mol Biol 1998;19(4):700–708.

126. van Iwaarden JF, Claassen E, Jeurissen SH, Haagsman HP, Kraal G. Alveolar macrophages, surfactant lipids, and surfactant protein B regulate the induction of immune responses via the airways. Am J Respir Cell Mol Biol 2001;24(4):452–458.

127. Wright JR. Immunomodulatory functions of surfactant. Physiol Rev 1997;77(4):931–962.

128. Wu H, Kuzmenko A, Wan S, Schaffer L, Weiss A, Fisher JH, et al. Surfactant proteins A and D inhibit the growth of Gram-negative bacteria by increasing membrane permeability. J Clin Invest 2003;111(10):1589–1602.

129. Lahti M, Marttila R, Hallman M. Surfactant protein C gene variation in the Finnish population—association with perinatal respiratory disease. Eur J Hum Genet 2004;12(4):312–320.

130. Lin Z, Pearson C, Chinchilli V, Pietschmann SM, Luo J, Pison U, et al. Polymorphisms of human SP-A, SP-B, and SP-D genes: association of SP-B Thr131Ile with ARDS. Clin Genet 2000;58(3):181–191.

131. Pantelidis P, Veeraraghavan S, du Bois RM. Surfactant gene polymorphisms and interstitial lung diseases. Respir Res 2002;3(1):14.

132. Wright JR. Immunoregulatory functions of surfactant proteins. Nat Rev Immunol 2005;5(1):58–68.

133. Floros J, Fan R. Surfactant protein A and B genetic variants and respiratory distress syndrome: allele interactions. Biol Neonate 2001;80 Suppl 1:22–25.

134. Floros J, Fan R, Diangelo S, Guo X, Wert J, Luo J. Surfactant protein (SP) B associations and interactions with SP-A in white and black subjects with respiratory distress syndrome. Pediatr Int 2001;43(6):567–576.

135. Floros J, Fan R, Matthews A, DiAngelo S, Luo J, Nielsen H, et al. Family-based transmission disequilibrium test (TDT) and case-control association studies reveal surfactant protein A (SP-A) susceptibility alleles for respiratory distress syndrome (RDS) and possible race differences. Clin Genet 2001;60(3):178–187.

136. Lofgren J, Ramet M, Renko M, Marttila R, Hallman M. Association between surfactant protein A gene locus and severe respiratory syncytial virus infection in infants. J Infect Dis 2002;185(3):283–289.

137. Clark JC, Wert SE, Bachurski CJ, Stahlman MT, Stripp BR, Weaver TE, et al. Targeted disruption of the surfactant protein B gene disrupts surfactant homeostasis, causing respiratory failure in newborn mice. Proc Natl Acad Sci USA 1995;92(17):7794–7798.

138. Floros J, Kala P. Surfactant proteins: molecular genetics of neonatal pulmonary diseases. Annu Rev Physiol 1998;60:365–384.

139. Whitsett JA, Nogee LM, Weaver TE, Horowitz AD. Human surfactant protein B: structure, function, regulation, and genetic disease. Physiol Rev 1995;75(4):749–757.

140. Tokieda K, Iwamoto HS, Bachurski C, Wert SE, Hull WM, Ikeda K, et al. Surfactant protein-B–deficient mice are susceptible to hyperoxic lung injury. Am J Respir Cell Mol Biol 1999;21(4):463–472.

141. Lin Z, deMello DE, Wallot M, Floros J. An SP-B gene mutation responsible for SP-B deficiency in fatal congenital alveolar proteinosis: evidence for a mutation hotspot in exon 4. Mol Genet Metab 1998;64(1):25–35.

142. Nogee LM, Garnier G, Dietz HC, Singer L, Murphy AM, deMello DE, et al. A mutation in the surfactant protein B gene responsible for fatal neonatal respiratory disease in multiple kindreds. J Clin Invest 1994;93(4):1860–1863.

143. Marttila R, Haataja R, Ramet M, Lofgren J, Hallman M. Surfactant protein B polymorphism and respiratory distress syndrome in premature twins. Hum Genet 2003;112(1):18–23.

144. Pryhuber GS, Hull WM, Fink I, McMahan MJ, Whitsett JA. Ontogeny of surfactant proteins A and B in human amniotic fluid as indices of fetal lung maturity. Pediatr Res 1991;30(6):597–605.

145. Greene KE, Wright JR, Steinberg KP, Ruzinski JT, Caldwell E, Wong WB, et al. Serial changes in surfactant-associated proteins in lung and serum before and after onset of ARDS. Am J Respir Crit Care Med 1999;160(6):1843–1850.

146. Gregory TJ, Longmore WJ, Moxley MA, Whitsett JA, Reed CR, Fowler AA 3rd, et al. Surfactant chemical composition and biophysical activity in acute respiratory distress syndrome. J Clin Invest 1991; 88(6):1976–1981.

147. Pison U, Obertacke U, Seeger W, Hawgood S. Surfactant protein A (SP-A) is decreased in acute parenchymal lung injury associated with polytrauma. Eur J Clin Invest 1992;22(11):712–718.

148. Pison U BJ, Pietschmann S, et al. The adult respiratory distress syndrome: pathophysiological concepts related to the pulmonary surfactant system. In Robertson BTH, ed. Surfactant Therapy for Lung Disease. New York: Marcel Dekker; 1995:167–197.

149. Willson DF, Thomas NJ, Markovitz BP, Bauman LA, DiCarlo JV, Pon S, et al. Effect of exogenous surfactant (calfactant) in pediatric acute lung injury: a randomized controlled trial. JAMA 2005;293(4):470–476.

150. Pilot-Matias TJ, Kister SE, Fox JL, Kropp K, Glasser SW, Whitsett JA. Structure and organization of the gene encoding human pulmonary surfactant proteolipid SP-B. DNA 1989;8(2):75–86.

151. Jacobs KA, Phelps DS, Steinbrink R, Fisch J, Kriz R, Mitsock L, et al. Isolation of a cDNA clone encoding a high molecular weight precursor to a 6-kDa pulmonary surfactant-associated protein. J Biol Chem 1987;262(20):9808–9811.

152. Wang G, Christensen ND, Wigdahl B, Guttentag SH, Floros J. Differences in N-linked glycosylation between human surfactant protein-B variants of the C or T allele at the single-nucleotide polymorphism at position 1580: implications for disease. Biochem J 2003;369(Pt 1):179–184.

153. Roberts SJ, Petropavlovskaja M, Chung KN, Knight CB, Elwood PC. Role of individual N-linked glycosylation sites in the function and intracellular transport of the human α folate receptor. Arch Biochem Biophys 1998;351(2):227–235.

154. Quasney MW, Waterer GW, Dahmer MK, Kron GK, Zhang Q, Kessler LA, et al. Association between surfactant protein B + 1580 polymorphism and the risk of respiratory failure in adults with community-acquired pneumonia. Crit Care Med 2004;32(5):1115–1119.

155. Idell S, Kueppers F, Lippmann M, Rosen H, Niederman M, Fein A. Angiotensin converting enzyme in bronchoalveolar lavage in ARDS. Chest 1987;91(1):52–56.

156. Wenz M, Steinau R, Gerlach H, Lange M, Kaczmarczyk G. Inhaled nitric oxide does not change transpulmonary angiotensin II formation in patients with acute respiratory distress syndrome. Chest 1997;112(2):478–483.

157. Marshall RP, Webb S, Bellingan GJ, Montgomery HE, Chaudhari B, McAnulty RJ, et al. Angiotensin converting enzyme insertion/deletion polymorphism is associated with susceptibility and outcome in acute respiratory distress syndrome. Am J Respir Crit Care Med 2002;166(5):646–650.

158. Gilliland HE, Armstrong MA, McMurray TJ. Tumour necrosis factor as predictor for pulmonary dysfunction after cardiac surgery. Lancet 1998;352(9136):1281–1282.

159. Wan S, LeClerc JL, Vincent JL. Inflammatory response to cardiopulmonary bypass: mechanisms involved and possible therapeutic strategies. Chest 1997;112(3):676–692.

160. Chenoweth DE, Cooper SW, Hugli TE, Stewart RW, Blackstone EH, Kirklin JW. Complement activation during cardiopulmonary bypass: evidence for generation of C3a and C5a anaphylatoxins. N Engl J Med 1981;304(9):497–503.

161. Kirklin JK, Westaby S, Blackstone EH, Kirklin JW, Chenoweth DE, Pacifico AD. Complement and the damaging effects of cardiopulmonary bypass. J Thorac Cardiovasc Surg 1983;86(6):845–857.

162. Lindal S, Gunnes S, Lund I, Straume BK, Jorgensen L, Sorlie D. Myocardial and microvascular injury following coronary surgery and its attenuation by mode of reperfusion. Eur J Cardiothorac Surg 1995;9(2):83–89.

163. Jansen NJ, van Oeveren W, Gu YJ, van Vliet MH, Eijsman L, Wildevuur CR. Endotoxin release and tumor necrosis factor formation during cardiopulmonary bypass. Ann Thorac Surg 1992;54(4):744–748.

164. Khabar KS, elBarbary MA, Khouqeer F, Devol E, al-Gain S, al-Halees Z. Circulating endotoxin and cytokines after cardiopulmonary bypass: differential correlation with duration of bypass and systemic inflammatory response/multiple organ dysfunction syndromes. Clin Immunol Immunopathol 1997;85(1):97–103.

165. Cremer J, Martin M, Redl H, Bahrami S, Abraham C, Graeter T, et al. Systemic inflammatory response syndrome after cardiac operations. Ann Thorac Surg 1996;61(6):1714–1720.

166. te Velthuis H, Jansen PG, Oudemans-van Straaten HM, Sturk A, Eijsman L, Wildevuur CR. Myocardial performance in elderly patients after cardiopulmonary bypass is suppressed by tumor necrosis factor. J Thorac Cardiovasc Surg 1995;110(6):1663–1669.

167. Yende S, Wunderink R. Causes of prolonged mechanical ventilation after coronary artery bypass surgery. Chest 2002;122(1):245–252.

168. Galley HF, Lowe PR, Carmichael RL, Webster NR. Genotype and interleukin-10 responses after cardiopulmonary bypass. Br J Anaesth 2003;91(3):424–426.

169. Gaudino M, Andreotti F, Zamparelli R, Di Castelnuovo A, Nasso G, Burzotta F, et al. The –174G/C interleukin-6 polymorphism influences postoperative interleukin-6 levels and postoperative atrial fibrillation. Is atrial fibrillation an inflammatory complication? Circulation 2003;108(Suppl 1):II195–II199.

170. Grunenfelder J, Umbehr M, Plass A, Bestmann L, Maly FE, Zund G, et al. Genetic polymorphisms of apolipoprotein E4 and tumor necrosis factor β as predisposing factors for increased inflammatory cytokines after cardiopulmonary bypass. J Thorac Cardiovasc Surg 2004;128(1):92–97.

171. Schroeder S, Borger N, Wrigge H, Welz A, Putensen C, Hoeft A, et al. A tumor necrosis factor gene polymorphism influences the inflammatory response after cardiac operation. Ann Thorac Surg 2003;75(2):534–537.

172. Tomasdottir H, Hjartarson H, Ricksten A, Wasslavik C, Bengtsson A, Ricksten SE. Tumor necrosis factor gene polymorphism is associated with enhanced systemic inflammatory response and increased cardiopulmonary morbidity after cardiac surgery. Anesth Analg 2003;97(4):944–949.

173. Yende S, Quasney MW, Tolley E, Zhang Q, Wunderink RG. Association of tumor necrosis factor gene polymorphisms and prolonged mechanical ventilation after coronary artery bypass surgery. Crit Care Med 2003;31(1):133–140.

174. Hill GE, Alonso A, Spurzem JR, Stammers AH, Robbins RA. Aprotinin and methylprednisolone equally blunt cardiopulmonary bypass-induced inflammation in humans. J Thorac Cardiovasc Surg 1995;110(6):1658–1662.

175. Jansen NJ, van Oeveren W, van den Broek L, Oudemans-van Straaten HM, Stoutenbeek CP, Joen MC, et al. Inhibition by dexamethasone of the reperfusion phenomena in cardiopulmonary bypass. J Thorac Cardiovasc Surg 1991;102(4):515–525.

176. Nakano M, Knowlton AA, Dibbs Z, Mann DL. Tumor necrosis factor-α confers resistance to hypoxic injury in the adult mammalian cardiac myocyte. Circulation 1998;97(14):1392–1400.

177. Sharma HS, Stahl J, Weisensee D, Low-Friedrich I. Cytoprotective mechanisms in cultured cardiomyocytes. Mol Cell Biochem 1996;160–161, 217–224.

178. Mestril R, Dillmann WH. Heat shock proteins and protection against myocardial ischemia. J Mol Cell Cardiol 1995;27(1):45–52.

179. LoCicero J, 3rd, Xu X, Zhang L. Heat shock protein suppresses the senescent lung cytokine response to acute endotoxemia. Ann Thorac Surg 1999;68(4):1150–1153.

180. Koh Y, Lim CM, Kim MJ, Shim TS, Lee SD, Kim WS, et al. Heat shock response decreases endotoxin-induced acute lung injury in rats. Respirology 1999;4(4):325–330.

181. Yang B, Li D, Phillips MI, Mehta P, Mehta JL. Myocardial angiotensin II receptor expression and ischemia-reperfusion injury. Vasc Med 1998;3(2):121–130.

182. Zughaib ME, Sun JZ, Bolli R. Effect of angiotensin-converting enzyme inhibitors on myocardial ischemia/reperfusion injury: an overview. Basic Res Cardiol 1993;88(Suppl 1):155–167.

183. Gorin AB, Liebler J. Changes in serum angiotensin-converting enzyme during cardiopulmonary bypass in humans. Am Rev Respir Dis 1986;134(1):79–84.

184. Volzke H, Engel J, Kleine V, Schwahn C, Dahm JB, Eckel L, et al. Angiotensin I–converting enzyme insertion/deletion polymorphism and cardiac mortality and morbidity after coronary artery bypass graft surgery. Chest 2002;122(1):31–36.

185. Yende S, Quasney MW, Tolley EA, Wunderink RG. Clinical relevance of angiotensin-converting enzyme gene polymorphisms to predict risk of mechanical ventilation after coronary artery bypass graft surgery. Crit Care Med 2004;32(4):922–927.

186. Beck C, Dubois J, Grignon A, Lacroix J, David M. Incidence and risk factors of catheter-related deep vein thrombosis in a pediatric intensive care unit: a prospective study. J Pediatr 1998;133(2):237–241.

187. Casado-Flores J, Barja J, Martino R, Serrano A, Valdivielso A. Complications of central venous catheterization in critically ill children. Pediatr Crit Care Med 2001;2(1):57–62.

188. DeAngelis GA, McIlhenny J, Willson DF, Vittone S, Dwyer SJ, 3rd, Gibson JC, et al. Prevalence of deep venous thrombosis in the lower extremities of children in the intensive care unit. Pediatr Radiol 1996;26(11):821–824.

189. Derish M, Smith D, Frankel L. Venous catheter thrombus formation and pulmonary embolism in children. Pediatr Pulmonol 1995;20: 349–354.

190. Donnelly KM. Venous thromboembolic disease in the pediatric intensive care unit. Curr Opin Pediatr 1999;11(3):213–217.

191. Gutierrez JA, Bagatell R, Samson MP, Theodorou AA, Berg RA. Femoral central venous catheter-associated deep venous thrombosis in children with diabetic ketoacidosis. Crit Care Med 2003;31(1): 80–83.

192. Massicotte MP, Dix D, Monagle P, Adams M, Andrew M. Central venous catheter related thrombosis in children: analysis of the Canadian Registry of Venous Thromboembolic Complications. J Pediatr 1998;133(6):770–776.

193. David M, Andrew M. Venous thromboembolic complications in children. J Pediatr 1993;123(3):337–346.

194. Krafte-Jacobs B, Sivit CJ, Mejia R, Pollack MM. Catheter-related thrombosis in critically ill children: comparison of catheters with and without heparin bonding. J Pediatr 1995;126(1):50–54.

195. Talbott GA, Winters WD, Bratton SL, O'Rourke PP. A prospective study of femoral catheter-related thrombosis in children. Arch Pediatr Adolesc Med 1995;149(3):288–291.

196. van Ommen CH, Heijboer H, Buller HR, Hirasing RA, Heijmans HS, Peters M. Venous thromboembolism in childhood: a prospective two-year registry in the Netherlands. J Pediatr 2001;139(5):676–681.

197. Dahlback B. Blood coagulation. Lancet 2000;355(9215):1627–1632.

198. De Stefano V, Finazzi G, Mannucci PM. Inherited thrombophilia: pathogenesis, clinical syndromes, and management. Blood 1996;87(9): 3531–3544.

199. Miletich JP, Prescott SM, White R, Majerus PW, Bovill EG. Inherited predisposition to thrombosis. Cell 1993;72(4):477–480.

200. Voetsch B, Loscalzo J. Genetics of thrombophilia: impact on atherogenesis. Curr Opin Lipidol 2004;15(2):129–143.

201. Bertina RM, Koeleman BP, Koster T, Rosendaal FR, Dirven RJ, de Ronde H, et al. Mutation in blood coagulation factor V associated with resistance to activated protein C. Nature 1994;369(6475):64–67.

202. Bertina RM. The prothrombin 20210 G to A variation and thrombosis. Curr Opin Hematol 1998;5(5):339–42.

203. Ceelie H, Bertina RM, van Hylckama Vlieg A, Rosendaal FR, Vos HL. Polymorphisms in the prothrombin gene and their association with plasma prothrombin levels. Thromb Haemost 2001;85(6):1066–1070.

204. Perez-Ceballos E, Corral J, Alberca I, Vaya A, Llamas P, Montes R, et al. Prothrombin A19911G and G20210A polymorphisms' role in thrombosis. Br J Haematol 2002;118(2):610–614.

205. Poort SR, Rosendaal FR, Reitsma PH, Bertina RM. A common genetic variation in the 3'-untranslated region of the prothrombin gene is associated with elevated plasma prothrombin levels and an increase in venous thrombosis. Blood 1996;88(10):3698–3703.

206. Caso R, Lane DA, Thompson EA, Olds RJ, Thein SL, Panico M, et al. Antithrombin Vicenza, Ala 384 to Pro (GCA to CCA) mutation, transforming the inhibitor into a substrate. Br J Haematol 1991;77(1): 87–92.

207. Erdjument H, Lane DA, Ireland H, Di Marzo V, Panico M, Morris HR, et al. Antithrombin Milano, single amino acid substitution at the reactive site, Arg393 to Cys. Thromb Haemost 1988;60(3):471–475.

208. Lane DA, Erdjument H, Thompson E, Panico M, Di Marzo V, Morris HR, et al. A novel amino acid substitution in the reactive site of a congenital variant antithrombin. Antithrombin pescara, ARG393 to pro, caused by a CGT to CCT mutation. J Biol Chem 1989;264(17): 10200–10204.

209. Lane DA, Olds RJ, Boisclair M, Chowdhury V, Thein SL, Cooper DN, et al. Antithrombin III mutation database: first update. For the Thrombin and its Inhibitors Subcommittee of the Scientific and Standardization Committee of the International Society on Thrombosis and Haemostasis. Thromb Haemost 1993;70(2):361–369.

210. Lane DA, Olds RJ, Thein SL. Antithrombin III: summary of first database update. Nucleic Acids Res 1994;22(17):3556–3559.

211. Aiach M, Nicaud V, Alhenc-Gelas M, Gandrille S, Arnaud E, Amiral J, et al. Complex association of protein C gene promoter polymorphism with circulating protein C levels and thrombotic risk. Arterioscler Thromb Vasc Biol 1999;19(6):1573–1576.

212. Spek CA, Greengard JS, Griffin JH, Bertina RM, Reitsma PH. Two mutations in the promoter region of the human protein C gene both cause type I protein C deficiency by disruption of two HNF-3 binding sites. J Biol Chem 1995;270(41):24216–24221.

213. Spek CA, Koster T, Rosendaal FR, Bertina RM, Reitsma PH. Genotypic variation in the promoter region of the protein C gene is associated with plasma protein C levels and thrombotic risk. Arterioscler Thromb Vasc Biol 1995;15(2):214–218.

214. Spek CA, Reitsma PH. Genetic risk factors for venous thrombosis. Mol Genet Metab 2000;71(1–2):51–61.

215. Reitsma PH, Bernardi F, Doig RG, Gandrille S, Greengard JS, Ireland H, et al. Protein C deficiency: a database of mutations, 1995 update. On behalf of the Subcommittee on Plasma Coagulation Inhibitors of the Scientific and Standardization Committee of the ISTH. Thromb Haemost 1995;73(5):876–889.

216. Duchemin J, Gandrille S, Borgel D, Feurgard P, Alhenc-Gelas M, Matheron C, et al. The Ser 460 to Pro substitution of the protein S α (PROS1) gene is a frequent mutation associated with free protein S (type IIa) deficiency. Blood 1995;86(9):3436–3443.

217. Koenen RR, Gomes L, Tans G, Rosing J, Hackeng TM. The Ser460Pro mutation in recombinant protein S Heerlen does not affect its APC-cofactor and APC-independent anticoagulant activities. Thromb Haemost 2004;91(6):1105–1114.

218. Koenen RR, Tans G, van Oerle R, Hamulyak K, Rosing J, Hackeng TM. The APC-independent anticoagulant activity of protein S in plasma is decreased by elevated prothrombin levels due to the prothrombin G20210A mutation. Blood 2003;102(5):1686–1692.

219. Reitsma PH, Ploos van Amstel HK, Bertina RM. Three novel mutations in five unrelated subjects with hereditary protein S deficiency type I. J Clin Invest 1994;93(2):486–492.

220. Gomez E, Poort SR, Bertina RM, Reitsma PH. Identification of eight point mutations in protein S deficiency type I—analysis of 15 pedigrees. Thromb Haemost 1995;73(5):750–755.

221. Gandrille S, Borgel D, Eschwege-Gufflet V, Aillaud M, Dreyfus M, Matheron C, et al. Identification of 15 different candidate causal point mutations and three polymorphisms in 19 patients with protein S deficiency using a scanning method for the analysis of the protein S active gene. Blood 1995;85(1):130–138.

222. Fukasawa M, Matsushita K, Kamiyama M, Mikami Y, Araki I, Yamagata Z, et al. The methylentetrahydrofolate reductase C677T point mutation is a risk factor for vascular access thrombosis in hemodialysis patients. Am J Kidney Dis 2003;41(3):637–642.

223. Heil SG, Den Heijer M, Van Der Rijt-Pisa BJ, Kluijtmans LA, Blom HJ. The 894 G > T variant of endothelial nitric oxide synthase (eNOS) increases the risk of recurrent venous thrombosis through interaction with elevated homocysteine levels. J Thromb Haemost 2004;2(5): 750–753.

224. Gorchakova O, Koch W, von Beckerath N, Mehilli J, Schomig A, Kastrati A. Association of a genetic variant of endothelial nitric oxide synthase with the 1 year clinical outcome after coronary stent placement. Eur Heart J 2003;24(9):820–827.

225. Shimasaki Y, Yasue H, Yoshimura M, Nakayama M, Kugiyama K, Ogawa H, et al. Association of the missense Glu298Asp variant of the endothelial nitric oxide synthase gene with myocardial infarction. J Am Coll Cardiol 1998;31(7):1506–1510.

226. Standeven KF, Ariens RA, Grant PJ. The molecular physiology and pathology of fibrin structure/function. Blood Rev 2005;19(5):275–288.

227. Standeven KF, Grant PJ, Carter AM, Scheiner T, Weisel JW, Ariens RA. Functional analysis of the fibrinogen α Thr312Ala polymorphism: effects on fibrin structure and function. Circulation 2003;107(18): 2326–2330.

228. Carter AM, Catto AJ, Kohler HP, Ariens RA, Stickland MH, Grant PJ. α-Fibrinogen Thr312Ala polymorphism and venous thromboembolism. Blood 2000;96(3):1177–1179.

229. Ozbek N, Atac FB, Yildirim SV, Verdi H, Yazici C, Yilmaz BT, et al. Analysis of prothrombotic mutations and polymorphisms in children who developed thrombosis in the perioperative period of congenital cardiac surgery. Cardiol Young 2005;15(1):19–25.

230. Ariens RA, Philippou H, Nagaswami C, Weisel JW, Lane DA, Grant PJ. The factor XIII V34L polymorphism accelerates thrombin activation of factor XIII and affects cross-linked fibrin structure. Blood 2000;96(3):988–995.

231. Balogh I, Szoke G, Karpati L, Wartiovaara U, Katona E, Komaromi I, et al. Val34Leu polymorphism of plasma factor XIII: biochemistry and epidemiology in familial thrombophilia. Blood 2000;96(7):2479–2486.

232. Wartiovaara U, Mikkola H, Szoke G, Haramura G, Karpati L, Balogh I, et al. Effect of Val34Leu polymorphism on the activation of the coagulation factor XIII-A. Thromb Haemost 2000;84(4):595–600.

233. Alhenc-Gelas M, Reny JL, Aubry ML, Aiach M, Emmerich J. The FXIII Val 34 Leu mutation and the risk of venous thrombosis. Thromb Haemost 2000;84(6):1117–1118.

234. Margaglione M, Bossone A, Brancaccio V, Ciampa A, Di Minno G. Factor XIII Val34Leu polymorphism and risk of deep vein thrombosis. Thromb Haemost 2000;84(6):1118–1119.

235. Van Hylckama Vlieg A, Komanasin N, Ariens RA, Poort SR, Grant PJ, Bertina RM, et al. Factor XIII Val34Leu polymorphism, factor XIII antigen levels and activity and the risk of deep venous thrombosis. Br J Haematol 2002;119(1):169–175.

236. Hagstrom JN, Walter J, Bluebond-Langner R, Amatniek JC, Manno CS, High KA. Prevalence of the factor V Leiden mutation in children and neonates with thromboembolic disease. J Pediatr 1998;133(6): 777–781.

237. Manco-Johnson MJ. Disorders of hemostasis in childhood: risk factors for venous thromboembolism. Thromb Haemost 1997;78(1): 710–714.

238. Nowak-Gottl U, Koch HG, Aschka I, Kohlhase B, Vielhaber H, Kurlemann G, et al. Resistance to activated protein C (APCR) in children with venous or arterial thromboembolism. Br J Haematol 1996;92(4):992–998.

239. Uttenreuther-Fischer MM, Vetter B, Hellmann C, Otting U, Ziemer S, Hausdorf G, et al. Paediatric thrombo-embolism: the influence of non-genetic factors and the role of activated protein C resistance and protein C deficiency. Eur J Pediatr 1997;156(4):277–281.

240. Evans WE, Relling MV. Pharmacogenomics: translating functional genomics into rational therapeutics. Science1999;286(5439):487–491.

241. Vesell ES. Pharmacogenetic perspectives gained from twin and family studies. Pharmacol Ther 1989;41(3):535–552.

242. Guengerich FP, Hosea NA, Parikh A, Bell-Parikh LC, Johnson WW, Gillam EM, et al. Twenty years of biochemistry of human P450s: purification, expression, mechanism, and relevance to drugs. Drug Metab Dispos 1998;26(12):1175–1178.

243. Meyer UA, Zanger UM. Molecular mechanisms of genetic polymorphisms of drug metabolism. Annu Rev Pharmacol Toxicol 1997;37:269–296.

244. Evans WE, Relling MV. Moving towards individualized medicine with pharmacogenomics. Nature 2004;429(6990):464–468.

245. Evans WE, Hon YY, Bomgaars L, Coutre S, Holdsworth M, Janco R, et al. Preponderance of thiopurine S-methyltransferase deficiency and heterozygosity among patients intolerant to mercaptopurine or azathioprine. J Clin Oncol 2001;19(8):2293–2301.

246. Evans WE, Horner M, Chu YQ, Kalwinsky D, Roberts WM. Altered mercaptopurine metabolism, toxic effects, and dosage requirement in a thiopurine methyltransferase-deficient child with acute lymphocytic leukemia. J Pediatr 1991;119(6):985–989.

247. Weinshilboum R. Inheritance and Drug Response. N Engl J Med 2003;348(6):529–537.

248. Barnes P, Lee T. Recent advances in asthma. Postgrad Med J 1992;68: 942–953.

249. Nelson HS. β-Adrenergic bronchodilators. N Engl J Med 1995;333(8): 499–501.

250. Drazen JM, Silverman EK, Lee TH. Heterogeneity of therapeutic responses in asthma. Br Med Bull 2000;56(4):1054–1070.

251. Small KM, McGraw DW, Liggett SB. Pharmacology and physiology of human adrenergic receptor polymorphisms. Annu Rev Pharmacol Toxicol 2003;43:381–411.

252. McGraw DW, Forbes S, Kramer L, Liggett SB. Polymorphisms of the 5' leader cistron of the human β2-adrenergic receptor regular receptor expression. J Clin Invest 1998;102:1927–1932.

253. Scott M, Swan C, Wheatley AP, Hall IP. Identification of novel polymorphisms within the promoter region of the human β2–adrenergic receptor. Br J Pharmacol 1999;126:841–844.

254. Drysdale CM, McGraw DW, Stack CB, Stephens JC, Judson RS, Nandabalan K, et al. Complex promoter and coding region β2-adrenergic receptor haplotypes alter receptor expression and predict in vivo responsiveness. Proc Natl Acad Sci USA 2000;97:10483–10488.

255. Holloway JW, Dunbar PR, Riley GA, Sawyer GM, Fitzharris PF, Pearce N, et al. Association of β2-adrenergic receptor polymorphisms with severe asthma. Clin Exp Allergy 2000;30:1097–1103.

256. Israel E, Drazen JM, Liggett SB, Boushey HA, Cherniack RM, Chinchilli VM, et al. The effect of polymorphisms of the β2-adrenergic receptor on the response to regular use of albuterol in asthma. Am J Respir Crit Care Med 2000;162(1):75–80.

257. Reihsaus E, Innis M, MacIntyre N, Liggett SB. Mutations in the gene encoding for the β2-adrenergic receptor in normal and asthmatic subjects. Am J Respir Cell Mol Biol 1993;8:334–339.

258. Tan S, Hall IP, Dewar J, Dow E, Lipworth B. Association between β2-adrenoreceptor polymorphism and susceptibility to bronchodilator desensitization in moderately severe stable asthmatics. Lancet 1997;350:995–999.

259. Taylor DR, Drazen JM, Herbison GP, Yandava C, Hancox RJ, Town GI. Asthma exacerbations during long term β agonist use: influence of β2 adrenoceptor polymorphism. Thorax 2000;55:762–767.

260. Turki J, Green S, Newman KB, Meyers MA, LIGGETT SB. Human lung cell β2-adrenergic receptors desensitize in response to in vivo administered β-agonist. Am J Physiol 1995;269:L709–L714.

261. Martinez FD, Graves PE, Baldini M, Solomon S, Erickson R. Association between genetic polymorphisms of the β2-adrenoceptor and response to albuterol in children with and without a history of wheezing. J Clin Invest 1997;100:3184–3188.

262. Elbahlawan MD, Binaei S, Christensen ML, Zhang Q, Quasney MW, Dahmer MK. β2-Adrenergic receptor polymorphisms in African

American children with status asthmaticus. Pediatr Crit Care Med 2006;7(1):15–18.

263. Moore PE, Laporte JD, Abraham JH, Schwartzman IN, Yandava CN, Silverman ES, et al. Polymorphism of the β2-adrenergic receptor gene and desensitization in human airway smooth muscle. Am J Respir Crit Care Med 2000;162(6):2117–2124.

264. Green SA, Turki J, Bejarano P, Hall IP, Liggett SB. Influence of β2-adrenergic receptor genotypes on signal transduction in human airway smooth muscle. Am J Respir Cell Mol Biol 1995;13:25–33.

265. Vitali SH, Randolph AG. Assessing the quality of case–control association studies on the genetic basis of sepsis. Pediatr Crit Care Med 2005;6(3 Suppl):S74–S77.

17

Signal Transduction Pathways in Critical Illness and Injury

Timothy T. Cornell and Thomas P. Shanley

Introduction

Among the most important biologic functions that cells perform is to sense and respond to an external stimulus. Physical, chemical, and ionic changes that occur in the extracellular environment or that are directly applied to the cell must be *sensed* at the cell surface. Such stimuli most often create the need for the cell to mount an adaptive response that commonly necessitates the initiation of transcriptional regulation of gene expression. For the signal to be sensed at the cell surface and subsequently be communicated to the nuclear transcriptional machinery requires the propagation or *transduction* of this signal through the cytosol to the nuclear compartment. Cells utilize some general mechanistic principles that have been highly conserved and have also adapted a broad array of specific pathways to accomplish this biologic task. The synonymous terms *signal transduction*, *cell signaling*, and *transmembrane signaling* have been used to define this conserved, fundamental cellular process. This field now comprises its own scientific entity [1] and a comprehensive review of all pertinent pathways is beyond the scope of this chapter. For this purpose, the reader is referred to recent, excellent, comprehensive texts [1,2]. The intent of the current chapter is to review some fundamental biologic processes involved in signal transduction and gene expression, introduce some of the key pathways currently focused on by investigators in critical care medicine, and emphasize the biologic relevance of these pathways to critical illness.

Historical Perspective of Signal Transduction

The science of signal transduction owes its origin to the field of endocrinology and hormonal biology. The concept of intracellular communication or *messaging* originated from Claude Bernard's work in the 1850s, which described how *internal secretions* of the thyroid and adrenal glands were released into the circulation and had distant effects on various organs. Later, this concept was refined by Bayliss and Starling [3], who described *secretin* as a member of a large group of chemical messengers that ultimately came to be called *hormones*, a term attributed to Dr. William B. Hardy in 1905 [4]. This work was the initial summary of the biologic function by which a secreted product could affect a specific response in distal cells of a target organ. With the subsequent explosion of biochemical and molecular research tools, the most recent decades have witnessed extraordinary advances in our understanding of signal transduction pathways. At every level of this biologic principle—cell surface receptors that sense a stimulus, identification of a myriad of second messengers that propagate the signal, and numerous nuclear factors that regulate gene expression—advances have helped us better understand the pathophysiology of critical illnesses and provided hope that novel targets will continue to increase our therapeutic armamentarium. It is the goal of this chapter to focus on some of these specific pathways, particularly as they pertain to inflammatory cell signaling and those disease states faced on a daily basis by pediatric critical care practitioners.

Basic Overview of Signal Transduction

Signal transduction schematically incorporates a series of mechanisms arranged in a pathway that function to transmit a signal (generally from the cell surface) to the nuclear compartment where the machinery capable of mounting an adaptive cellular response, usually by affecting gene expression, exists (Figure 17.1). Thus, the initial step involves a receptor to sense a stimulus or cell membrane change in response to a stimulus followed by the generation of a signal that must then be amplified and/or propagated. A myriad of receptor-to-protein and protein-to-protein signal propagating events ultimately transmit the signal to the nuclear transcriptional machinery to allow for de novo gene expression. To accomplish this

D.S. Wheeler et al. (eds.), *Science and Practice of Pediatric Critical Care Medicine*,
DOI 10.1007/978-1-84800-921-9_17, © Springer-Verlag London Limited 2009

FIGURE 17.1. Overview of signal transduction mechanisms.

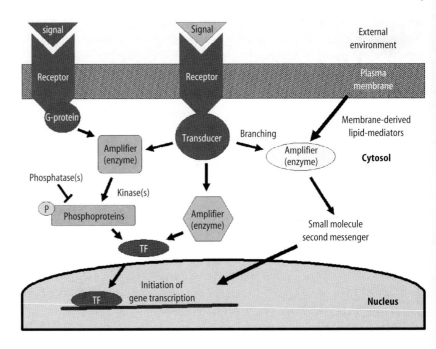

with both specificity and fidelity, a number of strategies are used, including reversible phosphorylation of proteins, mobilization of calcium and other ions, activation of lipid-derived mediators, accumulation and/or degradation of cyclic nucleotides, and stimulation of G-coupled proteins. Finally, in the nuclear compartment, transcription activating factors facilitate the process of transcribing DNA to mRNA which in turn can be subjected to post-transcriptional modifications (e.g. destabilization or degradation) that influence the amount of mRNA translated to protein [5]. In light of the vast numbers of proteins playing a role in signaling (receptors, adaptor proteins, kinases, phosphatases, and so forth), complete understanding of the complexity of even a single pathway can be daunting. In this chapter, we highlight those pathways that have specific relevance to the biology of critical illness.

Stimuli Triggering Signal Transduction

Signal transduction is initiated by any number of stimuli that influence cellular responses and activities. Among those stimuli relevant to critical care are circulating mediators (hormones, cytokines, and growth factors), osmolar changes, and mechanical stress (such as shear, stretch, and pathogens; Table 17.1). Of particular importance to the pediatric critical care practitioner are those responses observed in the setting of an invading pathogen that are commonly responsible for the pathophysiologic consequence of severe sepsis.

As reviewed elsewhere in this text, basic science investigators have identified an increasing number of molecular patterns expressed by pathogens, so-called *pathogen- associated molecular patterns* or *PAMPS* that distinguish them from the human host. To sense these PAMPS, the innate immune system has adapted a series of toll-like receptors (TLRs) that possess specific affinity for the various PAMPS [6] (see Chapters 15). As a prime example of receptors capable of initiating a signaling response, many but not all TLRs are cell membrane bound and possess an extracellular ligand-binding domain and usually an intracellular signaling domain or adapter protein that serves to transmit the signal across

the cell membrane [7]. A numbers of receptor-based or cell membrane—based systems possess the capacity to undergo ligand binding and/or conformational changes that result in the initiation of the signal that then requires propagation through the cytosolic compartment.

General Strategies for Signal Propagation

Upon initiation of the signal, a number of serial and/or parallel pathways that are comprised of transducing proteins or amplifiers regulate the amplification and/or propagation of the signal. One of the most common mechanisms employed by mammalian cells to

TABLE 17.1. Factors initiating signal transduction events.

Classes of factors	Examples
Circulating mediators	
Hormones	Cortisol, thyroid hormone, catecholamines
Cytokines/chemokines	TNF-α, IL-1, IL-6, CXCL-8/IL-8, CCL-2/MCP-1
Growth factors	Insulin growth factor, GM-CSF
Pathogens	Pathogen-associated molecular pattern
Gram-negative bacteria	Lipopolysaccharide, CpG DNA
Gram-positive bacteria	Lipotechoic acid
Viruses	Capsid proteins, viral DNA/RNA
Fungi	Mannose
Biologic stresses (biotrauma)	
Mechanical stress	Mechanical ventilation, vascular resistance, trauma
Shear stress	Vasculopathies, hypercoagulation, hypertension
Thermal stress	Heat shock, cold stress
Osmotic stress	Hyper-, hyponatremia, osmolar therapies
In vivo, endogenous ligands	
Extracellular matrix proteins	Heparin sulfate
Cell-to-cell interactions	Leukocyte/platelet–endothelial cell interaction

Note: GM-CSF, granulocyte-macrophage colony-stimulating factor; IL, interleukin; TNF, tumor necrosis factor.

propagate a signal is reversible phosphorylation of serine, threonine, and/or tyrosine residues on target proteins [8,9]. To accomplish this, protein kinases, one of the largest gene families known, facilitate the catalytic transfer of a γ-phosphate group from Mg^{2+}-ATP to these amino acid residues. An example of kinases that modulate inflammatory responses associated with sepsis and acute lung injury are the mitogen-activated protein (MAP) kinases, which includes the ERK, JNK, and p38 pathways, reviewed below [10,11].

The activity of a kinase is generally measured in one of two ways—by determining the presence of phosphorylation of the target substrate using Western blot analysis or by directly measuring kinase activity using an in vitro kinase assay. In the latter case, the kinase of interest is specifically immunoprecipitated and then combined with a substrate for the kinase and a radiolabeled source of phosphate (usually ^{32}P-ATP) so that phosphorylation of the substrate can be determined by subsequent radiography. It is imperative to note that, at any point in time, the phosphorylation state of a protein is maintained by a balance between the actions of kinases and possible dephosphorylation by enzymes called *protein phosphatases*. The phosphatases are proteins that hydrolyze the phosphoester bonds of phosphorylated serine, threonine, and tyrosine residues and thus provide the counterregulatory arm of reversible protein phosphorylation. Two large protein phosphatase families exist—serine (Ser)/threonine (Thr) and tyrosine (Tyr) phosphatases, which are reviewed later.

Several other mechanisms for signal propagation exist, including calcium mobilization, activation of lipid-derived mediators, changes in cyclic nucleotides (e.g., cAMP) and stimulation of G-coupled proteins, all of which have some relevance to critical care. For example, depolarization of the muscle cell opens membrane calcium channels that subsequently signal release of additional calcium stores in the sarcoplasmic reticulum to mediate optimal contraction of the myocyte. Recent data have suggested that a principle proinflammatory mediator, platelet activating factor, increases the expression of the cell membrane, sphingolipid product, ceramide resulting in activation of inflammatory signaling pathways resulting in pulmonary edema formation [12]. Endothelin-1 mediates potent vasoconstriction through a G-protein coupled, endothelin (ET_A) receptor [13]. Thus, numerous examples of these general signaling principles exist throughout diseases faced in the critical care unit.

Specific Pathways

During the historic evolution of signal transduction as a scientific entity, the focus has been on understanding its role in the homeostatic functions of the cell. As greater insight into multiple disease states has been achieved, our understanding of the role of signal transduction pathways in these pathologic states (e.g., cancer cell transformation, dysregulated proinflammation) has substantially increased over the more recent years. As they pertain to critical care, some of these pathways have been studied in both preclinical models and the clinical states such as sepsis and acute lung injury and have increasingly associated activation of certain pathways with such clinical pathophysiologic states. Some of the notable examples are described in the following sections.

Nuclear Factor-κ B Pathway

For signaling pathways to initiate a cellular change on the basis of de novo protein synthesis, transcription (DNA serving as the genetic template for mRNA production) must be initiated. Proteins that serve this function are called *transcriptional activation factors*. Among the important transcription factors examined in the context of critical care is nuclear factor-κ B (NFκB) because of the large number of inflammatory genes induced by its activation (Table 17.2). Nuclear factor-κ B really refers to a series of proteins categorized as the so-called Rel family of transcription activation factors [14,15], but the canonical NFκB is a heterodimer composed of two subunits, p50 and p65. This heterodimer, under most steady-state conditions, is anchored in the cytoplasm by an inhibitory subunit called *inhibitor of kappa B* (IκB), commonly the α-form, which is a member of a larger family of IκB-related proteins [16–18]. The NFκB pathway is activated in response to a variety of pathologic stimuli (e.g., lipopolysaccharide, biotrauma, and other PAMPs).

One of the best-studied examples with relevance to critical care is activation by lipopolysaccharide [19]. Binding of lipopolysaccharide to its receptor complex (TLR4/CD14/MD2), facilitated by lipopolysaccharide binding protein, results in the recruitment of the myeloid differentiation adapter protein, MyD88, to this receptor complex (Figure 17.2). This process results in the recruitment of the interleukin-1 (IL-1) receptor associated kinase, which undergoes autophosphorylation and recruits the additional adapter protein, TNF receptor associated factor-6 (TRAF-6) [20]. Tumor necrosis receptor associated factor-6 then phosphorylates and activates an upstream, heterotrimeric member of the NFκB pathway, the IκB protein kinase complex (IκK-α, -β and -γ [also called NEMO]), resulting in IκB-α phosphorylation [21]. Once phosphorylated, IκB-α is targeted for polyubiquitination, a process that targets proteins for proteasomic degradation via the 26S proteasome.

Upon degradation of IκB-α, the nuclear localization sequence of the p50 subunit is unmasked, and nuclear translocation of NFκB occurs (Figure 17.3) [22]. NFκB then binds to a DNA sequence (a so-called *consensus sequence*) on those portions of chromatin in the promoter regions that are specifically recognized by NFκB to

TABLE 17.2. Various genes regulated by nuclear factor-κB involved in critical illness.

Cytokines and chemokines
    Tumor necrosis factor-α
    Interleukins-1, -2, -3, -6, and -12
    CXCL8/interleukin-8
    CXCL1/Gro-α
    CXCL2/Gro-β
    CCL3/Macrophage inflammatory protein (MIP)-1α
    CCL2/Monocyte chemotactic protein (MCP)-1
    CCL5/RANTES
    CCL11/eotaxin

Growth factors
    Granulocyte-macrophage colony-stimulating factor (GM-CSF)
    Granulocyte colony-stimulating factor (G-CSF)
    Macrophage colony-stimulating factor (M-CSF)

Adhesion molecules
    E-selectin
    Intercellular adhesion molecule (ICAM)-1
    Vascular cell adhesion molecule 1 (VCAM-1)
    Miscellaneous
    Inducible nitric oxide synthase (iNOS)
    C-reactive protein
    5-Lipoxygenase
    Cyclooxygenase (COX)-2

Figure 17.2. Tumor necrosis factor-α and lipopolysaccharide signaling pathways. IRAK, interleukin-1 receptor-associated kinase; IκK, inhibitor of κB; LPS, lipopolysaccharide; MEKK, mitogen-activated protein kinase kinase kinase; MyD88, myeloid differentiation adapter protein; NFκB, nuclear factor-κB; TNF, tumor necrosis factor; TRAF, TNF receptor-associated factor; TLR, toll-like receptor.

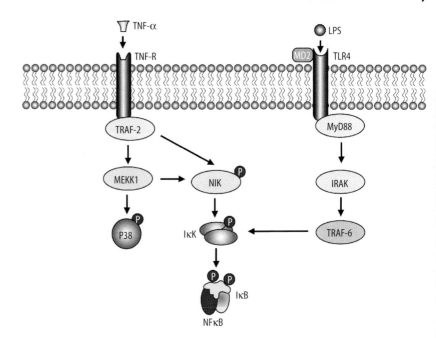

initiate transcription of a number of key inflammatory-related genes (see Table 17.2) [23]. Numerous clinical studies have associated certain disease states (e.g., sepsis, acute respiratory distress syndrome) with evidence of increased NFκB activation. For example, bronchoalveolar lavage–retrieved alveolar macrophages from patients with acute respiratory distress syndrome showed significantly greater activation of NFκB than did those of control patients [24]. In studies of septic shock in adults, increased binding activity of NFκB in circulating leukocytes positively correlated with severity of illness and also differentiated survivors from

nonsurvivors [25–27]. Thus, these observations provide increasing support for the concept that the NFκB pathway may be a valid therapeutic target in these disease states.

This description of the classic pathway of NFκB activation is probably simplistic as we continue to gain insight into the multiple levels of regulation of NFκB-driven gene activation. For example, the subunits of NFκB are subject to various post-translational modifications (e.g., phosphorylation and acetylation), with important consequences on subcellular localization, subunit composition, and interaction with co-activator and/or co-repressor proteins

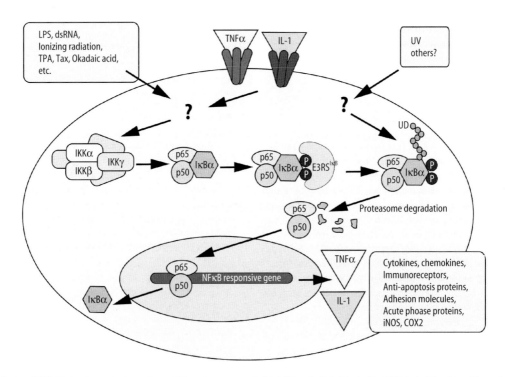

Figure 17.3. Nuclear factor-κB (NFκB) signal transduction pathway. COX, cyclooxygenase; IκK, inhibitor of κB; IL, interleukin; iNOS, inducible nitric oxide synthase.

[28]. In addition, alternative pathways from the IκK/IκB-α pathway have been shown to activate NFκB. As one example, the tyrosine phosphatase inhibitor pervanadate activated NFκB, but via tyrosine phosphorylation of IκB-α rather than serine phosphorylation and did not involve degradation of IκB-α [29].

An equally important task of the cell is to turn off activated pathways, and a well-described mechanism for deactivating NFκB involves its own inhibitor, IκB. Because the promoter region of the IκB-α gene contains NFκB consensus binding sites, NFκB activation induces de novo expression of its own inhibitor, IκB-α [30]. As a result, the newly synthesized IκBα can move to the cytosol and block ongoing NFκB activation by reforming the heterotrimeric complex with p50 and p65. In has also been shown that induced IκBα can bind activated NFκB in the nucleus and chaperone it to the cytoplasm to terminate NFκB-dependent transcription [31].

Mitogen-Activated Protein Kinase Pathways

Another transcription activating factor that mediates expression of a number of inflammation-related genes is activating protein-1 (AP-1). The AP-1 family consists of various homodimers and heterodimers of the Jun (e.g., c-Jun), Fos (e.g., c-fos), or activating transcription factor (e.g., ATF2) proteins [reviewed in 32]. Various combinations of these proteins have been described, although the most commonly described AP-1 *complex* is the heterodimer formed by c-jun and c-fos proteins. Activating protein-1 regulates a diverse set of cellular functions, including cell proliferation and growth, apoptosis, inflammation, and tissue morphogenesis. Activation of AP-1 occurs in response to propagation of the upstream signal by an interwoven cascade of pathways known as the mitogen-activated protein kinase (MAPK) pathways [reviewed in 33–35]. Three MAPK pathways exist: the c-Jun NH₂-terminal kinase (JNK) pathway (also called the *stress-activated MAPK* [SAPK] pathway); the extracellular-regulated protein kinase (ERK) pathway; and the p38 mitogen-activated kinase (p38 MAPK). All members of these MAPK families undergo activation via phosphorylation of threonine and tyrosine residues by upstream MAPK kinases (MKKs or MEKs), which are in turn activated via phosphorylation by upstream MKK kinase (MKKKs or MEKKs) (Figure 17.4) [36]. A diverse set of stimuli that activate these pathways can broadly influence a variety of cellular functions relevant to inflammation and critical illness.

p38 Mitogen-Activated Protein Kinase Pathway

The p38 family of MAPK is composed of various isoforms (two α isoforms and β1, β2, γ, and δ) whose expressions are dictated in large part by cellular and tissue localization. For example, leukocytes express predominantly p38α and p38δ isoforms. Similar to the NFκB pathway, a number of stimuli activate this pathway, notably lipopolysaccharide, TNF, IL-8, and platelet activating factor, which in turn mediates gene expression changes of several downstream targets described to play a critical role in numerous disease states (see Figure 17.4) [34]. One of the key occurrences in acute lung injury is the infiltration of leukocytes from the vascular space into the lung, which is mediated by a coordinated effort of cytokines, chemokines, integrins, and adhesion molecules. As a result of the genes regulated by p38, this pathway likely plays a central role in this pathogenesis. For example, lipopolysaccharide-induced expression of TNF-α from both neutrophils [37] and macrophages [38] is augmented by p38 activation

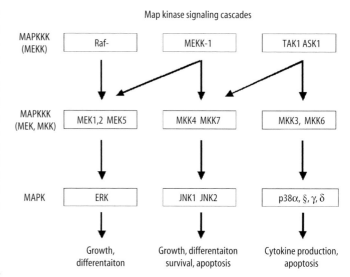

FIGURE 17.4. Mitogen-activated protein kinase (MAPK) signal transduction pathways. MAPKK (MEK, MKK), MAPK kinase; MAPKKK (MEKK), MAPK kinase kinase.

via a process of mRNA stabilization. Similarly, TNF-α-mediated upregulation of E-selectin, which initiates the *rolling* phase of the leukocyte–endothelial cell adhesion cascade, is regulated in part through p38 activation of the transcription factor ATF2 [39]. The migration of adherent neutrophils from the vascular endothelium to the alveolus in acute lung injury is mediated by chemokines, such as CXCL8/IL-8, often induced by lipopolysaccharide or TNF-α, which is also dependent on p38 activation. Finally, the lung injury associated with infiltration of neutrophils into the airspace is at least in part caused by release of toxic oxygen radical species. Production of reactive oxygen species is catalyzed by NADPH oxidase of which a necessary subunit is the p47^{phox} protein. Phosphorylation and subsequent activation of p47^{phox} by the p38 pathway appears necessary to the assembly of this complex [40]. One of the important endogenous counter-regulators of the p38 pathway is the dual-specific phosphatase MKP-1, which deactivates p38 via dephosphorylation as described below. Thus, given its ubiquitous role in mediating several events in leukocyte-mediated injury, the p38 MAPK pathway may be a valid target for inhibition in the hopes of attenuating inflammatory responses.

JNK Mitogen-Activated Protein Kinase Pathway

Three principal JNK protein kinases have been identified—JNK-1 and JNK-2, which are ubiquitously expressed, and JNK-3, which appears restricted to the brain. JNK protein kinases are also phosphorylated on threonine and tyrosine residues by upstream kinases (MKK4/SEK1 and MKK7 (see Figure 17.4) [33,35]. MKK4 is promiscuous in being capable of activating both the JNK and p38 MAPK pathways, while MKK7, which is primarily activated by proinflammatory cytokines, is generally restricted to JNK activation [41,42]. Upstream from MKK4/MKK7, the MKKK MEKK-1 appears to be responsible for downstream activation of the JNK pathway [43,44].

Using TNF-α as a stimulus, recent studies have elucidated the mechanisms by which initiation of the signal at the cell surface is transduced through MEKK-1, resulting in JNK activation. The use of TNF-α as a stimulus resulted in the identification of the role of TRAF adaptor proteins as it was observed that TNF-α binding to TRAF-2 caused receptor oligomerization with consequent binding to and activation of MEKK-1 [21,45]. Endotoxin [19] stimulation of monocytes also results in JNK activation with the observed downstream consequence of AP-1 complex formation and transcriptional activation of IL-1β expression [46,47]. Similar to the observed counterrelationship between p38 and MKP-1, lipopolysaccharide-induced JNK activation is negatively modulated by the endogenous serine-threonine phosphatase PP2A [47]. A physical association between JNK and the regulatory subunit PP2A-A/α, in addition to other reports of signal transduction complexes composed of MAP kinases and regulatory phosphatases in association with scaffolding proteins, suggests that these *signalosomes* may be critical regulatory components of inflammatory cell signal transduction pathways [48]. As on-going studies continue to unravel the mechanisms by which signals are transduced through these complex pathways, the precise roles of the JNK pathway in disease states such as sepsis and acute lung injury will be better understood to determine the validity of therapeutic measures aimed at its attenuation.

ERK Mitogen-Activated Protein Kinase Pathway

Although it was the first identified member of the MAPK pathways, less has been reported with regards to the potential role of the ERK pathway in inflammatory diseases such as sepsis and acute lung injury. Two ERK isoforms exist, denoted as ERK1 and ERK2. The principal MAPKKK that activates the ERK1/2 is Raf, which in turn activates the MAPKKs MEK1 and MEK2 (see Figure 17.4) [49,50]. Raf activation is initiated by the G-coupled protein Ras, which can be stimulated by a number of growth factors, including epidermal growth factor, platelet-derived growth factor, and transforming growth factor-β [51]. As a result, it is intuitive that ERK activation plays a primary role in cell growth and differentiation that may be vitally important to the repair process following tissue injury.

The role for ERK does not appear restricted to this function, as investigators have reported additional functional consequences of ERK activation. For example, ERK activation was described following respiratory syncytial virus infection of lung epithelial cells, and production of CXCL8/IL-8 from these cells was attenuated by ERK inhibition, suggesting a role for ERK in viral-induced chemokine production [52]. Thus, while data implicating the ERK MAPK pathway in critical illnesses remain limited, this pathway may ultimately play an important role in pathogen-mediated (e.g., viral) cell activation (Table 17.3).

Role of Phosphatases in Modulating Signal Transduction Pathways

From a historical perspective, the paradigm of reversible phosphorylation was initially described in the context of understanding the regulation of glycogen metabolism by phosphorylases a and b [53,54]. Since then, it is now understood that the phosphorylated state of a protein reflects a balance between phosphorylation mediated by protein kinases and dephosphorylation mediated by phosphatases. Protein phosphatases (PP) are categorized into three classes: those targeting serine and/or threonine residues (Ser/Thr phosphatases); those targeting tyrosine phosphorylated residues (Tyr phosphatases); and dual-specificity phosphatases that can

TABLE 17.3. Partial list of genes regulated by activating protein-1/mitogen-activated protein kinase pathways.

Inflammatory mediators
  Tumor necrosis factor-α
  Interleukins-1, -2, -4, and -18
  Inducible nitric oxide synthase (iNOS)
  Arginine transporter

Transcriptional activators
  c-fos/c-jun (self-activating mechanism)
  Nuclear factor AT4

Adhesion molecules
  E-selectin
  Intracellular adhesion molecule 1 (ICAM-1)
  Integrins ($\alpha_m\beta_2$ integrin)
  P-selectin glycoprotein ligand-1 (PSGL-1)

Others
  p47^{phox} (component of NADPH oxidase complex)
  Cyclooxygenase-2
  Fas ligand
  Tau (microtubule-associated protein)

target either tyrosine and/or threonine residues (e.g., mixed kinase phosphatases [MKPs]) (Table 17.4) [55].

Based on biochemical parameters, substrate specificity, and sensitivity to pharmacologic inhibitors, Ser/Thr protein phosphatases are further divided into two major classes. Type I phosphatases (e.g., PP1) can be inhibited by two heat-stable proteins known as Inhibitor-1 (I-1) and Inhibitor-2 (I-2) and preferentially dephosphorylate the β-subunit of phosphorylase kinase. In contrast, type II PPs are insensitive to heat-stable inhibitors and preferentially dephosphorylate the α-subunit of phosphorylase kinase. Type II phosphatases are subdivided into spontaneously active (PP2A), Ca^{2+}-dependent (PP2B), and Mg^{2+}-dependent (PP2C) classes. Subtle but important structural differences in and around the catalytic site provide one component of substrate specificity. Also, additional regulatory proteins that bind to the catalytic subunits and in some instances comprise larger phosphatase complexes or

TABLE 17.4. Classes of phosphatases.

Serine/threonine phosphatases	Tyrosine phosphatases
Protein phosphatase (PP) P family	Cytosolic protein tyrosine phosphatases
PP1	SHP-1
PP2A	SHP-2
PP2B	PTP-1B
PPM family	Receptor-like protein tyrosine phosphatases (RPTPs)
PP2C	CD45
Novel members	RPTPα
PP4/PPX	Low-molecular weight protein tyrosine phosphatases
PP6/PPV	T-cell protein tyrosine phosphatase
	Dual-specificity phosphatases
	MKP-1, MKP-2
	MKP-3/Pyst1
	CDC25
	MKP-5

Note: MKP, mixed kinase phosphatase; PP, protein phosphatase; PTP, protein tyrosine phosphatase.

holoenzymes afford additional substrate specificity [56]. Detailed structural and enzymatic biochemistries of the various phosphatases have been elucidated, but this discussion is beyond the objective of this chapter. Instead, for additional information on the formal biochemistry of these enzymes the reader is referred to other excellent reviews [57,58].

Given the importance of reversible protein phosphorylation to a myriad of cellular functions, it is likely that the various phosphatases regulate several key physiologic processes regulated by signal transduction pathways. For example, PP1 participates in glycogen metabolism, muscle contraction, protein synthesis, intracellular protein transport, and cell cycle (by regulating mitosis and chromosome segregation) [59]. Despite its ubiquitous role in these homeostatic cellular functions, whether PP1 plays a role in signaling pathways relevant to critical illness remains to be more completely defined. In contrast, much data suggest that PP2A plays a key role in the endogenous regulation of inflammation-related signaling pathways.

Cell stimulation by either TNF-α or IFN-γ has been shown to activate sphingomyelinase, leading to the formation of ceramide. Ceramide is capable of mimicking the cytotoxicity of TNF-α and Fas by activating caspases that lead to apoptosis [60]. Of note, ceramide formation has also been described to activate what was previously termed *ceramide-activated protein phosphatase*, which turns out to be the trimeric form of PP2A [61]. As reviewed above, the AP-1 transcriptional activation pathway regulates expression of a number of inflammatory mediators. The upstream kinases in the MAPK pathways are activated via phosphorylation principally of serine and threonine residues and as such are logical targets of Ser/Thr phosphatases [62]. Inhibition of PP2A by the small-t antigen [63], I-2 [64], or okadaic acid [47] has been shown to result in hyperphosphorylation and augmented activity of JNK. This increase in JNK activity was associated with increased AP-1–driven transcriptional activity and gene expression as evidenced by increased IL-1β expression [65]. The data with regards to PP2A regulation of the NF-κB pathway are less clear cut. Addition of phosphatase inhibitors to human T cells caused an increased activation of NFκB that correlated with hyperphosphorylation of IκB-α, and only recombinant PP2A, but not PP1 or PP2C, could dephosphorylate IκB-α [66].

In another biologic model, it was shown that respiratory syncytial virus infection of epithelial cells caused a persistent activation of NFκB that was mediated by expression of the viral phosphoprotein P, which was shown to sequester and inhibit PP2A [67]. Together, these data suggest that PP2A may be a crucial negative modulator of the NFκB pathway. In contrast, more recently Kray et al. [68] demonstrated that, in binding to the IκK-γ subunit, PP2A was necessary to fully achieve phosphorylation of IκK and activation of NFκB. Thus, although it appears certain that PP2A is a crucial modifier of important signal transduction cascades, what precise effects it has appears to depend on the stimulus, cell type, and pathway examined such that further investigation into the role of this Ser/Thr phosphatase is warranted.

One of the other families of phosphatases that are clearly important to regulation of inflammation-related signaling pathways is the dual-specificity phosphatases, which have been shown to be key negative modulators of the MAPK pathways, thus the term *MAPK phosphatases* (MKPs) [reviewed in 69,70]. At the time of this writing, 10 MKPs have now been cloned all of which share a conserved catalytic domain and an amino-terminal noncatalytic domain. Several notable characteristics distinguish the MKPs from previously reviewed phosphates. First, some of the MKPs (e.g., MKP-1) are transcriptionally induced by the same stimuli that activate the MAPKs, such as lipopolysaccharide [71]. Second, many of the MKPs show tremendous substrate specificity as exemplified by MKP-3 (Pyst1), which demonstrates nearly 100-fold more activity toward ERK2 than p38 [72]. Third, expression of some of the MKPs can be transient as shown for MKP-1, which can be targeted for ubiquitin-mediated proteasomal degradation similar to IκB-α [73]. Finally, MAPK inactivation may be governed by specific protein–protein interactions with MKPs as demonstrated for MKP-3 whose binding of its noncatalytic domain to ERK2 results in substantial enhancement of MKP-3 phosphatase activity [74]. Thus, the MKP family of dual-specificity phosphatases is anticipated to be key regulators of the MAP kinases that are known to mediate a number of proinflammatory events.

Regulation of mRNA Transcription

Alterations of the signal transduction pathways reviewed above will profoundly affect expression of numerous proinflammatory genes. However, mRNAs, particularly those of usually silent, but rapidly induced genes, are subject to *post-transcriptional* modification, ultimately affecting the amount of translation and therefore protein expression that can occur. One primary post-transcriptional mechanism that regulates gene expression is mRNA destabilization. Cytokines (e.g., TNF-α, IL-1β, IL-8) are among such genes that possess adenosine-uridine (AU)–rich elements (ARE) in the ribonucleotide sequence of the distal end of the untranslated region (3'-UTR) of their mRNA [75–77]. These ARE sequences are thus subject to both stabilizing and destabilizing proteins (e.g., ribonucleases) that can alter the half-life of the mRNA species, affecting the amount that can be translated to protein

One such example with relevance to sepsis and acute respiratory distress syndrome is the post-transcriptional regulation of TNF-α expression. There exist proteins (e.g., tristetraproin/TTP and AUF1) capable of binding to the AREs of the 3'-UTR to destabilize TNF-α mRNA and decrease TNF-α expression [78]. Conversely, other proteins such as HuR bind to the AREs to stabilize TNF-α mRNA [79]. Of note, activation of p38 MAPK appears critical to facilitating the interaction of these RNA binding proteins to stabilize lipopolysaccharide-induced TNF-α mRNA [80]. This highly sophisticated regulation explains the vast complexity faced in trying to mechanistically understand the myriad of pathways that can influence gene expression induced even by a single stimulus.

Conclusion

Signal transduction provides the cellular basis for sensing extracellular changes or pathologic stresses and transmitting this signal to the transcriptional machinery capable of mounting a response on the basis of gene expression. The vast complexity, remarkable interconnectedness, and substantial redundancy of the myriad of signal transduction pathways create an enormous challenge to deciphering their precise roles in biology, particularly in disease states as complex as those faced in the pediatric intensive care unit. In addition to this complexity, many of the scientific findings reported are often cell type, stimulus, and model specific with no direct relevance to an unrelated approach. Thus, the goal remains to strive to understand the molecular processes at play using both a reductionist (i.e., single pathway) and a more comprehensive (i.e., genomics, proteomics, clinical studies) approach to identify potential therapeutic targets within a relevant pathway. Surely as our methodologic approaches advance, our understanding of the molecular and biochemical regulation of signaling pathways will continue to grow at an extraordinary rate. The key will be translating this improved understanding into more effective therapeutic approaches directed toward improving the outcomes of critically ill children. Signal transduction is the language of the cells; to achieve this lofty goal, we too must become fluent in this sophisticated molecular language.

References

1. Bradshaw RA, Dennis EA. Handbook of Cell Signaling. San Diego, CA: Elsevier Academic Press; 2003.
2. Angus DC, Fink MP. Molecular biology for today's practicing intensivist. Crit Care Med 2005;33:S399.
3. Bayliss WM, Starling EH. The mechanism of pancreatic secretion. J Physiol 1902;28:325.
4. Wright RD. The origin of the term "hormone." Trends Biochem Sci 1978;3:275–277.
5. Wong HR. Translation. Crit Care Med 2005;33:S404–406.
6. Read RC, Wyllie DH. Toll receptors and sepsis. Curr Opin Crit Care 2001;7:371–375.
7. Dunne A, O'Neill LA. The interleukin-1 receptor/toll-like receptor superfamily: signal transduction during inflammation and host defense. Sci STKE 2003;171:re3.
8. Hunter T. Protein kinases and phosphatases: the yin and yang of protein phosphorylation and signaling. Cell 1995;80:225–236.
9. Hunter T. Protein modification: phosphorylation on tyrosine residues. Curr Opin Cell Biol 1989;1:1168–1181.
10. Chang L, Karin M. Mammalian MAP kinase signaling cascades. Nature 2001;410:37–45.
11. Johnson GL, Lapadat R. Mitogen-activated protein kinase pathways mediated by ERK, JNK and p38 kinases. Science 2002;298:1911–1912.
12. Goggel R, Winoto-Morbach S, Vielhaber G, Imai Y, Lindner K, Brade L, Brade H, Ehlers S, Slutsky AS, Schutze S, Gulbins E, Uhlig S. PAF-mediated pulmonary edema: a new role for acid sphingomyelinase and ceramide. Nat Med 2004;10:155–160.
13. Galie N, Manes A, Branzi A. The endothelin system in pulmonary arterial hypertension. Cardiovasc Res 2004;61:227–237.
14. Karin M. The NF-κB activation pathway: its regulation and role in inflammation and cell survival. Cancer J Sci Am 1998;4(Suppl 1):S92–S99.
15. Bonizzi G, Karin M. The two NF-κB activation pathways and their role in innate and adaptive immunity. Trends Immunol 2004;25:280–288.
16. Senftleben U, Karin M. The IKK/NF-κB pathway. Crit Care Med 2002;30:S18–S26.
17. Delhase M, Karin M. The I κ B kinase: a master regulator of NF-κB, innate immunity, and epidermal differentiation. Cold Spring Harbor Symp Quant Biol 1999;64:491–503.
18. Delhase M, Hayakawa M, Chen Y, Karin M. Positive and negative regulation of IκB kinase activity through IKKβ subunit phosphorylation. Science 1999;284:309–313.
19. Das AK, Helps NR, Cohen PT, Barford D. Crystal structure of the protein serine/threonine phosphatase 2C at 2.0 A resolution. EMBO J 1996;15:6798–6809.
20. Qian Y, Commane M, Ninomiya-Tsuji J, Matsumoto K, Li X. IRAK-mediated translocation of TRAF6 and TAB2 in the interleukin-1-induced activation of NFκ B. J Biol Chem 2001;276:41661–41667.
21. Baud V, Karin M. Signal transduction by tumor necrosis factor and its relatives. Trends Cell Biol 2001;11:372–377.
22. Karin M, Ben-Neriah Y. Phosphorylation meets ubiquitination: the control of NF-[kappa]B activity. Annu Rev Immunol 2000;18:621–663.
23. Wong HR, Shanley TP. Signal transduction pathways in acute lung injury: NF-κB and AP-1. In: Wong HR, Shanley TP, eds. Molecular Biology of Acute Lung Injury. Norwell, MA: Kluwer Academic Publishers; 2001:1–16.
24. Jarrar D, Kuebler JF, Rue LW, 3rd, Matalon S, Wang P, Bland KI, Chaudry IH. Alveolar macrophage activation after trauma-hemorrhage and sepsis is dependent on NF-κB and MAPK/ERK mechanisms. Am J Physiol Lung Cell Mol Physiol 2002;283:L799–L805.
25. Arnalich F, Garcia-Palomero E, Lopez J, Jimenez M, Madero R, Renart J, Vazquez JJ, Montiel C. Predictive value of nuclear factor κB activity and plasma cytokine levels in patients with sepsis. Infect Immun 2000;68:1942–1945.
26. Bohrer H, Qiu F, Zimmermann T, Zhang Y, Jllmer T, Mannel D, Bottiger BW, Stern DM, Waldherr R, Saeger HD, Ziegler R, Bierhaus A, Martin E, Nawroth PP. Role of NFκB in the mortality of sepsis. J Clin Invest 1997;100:972–985.
27. Paterson RL, Galley HF, Dhillon JK, Webster NR. Increased nuclear factor kappa B activation in critically ill patients who die. Crit Care Med 2000;28:1047–1051.
28. Hoberg JE, Popko AE, Ramsey CS, Mayo MW. IκB kinase α-mediated derepression of SMRT potentiates acetylation of RelA/p65 by p300. Mol Cell Biol 2006;26:457–471.
29. Imbert V, Rupec RA, Livolsi A, Pahl HL, Traenckner EB, Mueller-Dieckmann C, Farahifar D, Rossi B, Auberger P, Baeuerle PA, Peyron JF. Tyrosine phosphorylation of I kappa B-alpha activates NF-kappa B without proteolytic degradation of I kappa B-alpha. Cell 1996;86:787–798.
30. Ito CY, Kazantsev AG, Baldwin AS, Jr. Three NF-kappa B sites in the I kappa B-alpha promoter are required for induction of gene expression by TNF alpha. Nucleic Acids Res 1994;22:3787–3792.
31. Arenzana-Seisdedos F, Thompson J, Rodriguez MS, Bachelerie F, Thomas D, Hay RT. Inducible nuclear expression of newly synthesized I kappa B alpha negatively regulates DNA-binding and transcriptional activities of NF-kappa B. Mol Cell Biol 1995;15:2689–2696.
32. Karin M, Liu Z, Zandi E. AP-1 function and regulation. Curr Opin Cell Biol 1997;9:240–246.
33. Davis RJ. Signal transduction by the JNK group of MAP kinases. Cell 2000;103:239–252.
34. Herlaar E, Brown Z. p38 MAPK signaling cascades in inflammatory disease. Mol Med Today 1999;5:439–447.
35. Ip YT, Davis RJ. Signal transduction by the c-Jun N-terminal kinase (JNK)—from inflammation to development. Curr Opin Cell Biol 1998;10:205–219.
36. Su B, Karin M. Mitogen-activated protein kinase cascades and regulation of gene expression. Curr Opin Immunol 1996;8:402–411.
37. Nick JA, Avdi NJ, Young SK, Lehman LA, McDonald PP, Frasch SC, Billstrom MA, Henson PM, Johnson GL, Worthen GS. Selective activation and functional significance of p38α mitogen-activated protein kinase in lipopolysaccharide-stimulated neutrophils. J Clin Invest 1999;103:851–858.
38. Mahtani KR, Brook M, Dean JL, Sully G, Saklatvala J, Clark AR. Mitogen-activated protein kinase p38 controls the expression and posttranslational modification of tristetraprolin, a regulator of tumor necrosis factor alpha mRNA stability. Mol Cell Biol 2001;21:6461–6469.
39. Read MA, Whitley MZ, Gupta S, Pierce JW, Best J, Davis RJ, Collins T. Tumor necrosis factor α-induced E-selectin expression is activated by the nuclear factor-κB and c-JUN N-terminal kinase/p38 mitogen-activated protein kinase pathways. J Biol Chem 1997;272:2753–2761.
40. Brown GE, Stewart MQ, Bissonnette SA, Elia AE, Wilker E, Yaffe MB. Distinct ligand-dependent roles for p38 MAPK in priming and activation of the neutrophil NADPH oxidase. J Biol Chem 2004;279:27059–27068.

41. Tournier C, Whitmarsh AJ, Cavanagh J, Barrett T, Davis RJ. Mitogen-activated protein kinase kinase 7 is an activator of the c-Jun NH2-terminal kinase. Proc Natl Acad Sci USA 1997;94:7337–7342.

42. Tournier C, Dong C, Turner TK, Jones SN, Flavell RA, Davis RJ. MKK7 is an essential component of the JNK signal transduction pathway activated by proinflammatory cytokines. Genes Dev 2001;15:1419–1426.

43. Yujiri T, Sather S, Fanger GR, Johnson GL. Role of MEKK1 in cell survival and activation of JNK and ERK pathways defined by targeted gene disruption. Science 1998;282:1911–1914.

44. Xia Y, Makris C, Su B, Li E, Yang J, Nemerow GR, Karin M. MEK kinase 1 is critically required for c-Jun N-terminal kinase activation by pro-inflammatory stimuli and growth factor-induced cell migration. Proc Natl Acad Sci USA 2000;97:5243–5248.

45. Baud V, Liu ZG, Bennett B, Suzuki N, Xia Y, and Karin M. Signaling by proinflammatory cytokines: oligomerization of TRAF2 and TRAF6 is sufficient for JNK and IKK activation and target gene induction via an amino-terminal effector domain. Genes Dev 1999;13:1297–1308.

46. Hambleton J, Weinstein SL, Lem L, DeFranco AL. Activation of c-Jun N-terminal kinase in bacterial lipopolysaccharide-stimulated macrophages. Proc Natl Acad Sci USA 1996;93:2774–2778.

47. Shanley TP, Vasi N, Denenberg A, and Wong HR. The serine/threonine phosphatase, PP2A: endogenous regulator of inflammatory cell signaling. J Immunol 2001;166:966–972.

48. Burack WR, Shaw AS. Signal transduction: hanging on a scaffold. Curr Opin Cell Biol 2000;12:211–216.

49. Kolch W, Calder M, Gilbert D. When kinases meet mathematics: the systems biology of MAPK signalling. FEBS Lett 2005;579:1891–1895.

50. Kolch W. Coordinating ERK/MAPK signalling through scaffolds and inhibitors. Nat Rev Mol Cell Biol 2005;6:827–837.

51. Thompson N, Lyons J. Recent progress in targeting the Raf/MEK/ERK pathway with inhibitors in cancer drug discovery. Curr Opin Pharmacol 2005;5:350–356.

52. Chen W, Monick MM, Carter AB, Hunninghake GW. Activation of ERK2 by respiratory syncytial virus in A549 cells is linked to the production of interleukin 8. Exp Lung Res 2000;26:13–26.

53. Cori GT CC. The enzymatic conversion of phosphorylase b to a. J Biol Chem 1945;158:321–332.

54. Fischer EH, Krebs EG. Conversion of phosphorylase b to phosphorylase a in muscle extracts. J Biol Chem 1955;216.

55. Shanley TP. Phosphatases: counterregulatory role in inflammatory cell signaling. Crit Care Med 2002;30:S80–S88.

56. Schillace RV, Scott JD. Organization of kinases, phosphatases, and receptor signaling complexes. J Clin Invest 1999;103:761–765.

57. Mumby MC, Walter G. Protein serine/threonine phosphatases: structure, regulation, and functions in cell growth. Physiol Rev 1993;73:673–699.

58. Barford D, Das AK, Egloff MP. The structure and mechanism of protein phosphatases: insights into catalysis and regulation. Annu Rev Biophys Biomol Struct 1998;27:133–164.

59. Ceulemans H, Bollen M. Functional diversity of protein phosphatase-1, a cellular economizer and reset button. Physiol Rev 2004;84:1–39.

60. Kolesnick R, Golde DW. The sphingomyelin pathway in tumor necrosis factor and interleukin-1 signaling. Cell 1994;77:325–328.

61. Galadari S, Kishikawa K, Kamibayashi C, Mumby MC, Hannun YA. Purification and characterization of ceramide-activated protein phosphatases. Biochemistry 1998;37:11232–11238.

62. Chung H, Brautigan DL. Protein phosphatase 2A suppresses MAP kinase signalling and ectopic protein expression. Cell Signal 1999;11:575–580.

63. Sontag E, Sontag JM, Garcia A. Protein phosphatase 2A is a critical regulator of protein kinase C zeta signaling targeted by SV40 small t to promote cell growth and NF-κB activation. EMBO J 1997;16:5662–5671.

64. Al-Murrani SW, Woodgett JR, Damuni Z. Expression of I2PP2A, an inhibitor of protein phosphatase 2A, induces c-Jun and AP-1 activity. Biochem J 1999;341:293–298.

65. Shanley TP, Vasi N, Denenberg A, Wong HR. The serine/threonine phosphatase, PP2A: endogenous regulator of inflammatory cell signaling. J Immunol 2001;166:966–972.

66. Sun SC, Maggirwar SB, Harhaj E. Activation of NF-kappa B by phosphatase inhibitors involves the phosphorylation of I kappa B alpha at phosphatase 2A-sensitive sites. J Biol Chem 1995;270:18347–18351.

67. Bitko V, Barik S. Persistent activation of RelA by respiratory syncytial virus involves protein kinase C, underphosphorylated IκBβ, and sequestration of protein phosphatase 2A by the viral phosphoprotein. J Virol 1998;72:5610–5618.

68. Kray AE, Carter RS, Pennington KN, Gomez RJ, Sanders LE, Llanes JM, Khan WN, Ballard DW, Wadzinski BE. Positive regulation of IκB kinase signaling by protein serine/threonine phosphatase 2A. J Biol Chem 2005;280:35974–35982.

69. Camps M, Nichols A, Arkinstall S. Dual specificity phosphatases: a gene family for control of MAP kinase function. FASEB J 2000;14:6–16.

70. Keyse SM. Protein phosphatases and the regulation of mitogen-activated protein kinase signalling. Curr Opin Cell Biol 2000;12:186–192.

71. Nimah M, Zhao B, Denenberg AG, Bueno O, Molkentin J, Wong HR, Shanley TP. Contribution of MKP-1 regulation of p38 to endotoxin tolerance. Shock 2005;23:80–87.

72. Groom LA, Sneddon AA, Alessi DR, Dowd S, and Keyse SM. Differential regulation of the MAP, SAP and RK/p38 kinases by Pyst1, a novel cytosolic dual-specificity phosphatase. EMBO J 1996;15:3621–3632.

73. Brondello JM, Pouyssegur J, McKenzie FR. Reduced MAP kinase phosphatase-1 degradation after p42/p44MAPK-dependent phosphorylation. Science 1999;286:2514–2517.

74. Camps M, Nichols A, Gillieron C, Antonsson B, Muda M, Chabert C, Boschert U, Arkinstall S. Catalytic activation of the phosphatase MKP-3 by ERK2 mitogen-activated protein kinase. Science 1998;280:1262–1265.

75. Geanacopoulos M. An introduction to RNA-mediated gene silencing. Sci Prog 2005;88:49–69.

76. Guhaniyogi J, Brewer G. Regulation of mRNA stability in mammalian cells. Gene 2001;265:11–23.

77. Wilson GM, Sutphen K, Chuang K, Brewer G. Folding of A+U-rich RNA elements modulates AUF1 binding. Potential roles in regulation of mRNA turnover. J Biol Chem 2001;276:8695–8704.

78. Lai WS, Carballo E, Strum JR, Kennington EA, Phillips RS, Blackshear PJ. Evidence that tristetraprolin binds to AU-rich elements and promotes the deadenylation and destabilization of tumor necrosis factor alpha mRNA. Mol Cell Biol 1999;19:4311–4323.

79. Dean JL, Wait R, Mahtani KR, Sully G, Clark AR, Saklatvala J. The 3' untranslated region of tumor necrosis factor alpha mRNA is a target of the mRNA-stabilizing factor HuR. Mol Cell Biol 2001;21:721–730.

80. Carter AB, Monick MM, Hunninghake GW. Both Erk and p38 kinases are necessary for cytokine gene transcription. Am J Respir Cell Mol Biol 1999;20:751–758.

18
Proinflammatory and Antiinflammatory Mediators in Critical Illness

Daniel G. Remick

Introduction

There are several important pathways involved in critical illness. One aspect of these pathways is the inflammatory response, a response that may be generated in reaction to traumatic injury, acute pancreatitis, or severe infectious diseases. Many of the physiologic parameters that are traditionally measured in critically ill patients represent responses induced by the inflammatory mediators, which are discussed below. Therefore, understanding the nature of the inflammatory response aids our understanding of the physiologic response. A clear example of this is the altered body temperature, typically fever, which occurs in the setting of severe infections. The body's temperature is regulated by specific aspects of the inflammatory response [1–3]. Thus, the infection induces an inflammatory response that initiates the fever.

Among the important pathways altered in critical illness are the coagulation pathways, arachidonic acid metabolism pathways, and, the major topic of this chapter, the cytokine pathways. There are several reasons for focusing on the cytokine pathways. First, the body actively upregulates and downregulates cytokine production in response to numerous stimuli. Many of the stimuli have physiologic importance. Second, cytokines have been selected for therapeutic intervention in critical illnesses [4]. There was a belief that appropriate modulation of the cytokines would improve outcomes. Finally, the cytokines, and their naturally occurring inhibitors, are easily measured, which allows for correlation between cytokine levels and clinical outcome.

Cytokines are small peptides, usually produced by one cell, that exert biologic effects on another cell [5]. In virtually every case, the biologic activity is brought about by the cytokine interacting with a specific, or relatively specific, receptor. Cytokines may be regu-

lated at the level of induction of mRNA coding for the cytokine, modulation of release of the cytokine from the cell, altered cytokine binding to its receptor, or regulation of the receptor. Given the complexity of cytokine biology, it is not surprising that there have been numerous failures at attempts to modulate their biologic activity and improve disease outcome [4].

There are multiple ways that the cytokines and cytokine inhibitors can be organized. The approach used in this chapter is to divide them based on their broad biologic functions, although there could be other potential organizational schemes, such as grouping them based on the protein structure, phylogeny, or a simple chronological list of when they were discovered. Here, the division of these mediators into three broad groups, (1) proinflammatory, (2) inhibitors of synthesis of proinflammatory cytokines, and (3) molecules that block biological activity, aids in the understanding of how the interactions occur among the different pathways.

Mediators

Proinflammatory Cytokines

Tumor Necrosis Factor and Interleukin-1

There are numerous proinflammatory cytokines, and tumor necrosis factor (TNF) and interleukin (IL)–1 are considered to be classic proinflammatory mediators because they drive the inflammatory process forward. Typically, they will help initiate an acute inflammatory response by inducing production of other proinflammatory cytokines, recruiting acute inflammatory cells to the site of inflammation, and inducing an acute phase response by the liver. Additionally, TNF and IL-1 may directly cause organ injury and tissue damage when they are injected in high concentrations to either experimental animals or patients [6,7].

Tumor necrosis factor was originally described as a factor present in the serum of animals that had been injected with high doses of endotoxin [8]. When this serum was injected into an animal bearing an experimental tumor, there was a factor present that would cause necrosis of tumors. While TNF certainly does possess this biologic activity, it has other more relevant biologic activities when used at physiologic doses. Many of the other cytokines were originally named for their biologic activity, but there has been a strong attempt to unify and codify the naming of interleukins and

D.S. Wheeler et al. (eds.), *Science and Practice of Pediatric Critical Care Medicine*,
DOI 10.1007/978-1-84800-921-9_18, © Springer-Verlag London Limited 2009

cytokines. As a result, IL-1 was the first molecule to be given an official designation. It has been cloned into an α and β form, but the principal form that is secreted is the β form. Interleukin-1 is now considered part of a family of proteins that also includes interleukin-18. Interleukin-18 shares biologic activity with IL-12, including induction of γ-interferon [9] and clearance of intracellular pathogens [10].

Interleukin-2, -15, and -21

The IL-2, -15, and -21 cytokines are clustered together and share biologic activity. They signal to cells by binding to common receptor subunits located on the IL-2 receptor. These cytokines exert their effects primarily by activating T cells and natural killer (NK) cells [11,12].

Interleukin-6

Interleukin-6 is actively synthesized primarily by macrophages, although many other cell types have the capacity to synthesize and secrete this cytokine. Interleukin-6 is easily upregulated, and increased plasma levels may be found in a variety of conditions, such as cancer and severe bacterial infections, and even in normal individuals who have exercised vigorously. Interleukin-6 has been used frequently as a marker for the level of inflammation within experimental animals or patients [13]. It is somewhat controversial whether IL-6 is a marker of disease severity or if it actively participates in organ injury and altered pathophysiology. There are numerous reports documenting that IL-6 serves as a marker that closely correlates with clinical disease states [14].

Chemokines

Chemokines are divided into two broad families based on the protein structure. These two families are the CXC and the CC chemokines. The CXC chemokines have a total of four cysteine residues, indicated by the C, which are separated by an intervening amino acid, which is designated by the X. The first of these mediators to be well described was IL-8. The chief biologic properties of IL-8 include the recruitment and activation of neutrophils [15]. Interleukin-8 has been shown to recruit neutrophils to the site of an inflammatory response by generating a chemotactic gradient. The CXC chemokines also activate neutrophils to increase the production of reactive oxygen intermediates and proteases. The CC chemokines act principally on mononuclear cells such as monocytes and lymphocytes. Clues to the specificity of these molecules may be found in the very names that were assigned to them, such as monocyte chemotactic peptide. The chemokines are a very large family of proinflammatory molecules. As such they have undergone a name change, and each of the individual chemokines are now assigned a unique number [16]. The number is based on whether the chemokine belongs to the CC or the CXC family. The chemokine receptors have also been carefully numbered to include a CC or CXC designation. As an example, IL-8 has been renamed CXCL8.

The Interleukin 12 Family (Interleukin-12, -23, and -27)

Interleukin-12 is part of a family of cytokines that includes IL-23 and IL-27. Interleukin-12 is unusual among the cytokines because it is composed of two discrete subunits, a p40 and p35 subunit, which form a heterodimer [17]. Interleukin-23 is also a heterodimer composed of the p40 and a p19 subunit [18]. Interleukin-27 is also a heterodimer composed of an Epstein-Barr virus–induced protein and a p28 subunit [19]. Members of the IL-12 family are produced by monocytes, macrophages, and dendritic cells. Principal among the biologic activities of the IL-12 are the induction of the Th1-type response, including the induction of γ-interferon. Interleukin-23 has a similar γ-interferon effect [18] but also induces the proliferation and activation of T cells. The functional activity of IL-27 has yet to be fully developed.

γ-Interferon

γ-Interferon (γ-IFN) was one of the first cytokines to be cloned back in 1982 [20] and typically exists as a homodimer. Major activities of γ-IFN include induction of antiviral activities and macrophage activation [21].

Naturally Occurring Molecules That Inhibit the Action of Pre-Formed Cytokines

The cytokines have numerous potent biologic activities, as briefly described earlier. When the cytokines become increased at either the local or the systemic level, their biologic activity has the potential to alter inflammatory reactions as well as physiologic responses. At sufficiently high concentrations, cell, tissue, and organ injury may occur. Because these activities are so powerful, the body has developed regulatory mechanisms in order to appropriately modulate the biologic activities of these potent proteins. There are three broad classes of naturally occurring molecules that inhibit the biologic activity of pre-formed cytokines. The first of these representative molecules, and the first discovered, are soluble receptors that have been cleaved by proteolysis, and another group is the soluble binding proteins that are not receptors. The third group is composed of proteins that bind to the receptors on the surface of cells but do not transduce a signal, thereby acting as pure antagonists.

Soluble Receptors

One of the first-described cytokine inhibitors was the TNF soluble receptor [22]. There are two discrete receptors for TNF, and both may be cleaved from the surface of the cell by a specific enzyme. The receptors began as normal surface bound receptors where they function to transduce signals to the cell. However, once they have been released into the plasma or tissue culture supernatants, these soluble receptors retain their capacity to bind to their natural ligands. When the cytokine is bound to these soluble receptors, it is not available to bind to the receptor on the surface of the cell. In many respects, soluble receptors act like specific antibodies, as they couple with, and neutralize, a very discrete range of mediators. It must be mentioned that not all soluble receptors inhibit cytokine activity, because it has been reported that the soluble IL-6 receptor actually increases the biologic activity of IL-6 [23].

There is another class of receptors, the so-called decoy receptors. These receptors do not actually transduce the signal when present on the surface of the cell. The only apparent function for these receptors is to bind and inactivate the soluble cytokines. The type II IL-1 receptor is an example of this kind of receptor [24].

Soluble Binding Proteins

In contrast to soluble receptors, soluble binding proteins never function as receptors on the surface of cells. These are proteins that are synthesized and produced by cells, but their real function is to bind and inactivate circulating cytokines. An example of this type of protein is the IL-18 binding protein [25]. Although these proteins were never receptors originally, their biologic action is similar to the soluble receptors.

Receptor Antagonists

Receptor antagonists operate through a different mechanism of action to inhibit the action of cytokines. The previous two groups bound to the cytokines in solution to prevent them from binding to the receptors. The receptor antagonists bind to the receptor on the surface of the cell in a pure antagonist fashion. Since the antagonist is bound to the receptor, the stimulating cytokine is not able to bind to the receptor and stimulate the cell. The best example of this is the interleukin one receptor antagonist protein [26].

Naturally Occurring Molecules That Inhibit the Production of Cytokines

The previously discussed group of proteins functions by blocking the activity of cytokines after they have been formed. In contrast to blocking the activity of the preformed cytokines, there are several cytokines that prevent the synthesis of new, proinflammatory cytokines.

Interleukin-4

Interleukin-4 is produced by T cells as well as NK cells [27]. It has been demonstrated to block the lipopolysaccharide-induced production of several of the proinflammatory cytokines, such as those described above [28,29].

Interleukin-10

Interleukin-10 was originally described as cytokine synthesis inhibitory factor [30,31], which clearly indicates its range of biologic activity. It has been classically described as the TH2 cytokine that inhibits TH1 cytokine synthesis [32]. Viral IL-10 has also been described, and this molecule, secreted by viruses, shares functional properties with IL-10, such as the suppression of cytokine synthesis by cells [33]. This represents a novel way that viruses have discovered to evade the immune response. Based on protein structure homology, IL-20, IL-22, and IL-24 may be considered to be in the IL-10 family.

Interleukin-13

Interleukin-13 is another of the cytokines that has been documented to suppress the synthesis of other cytokines. It has been shown to specifically control the inflammation induced by excessively activated macrophages [32]. Additionally, it plays an important role in protective immunity against gastrointestinal nematodes [34].

Transforming Growth Factor-β

Transforming growth factor-β (TGF-β) was one of the first described cytokines, reported so early that it does not even have an interleukin number. The original description was based on the biologic activity by which it could transform the phenotype of cells [35]. Since these initial observations, it has been more fully defined in terms of its capacity to regulate the inflammatory response.

Determining the Status of the Inflammatory State

Many previous studies have documented that proinflammatory cytokines are frequently elevated following acute injury. For example, following injection of endotoxin there is frequently a substantial, brisk rise in cytokines, such as IL-6 and TNF. This elevation in the cytokines occurs in both experimental animals and humans [36]. For many years it was assumed that the biologic activity of the cytokines was dictated by their concentrations. These concentrations may be either in the local environment, such as the synovial space, cerebrospinal fluid, or bronchoalveolar lavage fluid, or in the systemic circulation, such as serum or plasma.

As our knowledge of the cytokines increased, it became apparent that this simple concept did not accurately reflect the interrelationship between cytokines and the physiologic response. It was reported over 10 years ago that an imbalance in the ratio of TNF to the soluble TNF receptors was associated with disease outcome [37]. Higher levels of TNF that were not matched by increases in the soluble receptors predicted a poor outcome. Such reports changed the perspective among cytokine biologists to view biologic activity as not dictated by a simple measurement of the concentration but rather as a ratio between the proinflammatory cytokines and the cytokine inhibitors. If cytokines became elevated, but an associated increase in the cytokine inhibitors also occurred, the net biologic effect would be the same. Thus, knowing only the level of the cytokine does not provide sufficient information to properly assess biologic impact.

Interleukin-1 and Interleukin-1 Receptor Antagonist

The data concerning the imbalance between the proinflammatory IL-1 and the cytokine inhibitors are quite strong. This information has been developed using the natural progression of many scientific investigations where initial studies were performed with in vitro cell cultures, followed by experimental animal data, progressing to clinical studies showing correlations and culminating in clinical trials with the inhibitors. There are numerous studies that have evaluated IL-1 and IL-1 receptor antagonist (RA) in patients with chronic inflammatory conditions [38,39]. In patients with inflammatory bowel disease, there is an imbalance between IL-1 and the IL-1 inhibitors [40]. The administration of exogenous IL-1 RA will improve disease outcome in patients with arthritis as demonstrated in clinical trials [41].

Interleukin-1 RA has been used to prevent lung injury in several experimental animal models, including injury induced by bleomycin or silica [42]. Lung injury observed after hindlimb ischemia–reperfusion injury was also blocked by IL-1 inhibitors [43]. Interleukin-1 RA has also been shown to reduce allergic responses within the lung [44]. In a very interesting study with patients with status asthmaticus it was determined that the bronchoalveolar lavage fluid had a ratio of IL-1 to IL-1 RA favoring a proinflammatory state [45]. The authors confirmed this proinflammatory phenotype by investigating the ability of the bronchoalveolar lavage fluid to induce adhesion molecule expression in a cultured cell line.

The bronchoalveolar lavage fluid levels of IL-1 RA and IL-1 were used to study patients with pulmonary sarcoidosis. In this study, patients were followed prospectively and longitudinally. The ratios of the IL-1 RA protein to inflammatory factors was a significant prognostic factor for predicting the course of the disease [46]. Among patients with meningitis, the cerebrospinal fluid ratios of IL-1 to IL-1 RA were significantly different in patients with bacterial compared with viral meningitis [47]. Interstitial pulmonary fibrosis results in excess deposition of collagen within the lung and may be considered the opposite end of the spectrum of an acute inflammatory response. In these situations, there are greater concentrations of IL-1 RA than IL-1 [48], which indicates that the ratio may be either proinflammatory or antiinflammatory.

It has been postulated that septic shock represents the physiologic response to the massive production of cytokines. In an experimental animal model of endotoxin, IL-1 RA was able to reduce mortality [49], and in a model of *Escherichia coli* infection mortality was also decreased [50]. However, as virtually all critical care physicians are aware, blockade of IL-1 with the IL-1 receptor antagonist did not demonstrate any survival benefit in large-scale clinical trials [51].

Tumor Necrosis Factor and Their Soluble Receptors

As described earlier, there are two different TNF receptors, both of which may exist in the soluble form [52]. High levels of TNF, IL-1, and the naturally produced TNF inhibitors have been found within the synovial fluid obtained from patients with temporomandibular joint disorders [53]. The use of TNF inhibitors has revolutionized the treatment of two chronic inflammatory conditions: rheumatoid arthritis and Crohn's disease. Both of these diseases are now successfully treated with either antibodies to TNF or soluble TNF receptors [54,55].

Several studies have measured the presence of both TNF and the TNF soluble receptors in human disease states. In a very interesting article, patients' self-rated health level correlated negatively with circulating cytokine levels, with higher cytokine levels being associated with lower ratings [56]. In children with viral infections, an imbalance between TNF and TNF soluble receptors has been reported [57]. Patients with Guillain-Barré syndrome have elevated levels of TNF, and treatment with intravenous immunoglobulin decreases plasma levels of TNF while increasing concentrations of TNF soluble receptors [58].

Within the bronchoalveolar lavage fluid of patients at increased risk for development of the acute respiratory distress syndrome (ARDS), concentrations of the proinflammatory TNF (and IL-1) are increased. However, once ARDS became manifest, the cytokine inhibitors increased, indicating that a dampening of the inflammatory response was taking place [59]. In another study, which evaluated the bronchoalveolar lavage fluid from patients with pneumonia, the cytokines/cytokine inhibitor ratios were altered such that the lung presented a relative proinflammatory state as the infectious process evolved [60]. Interestingly, these changes were not observed in the peripheral circulation but only in the bronchoalveolar lavage fluid.

In an experimental animal model of a parasitic infection, mice with cachexia had greater concentrations of TNF relative to the TNF soluble receptors [52]. The highest ratios were observed in mice that were about to die. The ratio of cytokines to cytokine inhibitors was carefully followed in an experimental animal study to document the progression of disease [61]. The model used was the well-described cecal litigation and puncture (CLP) model [62], which has been previously demonstrated to closely mimic many of the physiologic and pathologic changes observed in patients with sepsis [63,64]. In the recent paper, liver levels of cytokines and cytokine inhibitors were documented over the first 24 hours. The data show that, in a lethal model of sepsis, there is early production of proinflammatory cytokines followed by later production of antiinflammatory cytokines. Modulating the response by prior treatment with IL-1 RA resulted in increased bacterial load and greater mortality.

Altering the balance between the TNF and TNF soluble receptors alters the inflammatory response to diseases. The shedding of the soluble receptors of TNF has been demonstrated to control the threshold for activation of the innate immune response during infectious diseases [65]. In this study, a form of the TNF receptor was mutated so that it could not be shed. Mice with this mutant TNF receptor had increased resistance to intracellular infections but augmented autoimmune inflammatory type processes. In a similar manner, mice that lack the TNF soluble receptor were resistant to the toxic effects of TNF but more sensitive to bacterial infections [66]. Treatment of septic patients with TNF soluble receptors resulted in increasing concentrations of TNF in the plasma but did not alter the antiinflammatory response [67]. Additionally, blockade of TNF has not proven to be effective for the treatment of sepsis in several large trials [4,14].

Critical Interactions Among the Cytokines and Inhibitors

Now that we have briefly defined the principal mediators in the inflammatory response, we must attempt to detail how they interact with one another. The inflammatory response is multifactorial and complex. A simple, linear A ⇨ B ⇨ C probably does not fully reflect the multifaceted events that typically take place during the acute inflammatory response. A paradigm has arisen whereby it is believed that critically ill patients move through different phases. Shortly after the initiating event there is an acute phase of increased inflammation that is typically termed the *systemic inflammatory response syndrome* (SIRS) [68]. At the conclusion of this phase an antiinflammatory response arises, and the patients actually become immunosuppressed. This phase is typically termed the *compensatory antiinflammatory response syndrome* (CARS). This concept is usually graphed on a straight line [69,70], with the x-axis representing time and the y axis the level of inflammation. This oversimplifies a complex process. Many patients, and indeed even experimental animals, do not move in a straight line toward resolution of the inflammatory response or organ injury and death. Despite these caveats, the concept of different states of inflammation yielding different outcomes is attractive and worthy of pursuit.

There is some experimental data addressing the evolution of the inflammatory response. Several investigators have used a stimulated whole blood model to investigate regulation of the inflammatory response. In this model, human whole blood is combined with different stimuli and placed on a rocking platform in a 37° incubator. Numerous different stimuli may be used, including lipopoly-

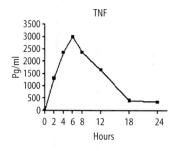
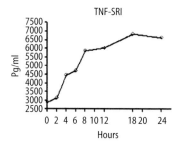
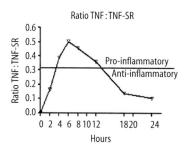

FIGURE 18.1. Production of tumor necrosis factor (TNF) and TNF soluble receptor I (TNF-SRI) following lipopolysaccharide stimulation of human whole blood. The TNF is rapidly produced, while the production and release of TNF-SRI is delayed and continued. The ratio of TNF to both soluble TNF receptors is displayed in the far-right graph. An arbitrary line is drawn at the 0.3 level to illustrate the concept that, as the level of TNF increases relative to the soluble receptors, the blood achieves a relative proinflammatory state.

saccharide, zymosan, and also some of the early proinflammatory cytokines such as TNF and IL-1. Samples may be collected at different time points following stimulation in order to document the evolution of the inflammatory response.

Using this system, changes in the pro- and antiinflammatory cytokines may be easily determined (Figure 18.1). At time zero, that is, before any stimulation, virtually no proinflammatory cytokines are detected. Specifically, TNF, IL-1, IL-6, and IL-8 are all below detection limits in the assay. In contrast, normal individuals have substantial plasma levels of cytokine inhibitors, such as the TNF soluble receptors and the IL-1 receptor antagonist protein. In fact, it is difficult to calculate a ratio between the proinflammatory and antiinflammatory cytokines because the proinflammatory cytokines are equal to zero. The situation changes dramatically within a few hours of stimulation. For these experiments, the blood is stimulated with lipopolysaccharide. The proinflammatory cytokines are quickly induced and achieve high plasma levels within 6 hours. Notably, the antiinflammatory molecules do not become induced during this early time frame. The antiinflammatory mediators increase in concentration at later time points.

If one calculates the ratio of the proinflammatory to the antiinflammatory mediators a clear pattern emerges. Using only TNF and the TNF soluble receptors, a kinetic graph may be drawn (see Figure 18.1). Starting at time zero, the antiinflammatory mediators are present in much greater excess than the proinflammatory mediators. This would favor the view that a normal person has a generally antiinflammatory state, characterized by an excess of the naturally occurring cytokine inhibitors. At 6 hours, the proinflammatory cytokine TNF has become significantly elevated while there has been little change in the levels of the TNF soluble receptors. At the 6-hour time point, the plasma may be considered to be proinflammatory as determined by the ratio between the cytokine and its naturally occurring cytokine inhibitors. By 24 hours, the ratio has reverted back to the original antiinflammatory state.

There are of course several limitations when using the ex vivo stimulated blood model. There is no clearance of the cytokines or the cytokine inhibitors such as would occur in normal circulating plasma. This results in much higher levels of the local cytokines. Additionally, the time to achieve peak cytokine synthesis occurs more slowly than that observed when endotoxin is infused into normal volunteers [36].

The concept concerning the ratios dictating biologic outcome extends beyond the proinflammatory and antiinflammatory cytokine inhibitors. Among the chemokines, the biologic activity may be dictated by the ratio of the local to the systemic concentrations.

Local levels need to exceed systemic levels in order to recruit inflammatory cells to the site of inflammation [71].

Conclusion

Multiple pathways dictate the clinical trajectory of individual patients. Previously, it was assumed that high levels of proinflammatory cytokines were responsible for the progression of disease. From this assumption evolved strategies to block the inflammatory response and attempt to improve survival and critical illnesses such as sepsis. As our knowledge of cytokine biology improved, the newer concept emerged that the biologic activity was dictated by the ratio of the proinflammatory to the antiinflammatory cytokines. Data are beginning to be developed to support this hypothesis. As these data evolve, a multiplex approach to measuring the inflammatory response in individual patients may be necessary in order to optimally direct therapy.

Acknowledgments. I wish to acknowledge the editorial assistance of Jill Granger and the technical assistance of Javed Siddiqui. This work was supported in part by grants from the National Institutes of Health and GM 44918 and GM 50401.

References

1. LeMay LG, Vander AJ, Kluger MJ. Role of interleukin 6 in fever in rats. Am J Physiol 1990;258(3 Pt 2):R798–R80.3
2. Leon LR, White AA, Kluger MJ. Role of IL-6 and TNF in thermoregulation and survival during sepsis in mice. Am J Physiol 1998;275(1 Pt 2): R269–R277.
3. Long NC, Otterness I, Kunkel SL, Vander AJ, Kluger MJ. Roles of interleukin 1 beta and tumor necrosis factor in lipopolysaccharide fever in rats. Am J Physiol 1990;259:R724–R728.
4. Remick DG. Cytokine therapeutics for the treatment of sepsis: why has nothing worked? Curr Pharm Design 2003;9(1):75–82.
5. Thomson AW, Lotze MT, eds. The Cytokine Handbook: 4th edition. New York: Academic Press, 2003.
6. Remick DG, Kunkel RG, Larrick JW, Kunkel SL. Acute in vivo effects of human recombinant tumor necrosis factor. Lab Invest 1987;56: 583–590.
7. Tracey KJ, Beutler B, Lowry SF, et al. Shock and tissue injury induced by recombinant human cachectin. Science 1986;234:470–474.
8. Carswell EA, Old LJ, Kassel RL, Green S, Fiore N, Williamson B. An endotoxin-induced serum factor that causes necrosis of tumors. Proc Natl Acad Sci USA 1975;72:3666–3670.

9. Okamura H, Tsutsi H, Komatsu T, et al. Cloning of a new cytokine that induces IFN-gamma production by T cells. Nature 1975;378(6552): 88–91.

10. Kobayashi K, Kai M, Gidoh M, et al. The possible role of interleukin (IL)-12 and interferon-gamma-inducing factor/IL-18 in protection against experimental *Mycobacterium leprae* infection in mice. Clin Immunol Immunopathol 1998;88(3):226–231.

11. Sivakumar PV, Foster DC, Clegg CH. Interleukin-21 is a T-helper cytokine that regulates humoral immunity and cell-mediated anti-tumour responses. Immunology 2004;112(2):177–182.

12. Waldmann T. The contrasting roles of IL-2 and IL-15 in the life and death of lymphocytes: implications for the immunotherapy of rheumatological diseases. Arthritis Res 2002;4(Suppl 3):S161–S167.

13. Remick DG, Bolgos GR, Siddiqui J, Shin J, Nemzek JA. Six at six: interleukin-6 measured 6h after the initiation of sepsis predicts mortality over 3 days. Shock 2002;17(6):463–467.

14. Remick DG. Mediators of sepsis. In: Dietch EA, Vincent JL, Windsor A, eds. Sepsis and Multiple Organ Dysfunction. New York: WB Saunders; 2002:63–72.

15. Moser B, Wolf M, Walz A, Loetscher P. Chemokines: multiple levels of leukocyte migration control. Trends Immunol 2004;25(2):75–84.

16. IUIS/Who Subcommittee on Chemokine Nomenclature. Chemokine/chemokine receptor nomenclature. Cytokine 2003;21(1):48–49.

17. Gately MK, Wilson DE, Wong HL. Synergy between recombinant interleukin 2 (rIL 2) and IL 2–depleted lymphokine-containing supernatants in facilitating allogeneic human cytolytic T lymphocyte responses in vitro. J Immunol 1986;136(4):1274–1282.

18. Oppmann B, Lesley R, Blom B, et al. Novel p19 protein engages IL-12p40 to form a cytokine, IL-23, with biological activities similar as well as distinct from IL-12. Immunity 2000;13(5):715–725.

19. Pflanz S, Timans JC, Cheung J, et al. IL-27, a heterodimeric cytokine composed of EBI3 and p28 protein, induces proliferation of naive CD4(+) T cells. Immunity 2002;16(6):779–790.

20. Gray PW, Goeddel DV. Structure of the human immune interferon gene. Nature 1982;298(5877):859–863.

21. Schreiber RD, Pace JL, Russell SW, Altman A, Katz DH. Macrophage-activating factor produced by a T cell hybridoma: physiochemical and biosynthetic resemblance to gamma-interferon. J Immunol 1983; 131(2):826–832.

22. Kohno T, Brewer MT, Baker SL, Schwartz PE, et al. A second tumor necrosis factor receptor gene product can shed a naturally occurring tumor necrosis factor inhibitor. Proc Natl Acad Sci USA 1990;87: 8331–8335.

23. Muller-Newen G, Kuster A, Hemmann U, Keul R, et al. Soluble IL-6 receptor potentiates the antagonistic activity of soluble gp130 on IL-6 responses. J Immunol 1998;161(11):6347–6355.

24. Sims JE, Giri JG, Dower SK. The two interleukin-1 receptors play different roles in IL-1 actions. Clin Immunol Immunopathol 1994;72: 9–14.

25. Dinarello CA. Novel targets for interleukin 18 binding protein. Ann Rheum Dis 2001;60 Suppl 3:iii18–iii24.

26. Carter DB, Deibel MR Jr, Dunn CJ, et al. Purification, cloning, expression and biological characterization of an interleukin-1 receptor antagonist protein [see comments]. Nature 1990;344:633–638.

27. Yokota T, Otsuka T, Mosmann T, et al. Isolation and characterization of a human interleukin cDNA clone, homologous to mouse B-cell stimulatory factor 1, that expresses B-cell- and T-cell–stimulating activities. Proc Natl Acad Sci USA 1986;83(16):5894–5898.

28. Hart PH, Vitti GF, Burgess DR, Whitty GA, Piccoli DS, Hamilton JA. Potential antiinflammatory effects of interleukin 4: suppression of human monocyte tumor necrosis factor alpha, interleukin 1, and prostaglandin E2. Proc Natl Acad Sci USA 1989;86(10):3803–3807.

29. Standiford TJ, Strieter RM, Chensue SW, et al. IL-4 inhibits the expression of IL-8 from stimulated human monocytes. J Immunol 1990; 145(5):1435–1439.

30. Fiorentino DF, Bond MW, Mosmann TR. Two types of mouse T helper cell. IV. Th2 clones secrete a factor that inhibits cytokine production by Th1 clones. J Exp Med 1989;170(6):2081–2095.

31. de Waal Malefyt R, Abrams J, Bennett B, Figdor CG, de Vries JE. Interleukin 10 (IL-10) inhibits cytokine synthesis by human monocytes: an autoregulatory role of IL-10 produced by monocytes. J Exp Med 1991;174:1209–1220.

32. de Waal Malefyt R, Figdor CG, Huijbens R, et al. Effects of IL-13 on phenotype, cytokine production, and cytotoxic function of human monocytes. Comparison with IL-4 and modulation by IFN-gamma or IL-10. J Immunol 1993;151(11):6370–6381.

33. McFadden G, Graham K, Ellison K, et al. Interruption of cytokine networks by poxviruses: lessons from myxoma virus. J Leukocyte Biol 1995;57(5):731–738.

34. Barner M, Mohrs M, Brombacher F, Kopf M. Differences between IL-4R alpha-deficient and IL-4–deficient mice reveal a role for IL-13 in the regulation of Th2 responses. Curr Biol 1998;8(11):669–672.

35. Moses HL, Branum EL, Proper JA, Robinson RA. Transforming growth factor production by chemically transformed cells. Cancer Res 1981; 41(7):2842–2848.

36. Copeland S, Warren HS, Lowry SF, Calvano SE, Remick D. Acute inflammatory response to endotoxin in mice and humans. Clin Diagn Lab Immunol 2005;12(1):60–67.

37. Girardin E, Roux-Lombard P, Grau GE, Suter P, Gallati H, Dayer JM. Imbalance between tumour necrosis factor-alpha and soluble TNF receptor concentrations in severe meningococcaemia. The J5 Study Group. Immunology 1992;76(1):20–23.

38. Arend WP. The balance between IL-1 and IL-1Ra in disease. Cytokine Growth Factor Rev 2002;13(4–5):323–340.

39. Arend WP, Gabay C. Cytokines in the rheumatic diseases. Rheum Dis Clin North Am 2004;30(1):41–67, v–vi.

40. Ludwiczek O, Vannier E, Borggraefe I, et al. Imbalance between interleukin-1 agonists and antagonists: relationship to severity of inflammatory bowel disease. Clin Exp Immunol 2004;138(2):323–329.

41. Cohen SB. The use of anakinra, an interleukin-1 receptor antagonist, in the treatment of rheumatoid arthritis. Rheum Dis Clin North Am 2004;30(2):365–380, vii.

42. Piguet PF, Vesin C, Grau GE, Thompson RC. Interleukin 1 receptor antagonist (IL-1ra) prevents or cures pulmonary fibrosis elicited in mice by bleomycin or silica. Cytokine 1993;5(1):57–61.

43. Seekamp A, Warren JS, Remick DG, Till GO, Ward PA. Requirements for tumor necrosis factor-alpha and interleukin-1 in limb ischemia/reperfusion injury and associated lung injury. Am J Pathol 1993;143: 453–463.

44. Selig W, Tocker J. Effect of interleukin-1 receptor antagonist on antigen-induced pulmonary responses in guinea pigs. Eur J Pharmacol 1992;213(3):331–336.

45. Tillie-Leblond I, Pugin J, Marquette CH, et al. Balance between proinflammatory cytokines and their inhibitors in bronchial lavage from patients with status asthmaticus. Am J Respir Crit Care Med 1999; 159(2):487–494.

46. Mikuniya T, Nagai S, Takeuchi M, et al. Significance of the interleukin-1 receptor antagonist/interleukin-1 beta ratio as a prognostic factor in patients with pulmonary sarcoidosis. Respiration 2000;67(4):389–396.

47. Akalin H, Akdis AC, Mistik R, Helvaci S, Kilicturgay K. Cerebrospinal fluid interleukin-1 beta/interleukin-1 receptor antagonist balance and tumor necrosis factor-alpha concentrations in tuberculous, viral and acute bacterial meningitis. Scand J Infect Dis 1994;26(6):667–674.

48. Smith D R, Kunkel SL, Standiford TJ, et al. Increased interleukin-1 receptor antagonist in idiopathic pulmonary fibrosis. A compartmental analysis. Am J Respir Crit Care Med 1995;151(6):1965–1973.

49. Ohlsson K, Bjork P, Bergenfeldt M, Hageman R, Thompson RC. Interleukin-1 receptor antagonist reduces mortality from endotoxin shock. Nature 1990;348(6301):550–552.

50. Wakabayashi G, Gelfand JA, Burke JF, Thompson RC, Dinarello CA. A specific receptor antagonist for interleukin 1 prevents *Escherichia coli*-induced shock in rabbits. FASEB J 1991;5:338–343.

51. Fisher CJ Jr, Dhainaut JF, Opal SM, Recombinant human interleukin 1 receptor antagonist in the treatment of patients with sepsis syndrome. Results from a randomized, double-blind, placebo-controlled trial. Phase III rhIL-1ra Sepsis Syndrome Study Group [see comments]. JAMA 1994;271:1836–1843.

52. Hehlgans T, Pfeffer K. The intriguing biology of the tumour necrosis factor/tumour necrosis factor receptor superfamily: players, rules and the games. Immunology 2005;115(1):1–20.

53. Kaneyama K, Segami N, Sun W, Sato J, Fujimura K. Analysis of tumor necrosis factor-alpha, interleukin-6, interleukin-1beta, soluble tumor necrosis factor receptors I and II, interleukin-6 soluble receptor, interleukin-1 soluble receptor type II, interleukin-1 receptor antagonist, and protein in the synovial fluid of patients with temporomandibular joint disorders. Oral Surg Oral Med Oral Pathol Oral Radiol Endod 2005;99(3);276–284.

54. Taylor PC. Anti-TNFalpha therapy for rheumatoid arthritis: an update. Internal Medicine. 2003;42(1):15–20.

55. Raza A. Anti-TNF therapies in rheumatoid arthritis, Crohn's disease, sepsis, and myelodysplastic syndromes. Microscopy Res Technique 2000;50(3):229–235.

56. Lekander M, Elofsson S, Neve IM, Hansson LO, Unden AL. Self-rated health is related to levels of circulating cytokines. Psychosom Med 2004;66(4):559–563.

57. Barash J, Dushnitzki D, Barak Y, Miron S, Hahn T. Tumor necrosis factor (TNF)alpha and its soluble receptor (sTNFR) p75 during acute human parvovirus B19 infection in children. Immunol Lett 2003;88(2):109–112.

58. Radhakrishnan VV, Sumi MG, Reuben S, Mathai A, Nair MD. Serum tumour necrosis factor-alpha and soluble tumour necrosis factor receptors levels in patients with Guillain-Barre syndrome. Acta Neurol Scand 2004;109(1):71–74.

59. Park WY, Goodman RB, Steinberg KP, et al. Cytokine balance in the lungs of patients with acute respiratory distress syndrome. Am J Respir Crit Care Med 2001;164(10 Pt 1):1896–1903.

60. Millo JL, Schultz MJ, Williams C, et al. Compartmentalisation of cytokines and cytokine inhibitors in ventilator-associated pneumonia. Intensive Care Med 2004;30(1):68–74.

61. Ashare A, Powers LS, Butler NS, Doerschug KC, Monick MM, Hunninghake GW. Anti-inflammatory response is associated with mortality and severity of infection in sepsis. Am J Physiol Lung Cell Mol Physiol 2005;288(4):L633–L640.

62. Wichterman KA, Baue AE, Chaudry IH. Sepsis and septic shock—a review of laboratory models and a proposal. J Surg Res 1980;29: 189–201.

63. Ebong SJ, Call DR, Bolgos G, et al. Immunopathologic responses to non-lethal sepsis. Shock 1999;12(2):118–126.

64. Ebong S, Call D, Nemzek J, Bolgos G, Newcomb D, Remick D. Immunopathologic alterations in murine models of sepsis of increasing severity. Infect Immun 1999;67(12):6603–6610.

65. Xanthoulea S, Pasparakis M, Kousteni S, et al. Tumor necrosis factor (TNF) receptor shedding controls thresholds of innate immune activation that balance opposing TNF functions in infectious and inflammatory diseases. J Exp Med 2004;200(3):367–376.

66. Rothe J, Lesslauer W, Lotscher H, et al. Mice lacking the tumour necrosis factor receptor 1 are resistant to TNF-mediated toxicity but highly susceptible to infection by *Listeria monocytogenes*. Nature 1993; 364(6440):798–802.

67. Butty VL, Roux-Lombard P, Garbino J, Dayer JM, Ricou B. Anti-inflammatory response after infusion of p55 soluble tumor necrosis factor receptor fusion protein for severe sepsis. Eur Cytokine Netw 2003;14(1):15–19.

68. Bone RC, Balk RA, Cerra FB, Dellinger RP, et al. Definitions for sepsis and organ failure and guidelines for the use of innovative therapies in sepsis. The ACCP/SCCM Consensus Conference Committee. American College of Chest Physicians/Society of Critical Care Medicine [see comments]. Chest 1992;101:1644–1655.

69. Hotchkiss RS, Karl IE. Medical progress: the pathophysiology and treatment of sepsis. N Engl J Med 2003;348(2):138–150.

70. Oberholzer A, Oberholzer C, Moldawer LL. Sepsis syndromes: understanding the role of innate and acquired immunity. Shock 2001;16(2): 83–96.

71. Call DR, Nemzek JA, Ebong SJ, Bolgos GL, Newcomb DE, Remick DG. Ratio of local to systemic chemokine concentrations regulates neutrophil recruitment. American Journal of Pathology 2001;158(2):715–721.

19
Endogenous Cytoprotective Mechanisms

Hector R. Wong

Introduction

A variety of fundamental endogenous cytoprotective mechanisms have evolved that impart mammalian adaptation and survival under highly adverse environmental and disease-related conditions. The number of potential mechanisms is vast and beyond the scope of this chapter. This chapter focuses on selected, major endogenous cytoprotective mechanisms that have been chosen for inclusion because of their broad cytoprotective effects. The mechanisms/pathways reviewed include heme oxygenase, the heat shock response, antioxidant systems, hypoxia inducible factor, and nitric oxide.

Heme Oxygenase

Heme oxygenase (HO) is responsible for catalyzing what is one of the most well-known and common colorimetric reactions in humans: the transformation of a common bruise through the spectrum of hues ranging from purple to green to yellow [1,2]. Heme oxygenase is the first and rate-limiting step in the degradation of heme (purple hue) to biliverdin (green hue), and finally to bilirubin (yellow hue). Three known isoforms of HO exist: HO-1, -2, and -3. In the context of cytoprotection, HO-1 appears to be the most relevant isoform. Heme oxygenase-1 is identical to heat shock protein 32 and is highly inducible by a variety of cellular stressors and stimuli, including heme, nitric oxide, cytokines, heavy metals, hyperoxia, hypoxia, endotoxin, heavy metals, and heat shock [3–5]. Heme oxygenase-1 activity is present in virtually all organs and is thought to primarily account for the cytoprotective properties of HO. The importance of HO-1 in human health and disease was recently demonstrated by the description of a 6-year-old boy with complete HO-1 deficiency [6]. Before the ultimate discovery of HO-1 deficiency, this patient came to medical attention because of severe growth retardation, hemolytic anemia, tissue iron deposits, widespread evidence of endothelial cell damage, and increased susceptibility to oxidant injury. Interestingly, despite the severe degree of hemolysis, the blood chemistry profiles of this patient revealed a low bilirubin level in the setting of a high haptoglobin level.

Since the discovery HO in 1968, several observations have provided notable indications that HO-1 may serve an important cytoprotective role. These include the ability of HO-1 to be highly induced in response to potentially cytotoxic stimuli, its relative high level of conservation throughout evolution, and its wide tissue distribution. The prediction that HO-1 would confer broad cytoprotection has been confirmed by a variety of in vitro and in vivo studies. In vitro studies involving gene transfection or gene transfer approaches have provided clear evidence that HO-1 confers cytoprotection. For example, overexpression of HO-1 conferred protection against oxygen toxicity (hyperoxia) in hamster fibroblasts [7], rat fetal lung cells [8], and human respiratory epithelial cells [9]. In a similar manner, overexpression of HO-1 in coronary endothelial cells conferred protection against heme and hemoglobin toxicity [10]. In cultured murine fibroblasts, regulated overexpression of HO-1 conferred protection against tumor necrosis factor-α–mediated apoptosis [11]. Finally, in a human respiratory epithelial cell line representative of lung epithelial cells found in patients with cystic fibrosis, overexpression of HO-1 conferred protection against *Pseudomonas*-mediated cellular injury and apoptosis [12].

Experiments in animal models, involving either pharmacologic induction of HO-1 or genetic overexpression of HO-1, have confirmed that these in vitro observations are also operative in vivo. For example, induction of HO-1 by intravenous hemoglobin protected rats against the lethal effects of endotoxemia. Protection in this model correlated with attenuation of endotoxin-mediated hypotension, renal dysfunction, hepatic dysfunction, and inflammation [13,14]. The direct role of HO-1 in conferring protection was further confirmed by co-administration of a competitive inhibitor of HO, tin protoporphyrin, which led to a substantial reduction of the protective effects induced by intravenous hemoglobin administration. Lung epithelial overexpression of HO-1, via an adenovirus vector, conferred protection in rats exposed to hyperoxia [15], and cardiac-specific overexpression conferred protection in a murine model of ischemia [16]. There is also a great deal of interest in HO-1–mediated cytoprotection in the field of transplant biology. In a cardiac xenograft transplantation model (mouse to rat),

D.S. Wheeler et al. (eds.), *Science and Practice of Pediatric Critical Care Medicine*,
DOI 10.1007/978-1-84800-921-9_19, © Springer-Verlag London Limited 2009

increased expression of HO-1 improved graft survival [17,18]. Analogous applications in transplantation-related biology have demonstrated that increased expression of HO-1 confers protection in hepatic and renal ischemia [19,20].

Gene knockout studies have provided further evidence of the cytoprotective properties of HO-1 and have been instrumental in further elucidating the biologic roles of HO-1. Heme oxygenase-1 null mutant mice generally do not survive to term, and animals that do survive die during the first year of life [21]. These animals also display severe growth retardation, anemia, iron deposition in the kidneys and liver, and evidence of chronic inflammation in a variety of organs. This murine phenotype is remarkably similar to that described in the aforementioned patient with documented HO-1 deficiency [6]. In other investigations involving HO-1 null mutant mice, the animals have been demonstrated to be more susceptible to (1) renovascular-related hypertension, renal failure, and cardiac hypertrophy [22]; (2) endotoxin-mediated lethality [23]; and (3) right ventricular dilation and infarction secondary to chronic hypoxia [24]. Collectively, the in vitro, in vivo, and gene deletion studies outlined above provide compelling evidence regarding the broad cytoprotective role of HO-1 in clinically relevant forms of cellular and tissue injury. What remains relatively elusive, however, is the mechanism(s) by which HO-1 confers this broad level of protection.

The byproducts of HO enzymatic activity include carbon monoxide (CO), bilirubin, and ferritin, and each of these byproducts has been postulated to play a role in cytoprotection [3–5]. For example, ferritin is known to protect against oxidant stress, and bilirubin can function as a potent antioxidant. Although it is likely that the three byproducts synergize in some way to confer cytoprotection, the most recent work in the field implicates CO-related cell signaling as the key component of HO-1–mediated cytoprotection [3,25,26].

Carbon monoxide shares a variety of properties with another gaseous molecule having ubiquitous biologic effects, nitric oxide. These properties include neurotransmission, regulation of vascular tone, and activation of soluble guanylate cyclase [26]. Other important connections between the CO pathway and the nitric oxide pathway include co-induction of inducible nitric oxide synthase and HO-1 by common stimuli (e.g., reactive oxygen species and cytokines), nitric oxide–dependent induction of HO-1 expression, and CO-dependent modulation of nitric oxide production [26–29]. The reported biologic effects of CO include potent antiinflammatory effects (via the mitogen-activated protein kinase pathway), antiapoptotic effects, and antioxidant effects [18,20, 30–35]. In the context of these biologic effects, the cytoprotective properties of CO have been demonstrated in a variety of experiments involving direct administration of CO. For example, exogenous administration of CO protected cultured fibroblasts from tumor necrosis factor-α–mediated apoptosis [11]. In vivo administration of low concentrations of inhaled CO protected rats from hyperoxia-mediated acute lung injury [33], and administration of exogenous CO to cardiac tissue protected the tissue from ischemia–reperfusion injury following transplantation [36]. These in vivo studies are particularly intriguing because the amount of CO administered is within the range administered to patients undergoing lung diffusion scans [25]. The rapidly evolving data strongly suggest that HO-1–derived CO is the key mechanism by which HO-1 confers cytoprotection, and further work in this area holds tremendous potential for therapeutic strategies involving HO-1 and/or CO.

Antioxidant Systems

A vast number of normal biologic processes make extensive use of oxygen. While requisite, this process inevitably leads to the production of reactive oxygen species (ROS), including hydrogen peroxide, superoxide, hydroxyl radicals, nitric oxide, and peroxynitrite. Within a specific context, the production of ROS serves important biologic roles such as intracellular signaling and antimicrobial functions [37]. When produced in large amounts, however, ROS can cause excessive oxidant stress for the host, leading to cellular and tissue injury. Reactive oxygen species–mediated cellular and tissue injury involves damage to genomic and mitochondrial DNA, lipid peroxidation, and protein modification [38,39]. In addition, cell death secondary to oxidant stress can be from either necrosis or apoptosis. To manage these potentially deleterious effects of ROS, all aerobic organisms have well-developed antioxidant systems to protect cells and tissues against high levels of ROS production.

The family of superoxide dismutases (SOD) include Mn-SOD, Cu/Zn-SOD, and Fe-SOD [40]. Superoxide dismutases can exist within the cytoplasmic and mitochondrial cellular compartments and in the extracellular compartment. It is capable of efficiently converting two superoxide molecules to hydrogen peroxide and oxygen (Figure 19.1). The importance of SOD in host defense against oxidant stress is illustrated by gene knockout studies and by numerous studies demonstrating that genetic overexpression of SOD confers protection against oxidant stress [41–44]. In addition, mutations of human SOD are strongly linked to development of amyotrophic lateral sclerosis [45].

Catalases convert hydrogen peroxide to water and oxygen (see Figure 19.1) [46] and thus synergize with SOD activity. In addition, by lowering intracellular levels of hydrogen peroxide, catalases can prevent formation of hydroxyl radicals that could occur via the Fenton reaction (see Figure 19.1). Glutathione (GSH) peroxidases consist of a least four isoforms in mammals and are widely distributed in many tissues [47]. Similar to catalases, all members of the GSH peroxidases can convert hydrogen peroxide to water by using glutathione as a substrate.

Hemoglobin is a known scavenger of nitric oxide in mammalian systems and is likely to be a central component for mammalian detoxification of nitric oxide [48]. Gardner et al, however, have recently discovered enzymatic systems within both aerobic and anaerobic bacteria that can efficiently detoxify and scavenge nitric oxide [49–53]. Similar systems appear to be present in mammalian cells [54,55].

Thioredoxin and thioredoxin reductase serve as another major antioxidant mechanism in mammals [56]. In conjunction with nicotinamide adenine dinucleotide (NADPH), thioredoxin reductase leads to the reduction of the active disulfide site of thioredoxin. Thioredoxin, in turn, can broadly function as a protein disulfide reductant. In addition, the thioredoxin system provides an efficient mechanism for the regeneration of various low-molecular-weight antioxidants such as vitamin E, vitamin C, selenium-related compounds, lipoic acid, and ubiquinones [56].

In summary, potent antioxidant systems have evolved to counterbalance the normal production of ROS that occurs during many cellular processes, as well as the excessive amounts of ROS that can occur during pathologic states. Despite this elegant counterregulatory system, ROS can lead to cellular injury when either a component of the antioxidant system is defective or when the high level production of ROS overwhelms an otherwise intact antioxidant

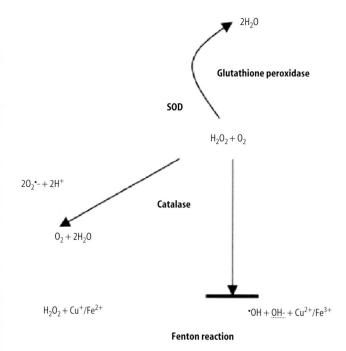

$$2H_2O$$

Glutathione peroxidase

SOD

$$H_2O_2 + O_2$$

$$2O_2^{\bullet-} + 2H^+$$

Catalase

$$O_2 + 2H_2O$$

$$H_2O_2 + Cu^+/Fe^{2+}$$

$$^{\bullet}OH + \underline{OH}\text{-} + Cu^{2+}/Fe^{3+}$$

Fenton reaction

FIGURE 19.1. Schematic depicting the activities of superoxide dismutase (SOD), catalase, and glutathione peroxidase. Superoxide dismutase converts two molecules of superoxide anion to form hydrogen peroxide and water. The hydrogen peroxide produced from this reaction can be further reduced by either catalase or glutathione peroxidase. Catalase converts two molecules of hydrogen peroxide to oxygen and water. Glutathione peroxidase converts hydrogen peroxide to two molecules of water using glutathione as a substrate. In addition, the reduction of hydrogen peroxide by catalase and glutathione peroxidase decreases the participation of hydrogen peroxide in the Fenton reaction, which can lead to the formation of hydroxyl radicals

system. Recognition of this critical balance and the mechanisms involved in defending against ROS holds tremendous potential for the design of therapeutic strategies directed toward restoring the balance between ROS production and endogenous antioxidant systems.

The Heat Shock Response

The heat shock response is another fundamental endogenous cytoprotective mechanism [57–59]. Originally described in *Drosophila*, it is now known to be highly conserved throughout virtually all known species. It is defined by the rapid expression of a class of proteins known as *heat shock proteins*, when a cell, tissue, or intact organism is exposed to elevated temperatures. In addition, heat shock proteins can be induced by a wide variety of nonthermal stressors and pharmacologic agents (Table 19.1).

One functional significance of the heat shock response, whether induced by thermal or nonthermal stress, is that it confers protection against subsequent and otherwise lethal hyperthermia. This phenomenon is referred to as *thermotolerance* [59,60]. Perhaps more interesting from a clinical standpoint is the phenomenon of cross-tolerance, whereby induction of the heat shock response confers protection against nonthermal cytotoxic stimuli. For example, in vitro experiments have demonstrated that induction of the heat shock response protects endothelial cells against endotoxin-mediated apoptosis [61]. Other examples include heat

shock response–dependent protection against nitric oxide [62], peroxynitrite [63], and hydrogen peroxide [64]. In vivo, induction of the heat shock response protects animals against endotoxemia/sepsis [65,66], acute lung injury [67,68], and ischemia–reperfusion injury [68].

The mechanisms by which the heat shock response confers such broad cytoprotection are not fully understood, but heat shock protein 70 (HSP70) certainly plays a central role in cytoprotection. Heat shock protein 70 is the most highly induced heat shock protein in cells and tissues undergoing the heat shock response [57], and it is known to be induced in patients with a variety of critical illnesses or injuries [69–72]. Microinjection of anti-HSP70 antibody into cells impairs their ability to achieve thermotolerance [73], and increased expression of HSP70 by gene transfer/transfection has been demonstrated to confer protection against in vitro toxicity secondary to lethal hyperthermia [74], endotoxin [61], nitric oxide [62], hyperoxia [75], and in vivo ischemia–reperfusion injury [76–78]. In addition, in vitro delivery of mature HSP70 into the intracellular compartment has been shown to protect fibroblasts against lethal thermal injury and hyperoxia [79], and neuronal cells against nitrosative stress and excitotoxicity [80].

Mice deficient in heat shock factor-1, the transcription factor responsible for high-level expression of HSP70, have a drastically reduced ability to express HSP70 [81,82]. Cell lines derived from these animals cannot achieve thermotolerance and are highly susceptible to oxidant stress compared with cells from wild-type mice [81–83]. When challenged with systemic endotoxin, heat shock factor-1–deficient mice have increased mortality compared with wild-type mice [82]. Collectively, these data demonstrate that HSP70 is central to the cytoprotective properties of the heat shock response. The mechanisms by which HSP70 and other heat shock proteins confer protection are not fully understood but most likely relate to the ability of heat shock proteins to serve as molecular chaperones by binding, refolding, transporting, and stabilizing damaged intracellular proteins.

Another potential mechanism by which the heat shock response may confer cytoprotection is by modulating inflammatory

TABLE 19.1. Nonthermal inducers of the heat shock response.

Inducer	Comments
Sodium arsenite	Used extensively in vitro and in vivo
Prostaglandin-A$_1$	Other prostaglandins also active
Dexamethasone	Variable effect
Bimoclomol	Hydroxylamine derivative, nontoxic
Herbimycin A	Tyrosine kinase inhibitor
Geldanamycin	Tyrosine kinase inhibitor and HSP90 inhibitor
Aspirin	Lowers temperature threshold for HSP induction
Nonsteroidal antiinflammatory drugs	Lowers temperature threshold for HSP induction
Serine protease inhibitors	Concomitant inhibition of NFκB
Pyrrolidine dithiocarbamate (PDTC)	Antioxidant; inhibitor of NFκB
Diethyldithiocarbamate	Similar to PDTC
Glutamine	Currently the most promising clinical application
Heavy metal ions	Cadmium, zinc
Phosphatase inhibitors	Tyrosine and serine/threonine phosphatases
Curcumin	Major constituent of turmeric; antiinflammatory
Geranylgeranylacetone	Antinuclear drug

Note: HSP, heat shock protein; NFκB, nuclear factor-κ B.

responses. The heat shock response has been demonstrated to inhibit the expression of a number of genes related to inflammation, including tumor necrosis factor-α, interleukin-1β, inducible nitric oxide synthase, interleukin-8, RANTES, C3, macrophage chemotactic protein-1, and intracellular adhesion molecule-1 [84–94]. In addition, it has been postulated that the inhibitory effects of the heat shock response are relatively selective for inflammation-associated genes [95]. The mechanisms by which the heat shock response inhibits proinflammatory gene expression involve inhibition of nuclear factor-κ B (NFκB). Several in vitro and in vivo studies have demonstrated that induction of the heat shock response inhibits activation of NFκB, a pluripotent transcription factor that regulates the expression of many genes associated with inflammation [95–97]. The latest work in the area has identified inhibitor of κ B (IκB) kinase (IKK) as the most upstream target through which the heat shock response modulates NFκB activity. It is the rate-limiting step in the activation of NFκB in that it phosphorylates the endogenous NFκB inhibitor IκBα. Phosphorylation of IκBα leads to its rapid degradation by a proteasome/ubiquitin-dependent mechanism, thus releasing NFκB to enter the nucleus. Induction of the heat shock response inhibits activation of IKK in part by an intracellular phosphatase-dependent mechanism [97–99]. Inhibition of IKK subsequently inhibits phosphorylation and degradation of IκBα [99], thus keeping NFκB in an inactive state.

Recent work suggests that the modulating effects of the heat shock response on inflammation-related signal transduction involve the de novo expression of proteins not traditionally considered to be classified as heat shock proteins. For example, it is now well established that the endogenous NFκB inhibitory protein IκBα is expressed in response to heat shock both in vitro and in vivo [94,100,101]. More recent work has demonstrated that the dual-specificity phosphatase MKP-1 (mitogen-activated protein kinase phosphatase) is also expressed in response to heat shock [102,103, and it is a potent counterregulator of many proinflammatory signal transduction pathways. Thus, heat shock response–associated induction of IκBα and MKP-1 gene expression serves as another mechanism by which the heat shock response can inhibit NFκB activity and inflammation-associated signal transduction.

The newest area of investigation in this field involves extracellular HSP70. Heretofore regarded as an exclusively intracellular protein, it is now well established that HSP70 is also found in the extracellular compartment. For example, extracellular HSP70 has been demonstrated in the cerebrospinal fluid of children with traumatic head injury [71], in children with septic shock [72], and in adult patients with severe trauma [70]. The exact function of extracellular HSP70, if any, remains to be defined. One potential function may be to serve as a *danger signal* for the innate immune system, because it has been demonstrated that extracellular HSP70 can activate mononuclear cells via toll-like receptors 2 and 4 [104,105]. In related work, Aneja, Wong, and colleagues (unpublished observations) have demonstrated that extracellular HSP70 can induce tolerance to subsequent endotoxin challenge in culture mononuclear cells.

Whether HSP70-mediated activation of toll-like receptors serves a cytoprotective function, a proinflammatory function, or both, depending on context, remains to be determined. The clinical data indirectly suggest that HSP70 may be a marker of injury severity, play a role in cytoprotection, or contribute to injury. For example, in children with traumatic head injury, cerebrospinal fluid levels of HSP70 were higher in children with inflicted head injury than in those with noninflicted head injury [71]. In children with septic

shock, higher HSP70 serum levels correlated with the severity of septic shock and mortality [72]. In contrast, higher levels of HSP70 correlated positively with survival in adult patients with severe trauma [70]. Future work in this area will determine if extracellular HSP70 plays a direct role in cytoprotection or pathophysiology.

In summary, the heat shock response serves a very broad cytoprotective role in virtually all organisms. Heat shock factor-1 and intracellular HSP70 play key roles in cytoprotection, and it would appear that the antiinflammatory effects of the heat shock response also play a prominent role in cytoprotection. The challenge remains to devise an effective and safe method (i.e., gene therapy or pharmacology) for inducing the heat shock response as a therapeutic strategy in the clinical setting. In this regard, the work of Wischmeyer and colleagues suggests that glutamine administration may be a feasible and safe approach for augmenting HSP70 expression in critically ill patients [106–109].

Hypoxia Inducible Factor

Hypoxia inducible factor (HIF) is thought to function in both cytoprotection and the pathophysiology of several diseases [110,111]. Hypoxia inducible factor-1 is a heterodimeric transcription factor containing the subunits HIF-1α and HIF-1β. In the context of cytoprotection, HIF-1 can be thought of as a major regulator of genes necessary for adaptation to hypoxia. The list of genes that are HIF-1 dependent include genes for vascularization], energy metabolism [113], vascular tone [114], and erythropoiesis (Table 19.2) [115]. In addition, HO-1 expression is, in part, dependent on HIF-1 activity [116].

The transcriptional activity of HIF-1 is primarily dependent on the intracellular level of the HIF-1α subunit, which is susceptible to continuous intracellular degradation [110,111]. Under conditions of normal oxygen tension, the HIF-1α protein subunit undergoes continuous ubiquitination and subsequent degradation by proteasome activity, thereby preventing formation of the HIF-1α/HIF-1β heterodimer [117,118]. In response to hypoxia, HIF-1α protein subunit degradation is terminated, thereby rapidly increasing intracellular levels of HIF-1α protein and allowing formation of the HIF-1α/HIF-1β heterodimer, which is then transcriptionally active and allows for the expression of HIF-1–dependent genes. This mechanism allows for a rapid means of expressing genes necessary for adaptation to hypoxia. The exact mechanism by which cells *sense* hypoxia and curtail the degradation of the HIF-1α protein subunit is not fully understood, but likely involves

TABLE 19.2. Genes regulated by hypoxia inducible factor-1 (adapted from Refs. 109, 110).

Adenylate kinase 3	α_{1B}-Adrenergic receptor
Adrenomedullin	Aldolases A and C
Endothelin-1	Enolase 1
Erythropoietin	Glucose transporters 1 and 3
Heme oxygenase-1	Glyceraldehyde phosphate dehydrogenase
Hexokinases 1 and 2	Insulin-like growth factor-II
Lactate dehydrogenase A	Insulin-like growth factor binding proteins 1 and 3
Nitric oxide synthase 2	p21
P35srj	Phosphofructokinase L
Phosphoglycerate kinase 1	Pyruvate kinase M
Transferrin	Transferrin receptor
Vascular endothelial growthfactor	Vascular endothelial growth factor receptor

Source: Adapted from Singleton et al. [109] and Semenza [110].

inhibition of ubiquitination and is related to the von Hippel-Lindau tumor suppressor protein [119,120].

As would be expected, the cytoprotective properties of HIF-1 relate primarily to the HIF-1–dependent genes that allow for adaptation to hypoxia. For example, induction of the HIF-1–dependent gene erythropoietin leads to increased production of red blood cells, thereby increasing the oxygen-carrying capacity of blood to compensate for hypoxia. This type of cytoprotective response is particularly important, for example, in children with cyanotic heart disease. Another example involves the HIF-1–dependent gene vascular endothelial growth factor (VEGF), which is a critical growth factor for the development of blood vessels. In tissues subjected to ischemia, such as the myocardium, expression of VEGF promotes the development of neovascularization as a potential means of increasing blood flow to the ischemic tissue [121]. Yet another role for HIF-1 involves HIF-1–dependent expression of inducible nitric oxide synthase (discussed in a subsequent section) and ischemic preconditioning of the myocardium [122,123].

The biologic importance of HIF-1 has been established in transgenic mice having targeted deletions of the HIF-1 subunits. Mice homozygous for deletions of either subunit (HIF-1α −/− and HIF-1β −/−) die during embryogenesis secondary to insufficient vascular development [113,124]. In contrast, heterozygote animals (HIF-1α +/−) seem to develop normally compared with wild-type animals. When exposed to hypoxia, however, heterozygote animals have impairment of the classic responses and adaptations to hypoxia. For example, these animals have a blunted increase in hematocrit and a blunted increase in right ventricular mass [125].

In summary, HIF-1–dependent gene expression warrants classification as an endogenous cytoprotective mechanism by allowing for adaptation to cellular hypoxia, whether it is secondary to low oxygen tension or caused by decreased blood flow (ischemia). Although some of the aforementioned cytoprotective mechanisms (e.g., the heat shock response) allow for more immediate forms of cytoprotection, the cytoprotective responses and adaptations associated with HIF-1 activation are comparatively slower to develop and allow for longer term adaptation. In addition, some of the responses induced by HIF-1 activation can be maladaptive/pathologic, depending on duration of activation. For example, HIF-1 activation is thought to play a role in the development of pulmonary hypertension in the setting of chronic hypoxia. Thus a greater understanding of HIF-1 regulation and activity will be necessary in order to manipulate HIF-1 activity as a therapeutic option.

Nitric Oxide

Nitric oxide (NO) is produced by the enzyme nitric oxide synthase (NOS), which converts L-arginine to citrulline and NO [126]. There are three known isoforms of NOS: endothelial NOS (eNOS), neuronal NOS (nNOS), and inducible NOS (iNOS). The terms *eNOS* and *nNOS* reflect the original tissues from which these isoforms were cloned. This is, however, a relative misnomer, because both isoforms are widely distributed beyond the endothelium and central nervous system. Both eNOS and nNOS are constitutively active, dependent on intracellular calcium for activity, and produce relatively small amounts of NO. Inducible NOS derives its name from the observation that it requires de novo gene expression for maximal activity. In addition, iNOS is calcium independent and is responsible for high level production of NO following proinflammatory and other forms of stimuli. Although historically these isoforms have

been classified as being *constitutive* and *inducible*, it is now recognized that the eNOS and nNOS genes can undergo regulation (i.e., induction) under certain conditions and that iNOS can also be constitutively active [126,127]. Finally, the human genes for the NOS isoforms are now categorized based on the order in which they were cloned: human nNOS is NOS1, human iNOS is NOS2, and human eNOS is NOS3 [128].

One of the primary mechanisms by which NO affects cellular function is through the activation of soluble guanylate cyclase leading to increased intracellular levels of cyclic guanosine monophosphate. Because NO is a free radical gas, other important NO mechanisms that affect cellular function include reactions with metal complexes, nitrosation, nitration, and oxidation reactions [129]. The degree to which any one of these mechanisms is operative in a given biologic process is, in turn, highly dependent on the amount of NO produced and the biologic milieu.

An abundance of quality data indicate that NO can function as a cytoprotective molecule. Assigning biologic significance to these data is difficult given that the literature suggests that a very broad spectrum of biologic processes are affected by NO and that equally abundant and quality data indicate that NO can be either directly cytotoxic or mediate cytotoxic/pathologic processes. Thus, NO appears to have dual properties as both a cytoprotective and a cytotoxic molecule. Examples of NO-dependent cytoprotection will be provided, but the reader is reminded that for virtually each example of cytoprotection, there is an example of NO functioning in an opposite manner (i.e., cytotoxicity).

Apoptosis, or programmed cell death, can be modulated by NO and is perhaps the most prominent and well-studied example of NO-mediated cytoprotection [130,131]. Various examples exist demonstrating that NO can either inhibit apoptosis or promote apoptosis. The antiapoptotic effects of NO have been demonstrated in various cultured cells such as human B lymphocytes [132], endothelial cells [133], splenocytes [134], and hepatocytes [135,136] and in whole-animal models [137,138]. In addition, NO has been demonstrated to prevent apoptosis secondary to diverse signals such as tumor necrosis factor, growth factor withdrawal, and Fas ligand [130,131]. The mechanisms by which NO inhibits apoptosis are also quite diverse. For example, NO can induce expression of the aforementioned cytoprotective proteins, HO-1 and HSP70 and thereby prevent apoptosis [135,139. because cyclic guanosine monophosphate can also prevent apoptosis, NO-mediated activation of cyclic guanosine monophosphate is another mechanism by which NO can prevent apoptosis, possibly by lowering intracellular calcium levels [134]. Nitric oxide has also been shown to inhibit caspase activity [136] and inhibit cytochrome c release [140], two key events in the proapoptotic pathway. Finally, NO has been demonstrated to maintain or preserve intracellular levels of Bcl-2, a key antiapoptotic protein [134,140].

Nitric oxide can also be protective for whole organs. It has been demonstrated to confer cytoprotection in the liver [141], kidney [142], brain [143], heart [144], and intestine [145]. The mechanisms by which NO protect these organs involves vascular dilation, prevention of platelet and neutrophil adherence, antioxidant effects by reactions with ROS, antiapoptotic effects, and induction of other cytoprotective mechanisms (e.g., HSP70 and HO-1). Thus, NO can protect organs during various forms of injury or stress by maintaining blood flow, preventing thrombosis, limiting inflammation, decreasing oxidant stress, and/or preventing apoptosis. Again, the degree to which any one of these mechanisms is operative, or predominant, is dependent on the type of injury/stress, the amount of

NO produced, and the biologic context in which the NO is produced.

The cytoprotective properties of NO are indisputable, and many biologically plausible mechanisms account for the observed cytoprotective effects. The availability of commonly used NO donors (e.g., sodium nitroprusside and nitroglycerin) and novel NO donors allows for the direct application of these principles in the clinical setting as a means of affording organ and tissue protection during a variety of disease states [125,131]. Enthusiasm for this approach must be tempered, however, by the known dual nature of NO as both a cytoprotective and cytotoxic molecule.

Conclusion

This chapter has attempted to describe some of the more powerful and ubiquitous endogenous mechanisms that exist to counteract the multitude of cytotoxic stimuli that can adversely affect the human host. Many of these mechanisms are ancient, and during disease states these mechanisms can either fail or be overwhelmed. The next formidable challenge is to devise therapeutic strategies (through either pharmacology or gene therapy) that will allow for the safe and efficacious manipulation of these endogenous mechanisms of cytoprotection.

References

1. Tenhunen R, Marver HS, Schmid R. The enzymatic conversion of heme to bilirubin by microsomal heme oxygenase. Proc Natl Acad Sci USA 1968;61(2):748–755.
2. Tenhunen R, Marver HS, Schmid R. Microsomal heme oxygenase. Characterization of the enzyme. J Biol Chem 1969;244(23):6388–6394.
3. Ryter SW, Otterbein LE, Morse D, Choi AM. Heme oxygenase/carbon monoxide signaling pathways: regulation and functional significance. Mol Cell Biochem 2002;234–235(1–2):249–263.
4. Morse D, Choi AM. Heme oxygenase-1: the "emerging molecule" has arrived. Am J Respir Cell Mol Biol 2002;27(1):8–16.
5. Otterbein LE, Choi AM. Heme oxygenase: colors of defense against cellular stress. Am J Physiol Lung Cell Mol Physiol 2000;279(6):L1029–L1037.
6. Yachie A, Niida Y, Wada T, Igarashi N, Kaneda H, Toma T, et al. Oxidative stress causes enhanced endothelial cell injury in human heme oxygenase-1 deficiency. J Clin Invest 1999;103(1):129–135.
7. Dennery PA, Sridhar KJ, Lee CS, Wong HE, Shokoohi V, Rodgers PA, et al. Heme oxygenase-mediated resistance to oxygen toxicity in hamster fibroblasts. J Biol Chem 1997;272(23):14937–14942.
8. Suttner DM, Sridhar K, Lee CS, Tomura T, Hansen TN, Dennery PA. Protective effects of transient HO-1 overexpression on susceptibility to oxygen toxicity in lung cells. Am J Physiol 1999;276(3 Pt 1):L443–L451.
9. Lee PJ, Alam J, Wiegand GW, Choi AM. Overexpression of heme oxygenase-1 in human pulmonary epithelial cells results in cell growth arrest and increased resistance to hyperoxia. Proc Natl Acad Sci USA 1996;93(19):10393–10398.
10. Abraham NG, Lavrovsky Y, Schwartzman ML, Stoltz RA, Levere RD, Gerritsen ME, et al. Transfection of the human heme oxygenase gene into rabbit coronary microvessel endothelial cells: protective effect against heme and hemoglobin toxicity. Proc Natl Acad Sci USA 1995;92(15):6798–6802.
11. Petrache I, Otterbein LE, Alam J, Wiegand GW, Choi AM. Heme oxygenase-1 inhibits TNF-alpha–induced apoptosis in cultured fibroblasts. Am J Physiol Lung Cell Mol Physiol 2000;278(2):L312–L319.
12. Zhou H, Lu F, Latham C, Zander DS, Visner GA. Heme oxygenase-1 expression in human lungs with cystic fibrosis and cytoprotective effects against *Pseudomonas aeruginosa* in vitro. Am J Respir Crit Care Med 2004;170(6):633–640.
13. Otterbein L, Sylvester SL, Choi AM. Hemoglobin provides protection against lethal endotoxemia in rats: the role of heme oxygenase-1. Am J Respir Cell Mol Biol 1995;13(5):595–601.
14. Otterbein L, Chin BY, Otterbein SL, Lowe VC, Fessler HE, Choi AM. Mechanism of hemoglobin-induced protection against endotoxemia in rats: a ferritin-independent pathway. Am J Physiol 1997;272(2 Pt 1):L268–L275.
15. Otterbein LE, Kolls JK, Mantell LL, Cook JL, Alam J, Choi AM. Exogenous administration of heme oxygenase-1 by gene transfer provides protection against hyperoxia-induced lung injury. J Clin Invest 1999;103(7):1047–1054.
16. Yet SF, Tian R, Layne MD, Wang ZY, Maemura K, Solovyeva M, et al. Cardiac-specific expression of heme oxygenase-1 protects against ischemia and reperfusion injury in transgenic mice. Circ Res 2001;89(2):168–173.
17. Soares MP, Lin Y, Anrather J, Csizmadia E, Takigami K, Sato K, et al. Expression of heme oxygenase-1 can determine cardiac xenograft survival. Nat Med 1998;4(9):1073–1077.
18. Sato K, Balla J, Otterbein L, Smith RN, Brouard S, Lin Y, et al. Carbon monoxide generated by heme oxygenase-1 suppresses the rejection of mouse-to-rat cardiac transplants. J Immunol 2001;166(6):4185–4194.
19. Camara NO, Soares MP. Heme oxygenase-1 (HO-1), a protective gene that prevents chronic graft dysfunction. Free Radic Biol Med 2005;38(4):426–435.
20. Ke B, Buelow R, Shen XD, Melinek J, Amersi F, Gao F, et al. Heme oxygenase 1 gene transfer prevents CD95/Fas ligand-mediated apoptosis and improves liver allograft survival via carbon monoxide signaling pathway. Hum Gene Ther 2002;13(10):1189–1199.
21. Poss KD, Tonegawa S. Heme oxygenase 1 is required for mammalian iron reutilization. Proc Natl Acad Sci USA 1997;94(20):10919–10924.
22. Wiesel P, Patel AP, Carvajal IM, Wang ZY, Pellacani A, Maemura K, et al. Exacerbation of chronic renovascular hypertension and acute renal failure in heme oxygenase-1-deficient mice. Circ Res 2001;88(10):1088–1094.
23. Wiesel P, Patel AP, DiFonzo N, Marria PB, Sim CU, Pellacani A, et al. Endotoxin-induced mortality is related to increased oxidative stress and end-organ dysfunction, not refractory hypotension, in heme oxygenase-1-deficient mice. Circulation 2000;102(24):3015–3022.
24. Yet SF, Perrella MA, Layne MD, Hsieh CM, Maemura K, Kobzik L, et al. Hypoxia induces severe right ventricular dilatation and infarction in heme oxygenase-1 null mice. J Clin Invest 1999;103(8):R23–R29.
25. Choi AM, Otterbein LE. Emerging role of carbon monoxide in physiologic and pathophysiologic states. Antioxid Redox Signal 2002;4(2):227–228.
26. Morse D, Sethi J, Choi AM. Carbon monoxide-dependent signaling. Crit Care Med 2001;30(1 Suppl):S12–S17.
27. Zuckerbraun BS, Billiar TR, Otterbein SL, Kim PK, Liu F, Choi AM, et al. Carbon monoxide protects against liver failure through nitric oxide-induced heme oxygenase 1. J Exp Med 2003;198(11):1707–1716.
28. Mayer RD, Wang X, Maines MD. Nitric oxide inhibitor N omega-nitro-L-arginine methyl ester potentiates induction of heme oxygenase-1 in kidney ischemia/reperfusion model: a novel mechanism for regulation of the oxygenase. J Pharmacol Exp Ther 2003;306(1):43–50.
29. Carter EP, Hartsfield CL, Miyazono M, Jakkula M, Morris KG, Jr., McMurtry IF. Regulation of heme oxygenase-1 by nitric oxide during hepatopulmonary syndrome. Am J Physiol Lung Cell Mol Physiol 2002;283(2):L346–L353.
30. Sethi JM, Otterbein LE, Choi AM. Differential modulation by exogenous carbon monoxide of TNF-alpha stimulated mitogen-activated protein kinases in rat pulmonary artery endothelial cells. Antioxid Redox Signal 2002;4(2):241–248.

31. Chapman JT, Otterbein LE, Elias JA, Choi AM. Carbon monoxide attenuates aeroallergen-induced inflammation in mice. Am J Physiol Lung Cell Mol Physiol 2001;281(1):L209–L216.

32. Otterbein LE, Bach FH, Alam J, Soares M, Tao Lu H, Wysk M, et al. Carbon monoxide has anti-inflammatory effects involving the mitogen-activated protein kinase pathway. Nat Med 2000;6(4):422–428.

33. Otterbein LE, Mantell LL, Choi AM. Carbon monoxide provides protection against hyperoxic lung injury. Am J Physiol 1999;276(4 Pt 1):L688–L694.

34. Liu XM, Chapman GB, Peyton KJ, Schafer AI, Durante W. Carbon monoxide inhibits apoptosis in vascular smooth muscle cells. Cardiovasc Res 2002;55(2):396–405.

35. Soares MP, Usheva A, Brouard S, Berberat PO, Gunther L, Tobiasch E, et al. Modulation of endothelial cell apoptosis by heme oxygenase-1-derived carbon monoxide. Antioxid Redox Signal 2002;4(2):321–329.

36. Akamatsu Y, Haga M, Tyagi S, Yamashita K, Graca-Souza AV, Ollinger R, et al. Heme oxygenase-1-derived carbon monoxide protects hearts from transplant associated ischemia reperfusion injury. FASEB J 2004;18(6):771–772.

37. Kamata H, Hirata H. Redox regulation of cellular signalling. Cell Signal 1999;11(1):1–14.

38. Marnett LJ. Oxyradicals and DNA damage. Carcinogenesis 2000;21(3):361–370.

39. Stadtman ER, Berlett BS. Reactive oxygen-mediated protein oxidation in aging and disease. Drug Metab Rev 1998;30(2):225–243.

40. McCord JM. Superoxide dismutase in aging and disease: an overview. Methods Enzymol 2002;349:331–341.

41. Tsan MF, White JE, Caska B, Epstein CJ, Lee CY. Susceptibility of heterozygous MnSOD gene-knockout mice to oxygen toxicity. Am J Respir Cell Mol Biol 1998;19(1):114–120.

42. Tsan MF. Superoxide dismutase and pulmonary oxygen toxicity: lessons from transgenic and knockout mice. Int J Mol Med 2001;7(1):13–19.

43. White CW, Avraham KB, Shanley PF, Groner Y. Transgenic mice with expression of elevated levels of copper-zinc superoxide dismutase in the lungs are resistant to pulmonary oxygen toxicity. J Clin Invest 1991;87(6):2162–2168.

44. Wispe JR, Warner BB, Clark JC, Dey CR, Neuman J, Glasser SW, et al. Human Mn-superoxide dismutase in pulmonary epithelial cells of transgenic mice confers protection from oxygen injury. J Biol Chem 1992;267(33):23937–23941.

45. Garcia-Redondo A, Bustos F, Juan YSB, Del Hoyo P, Jimenez S, Campos Y, et al. Molecular analysis of the superoxide dismutase 1 gene in Spanish patients with sporadic or familial amyotrophic lateral sclerosis. Muscle Nerve 2002;26(2):274–278.

46. Bai J, Cederbaum AI. Mitochondrial catalase and oxidative injury. Biol Signals Recept 2001;10(3–4):189–199.

47. Mates JM, Perez-Gomez C, Nunez de Castro I. Antioxidant enzymes and human diseases. Clin Biochem 1999;32(8):595–603.

48. Joshi MS, Ferguson TB, Jr., Han TH, Hyduke DR, Liao JC, Rassaf T, et al. Nitric oxide is consumed, rather than conserved, by reaction with oxyhemoglobin under physiological conditions. Proc Natl Acad Sci USA 2002;99(16):10341–10346.

49. Gardner PR, Costantino G, Salzman AL. Constitutive and adaptive detoxification of nitric oxide in Escherichia coli. Role of nitric-oxide dioxygenase in the protection of aconitase. J Biol Chem 1998;273(41):26528–26533.

50. Gardner PR, Gardner AM, Martin LA, Salzman AL. Nitric oxide dioxygenase: an enzymic function for flavohemoglobin. Proc Natl Acad Sci USA 1998;95(18):10378–10383.

51. Gardner PR, Gardner AM, Martin LA, Dou Y, Li T, Olson JS, et al. Nitric-oxide dioxygenase activity and function of flavohemoglobins. sensitivity to nitric oxide and carbon monoxide inhibition. J Biol Chem 2000;275(41):31581–31587.

52. Gardner AM, Gardner PR. Flavohemoglobin detoxifies nitric oxide in aerobic, but not anaerobic, Escherichia coli. Evidence for a novel inducible anaerobic nitric oxide-scavenging activity. J Biol Chem 2002;277(10):8166–81671.

53. Gardner AM, Helmick RA, Gardner PR. Flavorubredoxin, an inducible catalyst for nitric oxide reduction and detoxification in Escherichia coli. J Biol Chem 2002;277(10):8172–8177.

54. Gardner PR, Martin LA, Hall D, Gardner AM. Dioxygen-dependent metabolism of nitric oxide in mammalian cells. Free Radic Biol Med 2001;31(2):191–204.

55. Hallstrom CK, Gardner AM, Gardner PR. Nitric oxide metabolism in mammalian cells: substrate and inhibitor profiles of a NADPH-cytochrome P450 oxidoreductase-coupled microsomal nitric oxide dioxygenase. Free Radic Biol Med 2004;37(2):216–228.

56. Nordberg J, Arner ES. Reactive oxygen species, antioxidants, and the mammalian thioredoxin system. Free Radic Biol Med 2001;31(11):1287–1312.

57. Kregel KC. Heat shock proteins: modifying factors in physiological stress responses and acquired thermotolerance. J Appl Physiol 2002;92(5):2177–2186.

58. Hasday JD, Singh IS. Fever and the heat shock response: distinct, partially overlapping processes. Cell Stress Chaperones 2000;5(5):471–480.

59. Gerner EW, Schneider MJ. Induced thermal resistance in HeLa cells. Nature 1975;256(5517):500–502.

60. Li GC, Werb Z. Correlation between synthesis of heat shock proteins and development of thermotolerance in Chinese hamster fibroblasts. Proc Natl Acad Sci USA 1982;79(10):3218–3222.

61. Wong HR, Mannix RJ, Rusnak JM, Boota A, Zar H, Watkins SC, et al. The heat-shock response attenuates lipopolysaccharide-mediated apoptosis in cultured sheep pulmonary artery endothelial cells. Am J Respir Cell Mol Biol 1996;15(6):745–751.

62. Wong HR, Ryan M, Menendez IY, Denenberg A, Wispe JR. Heat shock protein induction protects human respiratory epithelium against nitric oxide-mediated cytotoxicity. Shock 1997;8(3):213–218.

63. Szabo C, Wong HR, Salzman AL. Pre-exposure to heat shock inhibits peroxynitrite-induced activation of poly(ADP) ribosyltransferase and protects against peroxynitrite cytotoxicity in J774 macrophages. Eur J Pharmacol 1996;315(2):221–226.

64. Wang YR, Xiao XZ, Huang SN, Luo FJ, You JL, Luo H, et al. Heat shock pretreatment prevents hydrogen peroxide injury of pulmonary endothelial cells and macrophages in culture. Shock 1996;6(2):134–141.

65. Ryan AJ, Flanagan SW, Moseley PL, Gisolfi CV. Acute heat stress protects rats against endotoxin shock. J Appl Physiol 1992;73(4):1517–1522.

66. Hauser GJ, Dayao EK, Wasserloos K, Pitt BR, Wong HR. HSP induction inhibits iNOS mRNA expression and attenuates hypotension in endotoxin-challenged rats. Am J Physiol 1996;271(6 Pt 2):H2529–H2535.

67. Villar J, Edelson JD, Post M, Mullen JB, Slutsky AS. Induction of heat stress proteins is associated with decreased mortality in an animal model of acute lung injury. Am Rev Respir Dis 1993;147(1):177–181.

68. Hiratsuka M, Yano M, Mora BN, Nagahiro I, Cooper JD, Patterson GA. Heat shock pretreatment protects pulmonary isografts from subsequent ischemia-reperfusion injury. J Heart Lung Transplant 1998;17(12):1238–1246.

69. Kindas-Mugge I, Hammerle AH, Frohlich I, Oismuller C, Micksche M, Trautinger F. Granulocytes of critically ill patients spontaneously express the 72 kD heat shock protein. Circ Shock 1993;39(4):247–252.

70. Pittet JF, Lee H, Morabito D, Howard MB, Welch WJ, Mackersie RC. Serum levels of Hsp 72 measured early after trauma correlate with survival. J Trauma 2002;52(4):611–617.

71. Lai Y, Kochanek PM, Adelson PD, Janesko K, Ruppel RA, Clark RS. Induction of the stress response after inflicted and non-inflicted traumatic brain injury in infants and children. J Neurotrauma 2004;21(3):229–237.

72. Wheeler DS, Fisher Jr LE, Catravas JD, Jacobs BR, Carcillo JA, Wong HR. Extracellular hsp70 levels in children with septic shock. Pediatr Crit Care Med 2005;6(3):308–311.

73. Riabowol KT, Mizzen LA, Welch WJ. Heat shock is lethal to fibroblasts microinjected with antibodies against hsp70. Science 1988;242(4877):433–436.

74. Li GC, Li LG, Liu YK, Mak JY, Chen LL, Lee WM. Thermal response of rat fibroblasts stably transfected with the human 70-kDa heat shock protein-encoding gene. Proc Natl Acad Sci USA 1991;88(5):1681–1685.

75. Wong HR, Menendez IY, Ryan MA, Denenberg AG, Wispe JR. Increased expression of heat shock protein-70 protects A549 cells against hyperoxia. Am J Physiol 1998;275(4 Pt 1):L836–L841.

76. Hiratsuka M, Mora BN, Yano M, Mohanakumar T, Patterson GA. Gene transfer of heat shock protein 70 protects lung grafts from ischemia–reperfusion injury. Ann Thorac Surg 1999;67(5):1421–1427.

77. Marber MS, Mestril R, Chi SH, Sayen MR, Yellon DM, Dillmann WH. Overexpression of the rat inducible 70-kD heat stress protein in a transgenic mouse increases the resistance of the heart to ischemic injury. J Clin Invest 1995;95(4):1446–1456.

78. Plumier JC, Ross BM, Currie RW, Angelidis CE, Kazlaris H, Kollias G, et al. Transgenic mice expressing the human heat shock protein 70 have improved post-ischemic myocardial recovery. J Clin Invest 1995;95(4):1854–1860.

79. Wheeler DS, Dunsmore KE, Wong HR. Intracellular delivery of HSP70 using HIV-1 Tat protein transduction domain. Biochem Biophys Res Commun 2003;301(1):54–59.

80. Lai Y, Du L, Dunsmore KE, Jenkins LW, Wong HR, Clark RS. Selectively increasing inducible heat shock protein 70 via TAT-protein transduction protects neurons from nitrosative stress and excitotoxicity. J Neurochem 2005;94(2):360–366.

81. McMillan DR, Xiao X, Shao L, Graves K, Benjamin IJ. Targeted disruption of heat shock transcription factor 1 abolishes thermotolerance and protection against heat-inducible apoptosis. J Biol Chem 1998;273(13):7523–7528.

82. Xiao X, Zuo X, Davis AA, McMillan DR, Curry BB, Richardson JA, et al. HSF1 is required for extra-embryonic development, postnatal growth and protection during inflammatory responses in mice. EMBO J 1999;18(21):5943–5952.

83. Malhotra V, Kooy NW, Denenberg AG, Dunsmore KE, Wong HR. Ablation of the heat shock factor-1 increases susceptibility to hyperoxia-mediated cellular injury. Exp Lung Res 2002;28(8):609–622.

84. Schmidt JA, Abdulla E. Down-regulation of IL-1 beta biosynthesis by inducers of the heat-shock response. J Immunol 1988;141(6):2027–2034.

85. Snyder YM, Guthrie L, Evans GF, Zuckerman SH. Transcriptional inhibition of endotoxin-induced monokine synthesis following heat shock in murine peritoneal macrophages. J Leukocyte Biol 1992;51(2):181–187.

86. Wong HR, Finder JD, Wasserloos K, Pitt BR. Expression of iNOS in cultured rat pulmonary artery smooth muscle cells is inhibited by the heat shock response. Am J Physiol 1995;269(6 Pt 1):L843–L848.

87. Thomas SC, Ryan MA, Shanley TP, Wong HR. Induction of the stress response with prostaglandin A1 increases I-kappaBalpha gene expression. FASEB J 1998;12(13):1371–1378.

88. Ayad O, Stark JM, Fiedler MM, Menendez IY, Ryan MA, Wong HR. The heat shock response inhibits RANTES gene expression in cultured human lung epithelium. J Immunol 1998;161(5):2594–2599.

89. Moon R, Pritts TA, Parikh AA, Fischer JE, Salzman AL, Ryan M, et al. Stress response decreases the interleukin-1beta-induced production of complement component C3 in human intestinal epithelial cells. Clin Sci (Lond) 1999;97(3):331–337.

90. Malhotra V, Eaves-Pyles T, Odoms K, Quaid G, Shanley TP, Wong HR. Heat shock inhibits activation of NF-kappaB in the absence of heat shock factor-1. Biochem Biophys Res Commun 2002;291(3):453–457.

91. Kohn G, Wong HR, Bshesh K, Zhao B, Vasi N, Denenberg A, et al. Heat shock inhibits TNF-induced ICAM-1 expression in human endothelial cells via I kappa kinase inhibition. Shock 2002;17(2):91–97.

92. Wong HR, Ryan M, Gebb S, Wispe JR. Selective and transient in vitro effects of heat shock on alveolar type II cell gene expression. Am J Physiol 1997;272(1 Pt 1):L132–L138.

93. Wong HR, Ryan M, Wispe JR. The heat shock response inhibits inducible nitric oxide synthase gene expression by blocking I kappa-B degradation and NF-kappa B nuclear translocation. Biochem Biophys Res Commun 1997;231(2):257–263.

94. Pritts TA, Wang Q, Sun X, Fischer DR, Hungness ES, Fischer JE, et al. The stress response decreases NF-kappaB activation in liver of endotoxemic mice. Shock 2002;18(1):33–37.

95. Malhotra V, Wong HR. Interactions between the heat shock response and the nuclear factor-kappa B signaling pathway. Crit Care Med 2002;30(1 Suppl):S89–S95.

96. Curry HA, Clemens RA, Shah S, Bradbury CM, Botero A, Goswami P, et al. Heat shock inhibits radiation-induced activation of NF-kappaB via inhibition of I-kappaB kinase. J Biol Chem 1999;274(33):23061–23067.

97. Yoo CG, Lee S, Lee CT, Kim YW, Han SK, Shim YS. Anti-inflammatory effect of heat shock protein induction is related to stabilization of I kappa B alpha through preventing I kappa B kinase activation in respiratory epithelial cells. J Immunol 2000;164(10):5416–5423.

98. Grossman BJ, Shanley TP, Odoms K, Dunsmore KE, Denenberg AG, Wong HR. Temporal and mechanistic effects of heat shock on LPS-mediated degradation of IkappaBalpha in macrophages. Inflammation 2002;26(3):129–137.

99. Shanley TP, Ryan MA, Eaves-Pyles T, Wong HR. Heat shock inhibits phosphorylation of I-kappaBalpha. Shock 2000;14(4):447–450.

100. Wong HR, Ryan M, Wispe JR. Stress response decreases NF-kappaB nuclear translocation and increases I-kappaBalpha expression in A549 cells. J Clin Invest 1997;99(10):2423–2428.

101. Wong HR, Ryan MA, Menendez IY, Wispe JR. Heat shock activates the I-kappaBalpha promoter and increases I-kappaBalpha mRNA expression. Cell Stress Chaperones 1999;4(1):1–7.

102. Wong HR, Dunsmore KE, Page K, Shanley TP. Heat shock-mediated regulation of MKP-1. Am J Physiol Cell Physiol 2005;289(5):C1152–1158.

103. Sanlorenzo L, Zhao B, Spight D, Denenberg AG, Page K, Wong HR, et al. Heat shock inhibition of lipopolysaccharide-mediated tumor necrosis factor expression is associated with nuclear induction of MKP-1 and inhibition of mitogen-activated protein kinase activation. Crit Care Med 2004;32(11):2284–2292.

104. Asea A, Rehli M, Kabingu E, Boch JA, Bare O, Auron PE, et al. Novel signal transduction pathway utilized by extracellular HSP70: role of toll-like receptor (TLR) 2 and TLR4. J Biol Chem 2002;277(17):15028–15034.

105. Asea A, Kraeft SK, Kurt-Jones EA, Stevenson MA, Chen LB, Finberg RW, et al. HSP70 stimulates cytokine production through a CD14-dependant pathway, demonstrating its dual role as a chaperone and cytokine. Nat Med 2000;6(4):435–442.

106. Ziegler TR, Ogden LG, Singleton KD, Luo M, Fernandez-Estivariz C, Griffith DP, et al. Parenteral glutamine increases serum heat shock protein 70 in critically ill patients. Intensive Care Med 2005;31(8):1079–1086.

107. Singleton KD, Serkova N, Beckey VE, Wischmeyer PE. Glutamine attenuates lung injury and improves survival after sepsis: role of enhanced heat shock protein expression. Crit Care Med 2005;33(6):1206–1213.

108. Wischmeyer PE. Can glutamine turn off the motor that drives systemic inflammation? Crit Care Med 2005;33(5):1175–1178.

109. Singleton KD, Serkova N, Banerjee A, Meng X, Gamboni-Robertson F, Wischmeyer PE. Glutamine attenuates endotoxin-induced lung metabolic dysfunction: potential role of enhanced heat shock protein 70. Nutrition 2005;21(2):214–223.

110. Semenza GL. Surviving ischemia: adaptive responses mediated by hypoxia-inducible factor 1. J Clin Invest 2000;106(7):809–812.

111. Semenza GL. HIF-1, O(2), and the 3 PHDs: how animal cells signal hypoxia to the nucleus. Cell 2001;107(1):1–3.

112. Carmeliet P, Dor Y, Herbert JM, Fukumura D, Brusselmans K, Dewerchin M, et al. Role of HIF-1alpha in hypoxia-mediated apoptosis, cell proliferation and tumour angiogenesis. Nature 1998;394(6692):485–490.

113. Iyer NV, Kotch LE, Agani F, Leung SW, Laughner E, Wenger RH, et al. Cellular and developmental control of O2 homeostasis by hypoxia-inducible factor 1 alpha. Genes Dev 1998;12(2):149–162.

114. Hu J, Discher DJ, Bishopric NH, Webster KA. Hypoxia regulates expression of the endothelin-1 gene through a proximal hypoxia-inducible factor-1 binding site on the antisense strand. Biochem Biophys Res Commun 1998;245(3):894–899.

115. Jiang BH, Rue E, Wang GL, Roe R, Semenza GL. Dimerization, DNA binding, and transactivation properties of hypoxia-inducible factor 1. J Biol Chem 1996;271(30):17771–17778.

116. Lee PJ, Jiang BH, Chin BY, Iyer NV, Alam J, Semenza GL, et al. Hypoxia-inducible factor-1 mediates transcriptional activation of the heme oxygenase-1 gene in response to hypoxia. J Biol Chem 1997;272(9):5375–5381.

117. Huang LE, Arany Z, Livingston DM, Bunn HF. Activation of hypoxia-inducible transcription factor depends primarily upon redox-sensitive stabilization of its alpha subunit. J Biol Chem 1996;271(50):32253–32259.

118. Huang LE, Gu J, Schau M, Bunn HF. Regulation of hypoxia-inducible factor 1alpha is mediated by an O2-dependent degradation domain via the ubiquitin-proteasome pathway. Proc Natl Acad Sci USA 1998;95(14):7987–7992.

119. Jaakkola P, Mole DR, Tian YM, Wilson MI, Gielbert J, Gaskell SJ, et al. Targeting of HIF-alpha to the von Hippel-Lindau ubiquitylation complex by O2-regulated prolyl hydroxylation. Science 2001;292(5516):468–472.

120. Mole DR, Maxwell PH, Pugh CW, Ratcliffe PJ. Regulation of HIF by the von Hippel-Lindau tumour suppressor: implications for cellular oxygen sensing. IUBMB Life 2001;52(1–2):43–47.

121. Lee SH, Wolf PL, Escudero R, Deutsch R, Jamieson SW, Thistlethwaite PA. Early expression of angiogenesis factors in acute myocardial ischemia and infarction. N Engl J Med 2000;342(9):626–633.

122. Melillo G, Musso T, Sica A, Taylor LS, Cox GW, Varesio L. A hypoxia-responsive element mediates a novel pathway of activation of the inducible nitric oxide synthase promoter. J Exp Med 1995;182(6):1683–1693.

123. Bolli R, Dawn B, Tang XL, Qiu Y, Ping P, Xuan YT, et al. The nitric oxide hypothesis of late preconditioning. Basic Res Cardiol 1998;93(5):325–338.

124. Maltepe E, Schmidt JV, Baunoch D, Bradfield CA, Simon MC. Abnormal angiogenesis and responses to glucose and oxygen deprivation in mice lacking the protein ARNT. Nature 1997;386(6623):403–407.

125. Yu AY, Shimoda LA, Iyer NV, Huso DL, Sun X, McWilliams R, et al. Impaired physiological responses to chronic hypoxia in mice partially deficient for hypoxia-inducible factor 1alpha. J Clin Invest 1999;103(5):691–696.

126. Michel T, Feron O. Nitric oxide synthases: which, where, how, and why? J Clin Invest 1997;100(9):2146–2152.

127. Guo FH, De Raeve HR, Rice TW, Stuehr DJ, Thunnissen FB, Erzurum SC. Continuous nitric oxide synthesis by inducible nitric oxide synthase in normal human airway epithelium in vivo. Proc Natl Acad Sci USA 1995;92(17):7809–7813.

128. Moncada S, Higgs A, Furchgott R. International Union of Pharmacology Nomenclature in Nitric Oxide Research. Pharmacol Rev 1997;49(2):137–142.

129. Wink DA, Mitchell JB. Chemical biology of nitric oxide: Insights into regulatory, cytotoxic, and cytoprotective mechanisms of nitric oxide. Free Radic Biol Med 1998;25(4–5):434–456.

130. Kim YM, Bombeck CA, Billiar TR. Nitric oxide as a bifunctional regulator of apoptosis. Circ Res 1999;84(3):253–256.

131. Dimmeler S, Zeiher AM. Nitric oxide and apoptosis: another paradigm for the double-edged role of nitric oxide. Nitric Oxide 1997;1(4):275–281.

132. Mannick JB, Asano K, Izumi K, Kieff E, Stamler JS. Nitric oxide produced by human B lymphocytes inhibits apoptosis and Epstein-Barr virus reactivation. Cell 1994;79(7):1137–1146.

133. Dimmeler S, Haendeler J, Nehls M, Zeiher AM. Suppression of apoptosis by nitric oxide via inhibition of interleukin-1beta-converting enzyme (ICE)-like and cysteine protease protein (CPP)-32-like proteases. J Exp Med 1997;185(4):601–607.

134. Genaro AM, Hortelano S, Alvarez A, Martinez C, Bosca L. Splenic B lymphocyte programmed cell death is prevented by nitric oxide release through mechanisms involving sustained Bcl-2 levels. J Clin Invest 1995;95(4):1884–1890.

135. Kim YM, de Vera ME, Watkins SC, Billiar TR. Nitric oxide protects cultured rat hepatocytes from tumor necrosis factor-alpha-induced apoptosis by inducing heat shock protein 70 expression. J Biol Chem 1997;272(2):1402–1411.

136. Li J, Bombeck CA, Yang S, Kim YM, Billiar TR. Nitric oxide suppresses apoptosis via interrupting caspase activation and mitochondrial dysfunction in cultured hepatocytes. J Biol Chem 1999;274(24):17325–17333.

137. Ou J, Carlos TM, Watkins SC, Saavedra JE, Keefer LK, Kim YM, et al. Differential effects of nonselective nitric oxide synthase (NOS) and selective inducible NOS inhibition on hepatic necrosis, apoptosis, ICAM-1 expression, and neutrophil accumulation during endotoxemia. Nitric Oxide 1997;1(5):404–416.

138. Saavedra JE, Billiar TR, Williams DL, Kim YM, Watkins SC, Keefer LK. Targeting nitric oxide (NO) delivery in vivo. Design of a liver-selective NO donor prodrug that blocks tumor necrosis factoralpha-induced apoptosis and toxicity in the liver. J Med Chem 1997;40(13):1947–1954.

139. Kim YM, Bergonia H, Lancaster JR, Jr. Nitrogen oxide–induced autoprotection in isolated rat hepatocytes. FEBS Lett 1995;374(2):228–232.

140. Kim YM, Kim TH, Seol DW, Talanian RV, Billiar TR. Nitric oxide suppression of apoptosis occurs in association with an inhibition of Bcl-2 cleavage and cytochrome c release. J Biol Chem 1998;273(47):31437–31441.

141. Wang Y, Vodovotz Y, Kim PK, Zamora R, Billiar TR. Mechanisms of hepatoprotection by nitric oxide. Ann N Y Acad Sci 2002;962:415–422.

142. Heeringa P, Steenbergen E, van Goor H. A protective role for endothelial nitric oxide synthase in glomerulonephritis. Kidney Int 2002;61(3):822–825.

143. Lipton SA. Neuronal protection and destruction by NO. Cell Death Differ 1999;6(10):943–951.

144. Dawn B, Bolli R. Role of nitric oxide in myocardial preconditioning. Ann N Y Acad Sci 2002;962:18–41.

145. Lefer AM, Lefer DJ. Nitric oxide. II. Nitric oxide protects in intestinal inflammation. Am J Physiol 1999;276(3 Pt 1):G572–G575.

20
Ischemia–Reperfusion Injury

Basilia Zingarelli

Introduction

Ischemia and reperfusion injury plays a critical role in several clinical conditions, including myocardial infarction, cerebral ischemia, stroke, solid organ transplantation, soft tissue flaps and extremities reimplantation, and hemorrhagic and other cardiovascular shock conditions with low cardiac output, that may require organ fluid maintenance. A dramatic reduction of oxygen supply may cause ischemia in a whole organ (global ischemia) or in defined tissue territories (focal ischemia) and rapidly results in cell metabolic derangement, molecular alterations, and dysfunction sequelae. If not reversed within a short period of time, the cellular dysmetabolism progresses to complete depletion of the energetic pools, accumulation of toxic substances, and eventually to cell death.

In all clinical conditions of ischemia, the main therapeutic intervention requires restoration of the blood flow (reperfusion) and/or recovery of the normal oxygen levels (reoxygenation). Once perfusion is reestablished, tissue ischemia is generally reversed. However, a paradoxical injury process is elicited that can be characterized simply as an exaggerated inflammatory response leading to cellular death and organ dysfunction. Although the mechanisms underlying the phenomenon of ischemia and reperfusion injury have not been precisely defined, toxicity by reactive oxygen free radicals and oxidants, leukocyte–endothelial cell adhesion, and a marked inflammatory reaction have been implicated in the process of injury. The endothelium is damaged in the early minutes after reperfusion, that is, before neutrophils accumulate and before tissue necrosis fully develops, and this suggests that endothelial injury is a crucial event in the postischemic inflammatory cascade. Neutrophil adherence to vascular endothelium is then an important event, initiating further leukocyte activation and release of cytodestructive agents (reactive species or enzymes), which in turn leads to amplification of the endothelial damage and to parenchyma or tissue injury.

Metabolic Derangements of Ischemia

Alteration of Oxygen Supply

Cells of all tissues undergo irreversible injury and death when deprived of oxygen and other nutrients. As described by Fick's equation, oxygen delivery (DO_2) depends on two variables: volume flow rate of blood (as determined by the cardiac output [CO]) and arterial oxygen content (CaO_2) [1]. Therefore, tissue *ischemia* may result as a consequence of arterial occlusion within the perfusion territory of an affected vessel or may be induced by insufficient tissue perfusion because of limited pump flow (Table 20.1). However, in some clinical conditions inadequate tissue energetic metabolism may derive by increase of total body oxygen consumption (VO_2) (see Table 20.1). For example, during septic shock, oxygenation of the splanchnic territory may be inadequate even in the presence of normal hepatic–splanchnic blood flow. This event is caused by a major increase in metabolic demand and impaired oxygen extraction [2]. Tissue *hypoxia* may also occur as a result of reduced content or saturation of hemoglobin (i.e., severe anemia) (see Table 20.1). In conditions of ischemia, energy failure develops rapidly and removal of toxic metabolites is often compromised. On the contrary, in conditions of hypoxia, metabolic substrate delivery and energy production can continue and waste removal is maintained. Therefore, ischemia is a more deleterious event than hypoxia.

Energy Failure and Calcium Overload During Ischemia

Although quantitative and kinetic features of ischemic injury are different for each specialized cell type, several metabolic responses are shared among all cell types (Figure 20.1). Immediately upon ischemia, a time-dependent cascade of metabolic events occurs. The first event is a rapid depletion of intracellular adenosine triphosphate (ATP) stores and other high-energy phosphate compounds (such as creatine phosphate in the heart). The cell shifts from oxidative metabolism to an inefficient anaerobic glycolysis, producing only 2 moles of ATP/mole of glucose instead of the 38 moles of ATP normally produced during aerobic metabolism. This collapse of high-energy phosphate compounds impairs the energy-dependent cell processes, such as membrane ion pumps (Na^+/H^+ exchanger) and protein synthesis. Within seconds or minutes, these abnormalities become sufficiently severe to reduce

D.S. Wheeler et al. (eds.), *Science and Practice of Pediatric Critical Care Medicine*,
DOI 10.1007/978-1-84800-921-9_20, © Springer-Verlag London Limited 2009

TABLE 20.1. Clinical conditions of cell hypoxia/ischemia.

Reduction of DO₂		
Reduction of CaO₂	Reduction of CO	Increase of VO₂
Artery occlusion	Hypovolemic shock	Sepsis
Solid organ transplantation	Cardiogenic shock	Septic shock
Tissue and limb reimplantation	Cardiopulmonary bypass	
Severe hypotension	Congestive heart failure	
Hypobaric conditions	Dysrhythmias	
Drug-induced vasoconstriction		
Anemia		
Hemorrhage		

cell function. For example, in the heart this metabolic derangement translates into reduction of the contractile force generated by actin–myosin cross-bridge formation; in the gut altered intestinal absorptive function is associated with translocation of bacteria from the intestine to the lymphatic vessels and bloodstream.

Anaerobic glycolysis leads to glycogen depletion and lactate accumulation, which, in conjunction with increased inorganic phosphates from ATP hydrolysis, reduce intracellular and extracellular pH. Membrane depolarization and failure of ATP-dependent ion pumps leads to efflux of potassium and influx of sodium and calcium. Increase of intracellular sodium concentration is accompanied by water influx into the cell, leading to swelling of the cytoplasm and organelles, such as mitochondria and endoplasmic reticulum. At this point, if oxygen supply is restored, cell injury is

reversible. However, if ischemia persists, cell injury may become irreversible. Increase of cytosol and mitochondrial concentration of calcium overcomes the cell calcium-exporting capacity. Mitochondria show amorphous matrix densities and granular dense bodies of calcium phosphate, which are considered the earliest sign of irreversible ischemic cell injury. Mitochondria play an important role in ischemic damage. Indeed, the excessive energy demand is likely to represent a crucial factor in the ensuing irreversible damage of cells, especially in cardiomyocytes, where the cell volume occupied by mitochondria is the greatest among all the cell types. A major role in the progression toward cell death might be attributed to the opening of the *mitochondrial permeability transition pore*, which, besides abolishing mitochondrial ATP production, amplifies the damage by causing NAD⁺ release.

The cytosol and mitochondrial calcium overload causes activation of a number of enzymes (proteases, phospholipase, ATPase) and disrupts mitochondrial and lysosomal membranes, further uncoupling mitochondrial oxidative phosphorylation and promoting the release of other acid hydrolases [3].

Cell death then occurs mainly by necrosis and is associated with widespread leakage of cellular enzymes or proteins across the cell membrane and into the plasma, which may provide important diagnostic tools of cell damage (such as the serum increase of creatine kinase and troponin levels for the diagnosis of myocardial infarction). However, apoptosis is also a major contributor of cell death and is activated by release of proapoptotic components from the altered mitochondria.

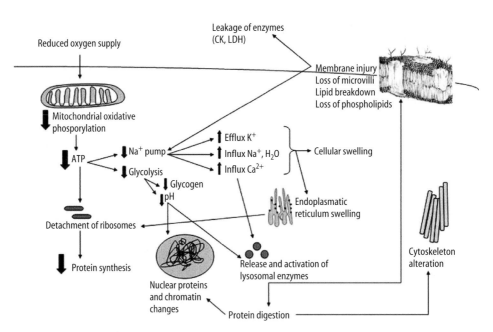

FIGURE 20.1. Metabolic events and cellular derangement during ischemia. After reduction of oxygen supply, mitochondrial oxidative phosphorylation is decreased with subsequent decrease in adenosine triphosphate (ATP) generation and rate of glycolysis, a progressive loss of glycogen content, and a decrease of protein synthesis. Accumulation of lactate and increased inorganic phosphates from ATP hydrolysis reduce intracellular and extracellular pH and cause membrane depolarization. This energy collapse impairs the membrane ion pumps, resulting in increases in intracellular levels of Na⁺, Ca²⁺, an influx of water, and a decrease of intracellular levels of K⁺. Water influx into the cell leads to swelling of the cytoplasm and organelles, such as mitochondria and endoplasmic reticulum, further impairing mitochondrial oxidative phosphorylation and protein synthesis. The cytosol calcium overload causes activation of a number of enzymes (proteases, phospholipase, ATPase) and disrupts lysosomal membranes, further promoting the release of other acid hydrolases. Protein digestion by these lysosomal enzymes causes cellular damage at the cytoskeleton, nucleus, and plasma membrane. After cell death, disruption of cell membrane leads to leakage of intracellular enzymes and proteins into the extracellular milieu, such as creatine kinase (CK) and lactate dehydrogenase (LDH).

The Reperfusion Injury

Restoration of blood flow or oxygen supply is a mandatory therapeutic approach to resuscitate an ischemic tissue and can result in
recovery of cell function if the cell is reversibly injured. Paradoxi-
cally, reoxygenation initiates a cascade of events that may lead to
additional cell injury, known as *reperfusion injury*. At least four
major components contribute to reperfusion injury: oxidative and
nitrosative stress, endothelial dysfunction, neutrophil activation,
and complement activation.

Oxidative and Nitrosative Stress

A delicate balance between intracellular oxidants and antioxidants
likely influences many physiologic functions of the cell. However,
this balance is altered during reperfusion. The restoration of
oxygen supply to the ischemic tissue is responsible for a further
cellular dysmetabolism because it induces the production of potent
reactive species. Endothelial cells represent the first target of this
event. The reactive species include reactive oxygen and nitrogen
species such as superoxide (O_2^-), hydrogen peroxide (H_2O_2), oxidized lipoproteins, lipid peroxides, nitric oxide (NO), and peroxynitrite (ONOO) [4,5]. Reactive species can be formed by several
mechanisms; they can be produced by reduction of molecular
oxygen in altered mitochondria; by enzymes such as xanthine
oxidase (XO), NAD(P)H oxidase, cytochrome P450, nitric oxide
synthetase (NOS), and cyclooxygenase (COX); and by autooxidation of catecholamines.

Briefly, the production of oxyradicals starts early in the ischemic
period in mitochondria with altered redox balance in endothelial
or parenchymal cells and is further enhanced during reperfusion
by a massive activation of XO in endothelial cells and NAD(P)H
oxidase in infiltrated neutrophils [4]. These reactive species
mediate tissue injury by two main mechanisms: directly by inducing damage of important cellular macromolecules and indirectly
by activating signal transduction pathways, which are responsible
of the production of inflammatory mediators and/or apoptotic
mediators.

Direct Oxidative and Nitrosative Injury: Damage of Macromolecules, DNA, and Activation of Poly (ADP-Ribose) Polymerase-1

As highly reactive species, free radicals and oxidants induce oxidation of sulfhydryl groups and thioethers, as well as nitration and
hydroxylation of aromatic compounds, thus influencing the structure and function of many enzymes, proteins, lipids, and DNA
[6,7]. For instance, lipid peroxidation results in disruption of the
cell membrane as well as the membranes of cellular organelles and
causes the release of highly cytotoxic products such as malondial-
dehyde. Modification of proteins by reactive oxygen and nitrogen
species can cause inactivation of critical enzymes and can induce
denaturation that renders proteins nonfunctional. For instance,
tyrosine nitration induced by ONOO or nitrogen derivatives may
lead to dysfunction of superoxide dismutase and cytoskeletal actin
[6]. Oxidation of sulfhydryl groups is responsible for the inhibition
of critical mitochondrial enzymes (Figure 20.2) [8].

Another important interaction occurs with nucleic acids, with
the production of 8-hydroxydeoxyguanosine and 8-nitroguanine
and the occurrence of DNA fragmentation [9]. The occurrence of
DNA breakage results in the activation of the nuclear enzyme poly
(ADP-ribose) polymerase-1 (PARP-1), which further amplifies
tissue damage (see Figure 20.2) [10,11]. It is a chromatin-associated
nuclear enzyme, which possesses putative DNA repair function in
eukaryotic cells. The enzyme is composed of three functional
domains: an N-terminal DNA binding domain that binds to DNA
strand breaks, a central automodification domain containing auto-
poly (ADP-ribosyl)ation sites, and a C-terminal catalytic domain.
Binding of the N-terminal domain to DNA nicks and breaks activates the C-terminal catalytic domain that, in turn, cleaves NAD^+
into ADP-ribose and nicotinamide. Poly (ADP-ribose) polymerase-
1 covalently attaches ADP-ribose to various nuclear proteins and
to PARP-1 itself and then extends the initial ADP-ribose group into
a nucleic acid-like polymer, poly-(ADP)ribose. Extensive poly(ADP-
ribosyl)ation can be induced by a wide variety of inflammatory
stimuli, including reactive species [12,13]. Although poly(ADP-
ribosyl)ation is an attempt of the cell to repair DNA, it appears that
this process may be more harmful than beneficial. Once activated

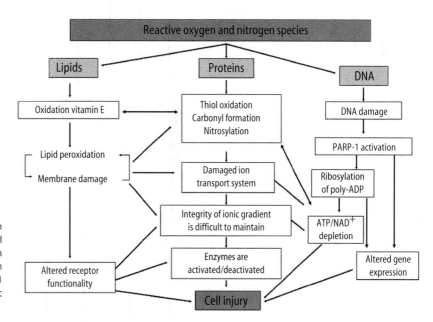

FIGURE 20.2. Direct cellular injury by reactive oxygen and nitrogen
species. Free radicals and oxidants may induce oxidation, carbonyl
formation, and nitrosylation, influencing the structure and function
of many enzymes, proteins, lipids, and DNA. DNA damage results in
the activation of the nuclear enzyme poly (ADP-ribose) polymerase-1
(PARP-1), which causes depletion of the NAD^+ and ATP energetic
pools and alteration of gene expression.

in response to nicks and breaks in the strand DNA, PARP-1 initiates an energy-consuming cycle, which rapidly depletes the intracellular NAD$^+$ and ATP energetic pools, slows the rate of glycolysis and mitochondrial respiration, and progresses to a loss of cellular viability postulated as a *suicide phenomenon* [13].

Several experimental reports have demonstrated that activation of PARP-1 is a major cytotoxic pathway of tissue injury in different pathologies associated with ischemia and reperfusion injury and inflammation. Genetic deletion and pharmacologic inhibition of PARP-1 has been shown to attenuate tissue injury in rodents after myocardial, cerebral, and splanchnic infarction; cardiopulmonary bypass; sepsis; hemorrhagic shock; diabetes; and other conditions of inflammation [10–15]. In addition to the energetic failure, PARP-1 activation and poly(ADP-ribosyl)ation may also cause tissue damage by playing a role in gene expression. Experimental reports have suggested that PARP-1, by direct protein interaction and/or by poly(ADP-ribosyl)ation, alters the function of a variety of transcription factors, including the proinflammatory factors nuclear factor κB (NFκB) and activator protein-1 (AP-1) and the cytoprotective heat shock factor-1 (HSF1), thus modulating the gene expression of several inflammatory mediators [12,16,17] .

Indirect Oxidative and Nitrosative Injury: The Interactive Role of Oxidants with Protein Kinases, Phosphatases, and Transcription Factors

Another mechanism by which reactive oxygen and nitrogen species can induce tissue damage is via regulation of transcription pathways that regulate the proinflammatory profile of the cell. The exact intracellular molecular signaling mechanism of action of reactive oxygen and nitrogen species has not been completely characterized. However, it appears that reactive species may regulate cellular function through changes of critical thiol groups or amino acid residues of mitogen-activated protein kinases and their regulatory phosphatases, which are important components of an extensive network of interconnected signal transduction pathways [18,19].

Mitogen-activated protein kinases mediate the transduction of extracellular signals from the receptor levels to the nuclear tran-

scription factors. These kinases activate each other by sequential steps of phosphorylation; whereas their inactivation is mediated by phosphatases through dephosphorylation. At the downstream of this cascade, oxidant-sensitive kinases include the extracellular signal-regulated kinase 1 and 2 (ERK 1/2), c-Jun N-terminal kinase (JNK), p38, and inhibitor κB kinase (IKK) [20]. Phosphorylation of ERK, JNK, p38, and IKK activates nuclear proteins and transcription factors.

At the nuclear level, one critical transcription factor is NFκB. It is ubiquitously found in all mammalian cells and is central to the activation of several cytokines and inflammatory modulators in ischemia and reperfusion. Nuclear factor κB is usually present in the cytoplasm of the cell in an inactive state bound to a related inhibitory protein known as inhibitor κBα (IκBα). A common pathway for the activation of NFκB occurs when its inhibitor protein IκBα is phosphorylated by IKK [21]. Phosphorylated IκBα is targeted for rapid ubiquitination, and then degraded by the 26S proteasome. Degradation of IκBα unmasks the nuclear translocation sequence of NFκB, allowing NFκB to enter the nucleus and direct transcription of target genes [21].

Activator protein-1, another nuclear transcription factor, is also purportedly regulated by reactive species and is involved in the transcriptional expression of several genes involved in inflammation. Activator protein-1 is a collective term referring to dimeric transcription factors commonly composed of c-Jun and c-Fos or other activating subunits. Activator protein-1 activation also requires phosphorylation of its subunits by JNK [22].

These signaling cascades are rapid and enable the cells to respond to environmental changes by inducing a prompt production of inflammatory mediators, such as cytokines, adhesion molecules, chemokines, and metabolic enzymes, thus determining the functional outcome in response to stress. It is important to note that several of the inflammatory mediators, which are regulated by NFκB (e.g., tumor necrosis factor-α and interleukin-1), and/or AP-1 can in turn further activate these transcription factors, thus creating a self-maintaining inflammatory cycle that increases the severity and the duration of the inflammatory response (Figure 20.3) [21–23].

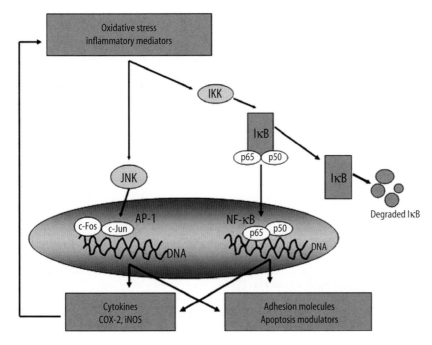

FIGURE 20.3. Activation of signal transduction pathways. Oxygen and nitrogen reactive species and several inflammatory mediators are potent stimuli for the activation of a cascade of mitogen-activated kinases. At the downstream of this cascade, the inhibitor κB kinase (IKK) phosphorylates inhibitor αkB (IκBα), allowing its ubiquitination and degradation. This event unmasks the nuclear factor-κB (NFκB), which is free to translocate into the nucleus to initiate gene transcription. Similarly, once activated, c-Jun N-terminal kinase (JNK) phosphorylates c-Jun, allowing its dimerization with c-Fos, thus forming the transcription factor activator protein-1 (AP-1). Activation of both NFκB and AP-1 induces production of inflammatory mediators, such as cytokines, adhesion molecules, enzymes (i.e., cyclooxygenase-2 [COX-2] and inducible nitric oxide synthase [iNOS]), and apoptotic modulators.

Activation of NFκB and AP-1 has been demonstrated during reperfusion in ischemic brain, heart, and liver and in conditions of sepsis and hemorrhagic shock in several experimental studies [16,17,24–26]. These data have been further confirmed in humans because nuclear translocation of NFκB, in correlation with increase of AP-1 has been found in cardiac biopsy specimens from patients with unstable angina [27]. These findings suggest that both NFκB and AP-1 work cooperatively to produce the specific inflammatory response of oxidant-induced injury [23].

The potential causative role of NFκB activation in reperfusion injury is also supported by several studies in rodents demonstrating that pharmacologic inhibitors of NFκB exerts beneficial effects in models of myocardial ischemia and reperfusion injury, hemorrhagic shock, and sepsis [21,28]. These reports suggest that targeting nuclear transcription factors may represent an effective therapeutic approach in the treatment of ischemia and reperfusion. However, this hypothesis remains to be confirmed in human studies.

Sources of Reactive Oxygen and Nitrogen Species

Mitochondrial Production

The production of oxyradicals starts early in the ischemic period in mitochondria with altered redox balance. During ischemia, the metabolic reduction of the adenine nucleotide pool leaves the mitochondrial carrier in a more fully reduced state, which results in electron leakage from the respiratory chain. This increase in electron leakage reacts with residual molecular oxygen entrapped within the inner mitochondrial membrane, yielding to superoxide radical production. Reintroduction of oxygen with reperfusion reenergizes the mitochondria, but electron leakage further increases because of ADP low content, enabling more reactions with molecular oxygen [4].

Xanthine Oxidase

The xanthine oxido-reductase enzyme system plays an important role in the catabolism of the purine. It is mostly localized in the vascular endothelial and smooth muscle cells and in epithelial cells and exists in two interconvertible forms, xanthine dehydrogenase (XDH) and XO [29–31]. During ischemia, XDH is converted to the oxidase form by a protease activated by the intracellular overload of calcium. At the same time, ATP is degraded to hypoxanthine, which accumulates in the ischemic tissue. During reperfusion, with the presence of large quantities of molecular oxygen and high concentrations of hypoxanthine, XO yields to a burst of superoxide (Figure 20.4). The hypothesis that generation of superoxide by XO may play an important pathogenetic role in reperfusion injury has been supported by studies demonstrating that inactivation of XO with allopurinol ameliorates reperfusion-induced tissue damage [32].

Recently, the xanthine oxido-reductase enzyme system has been shown to catalyze the reduction of nitrates and nitrites to nitrites and NO, respectively, thus also contributing to NO generation during ischemic conditions and during reperfusion [33,34]. However, the role of XO in reperfusion injury is not fully confirmed. For example, it appears that the conversion of XDH to XO is too slow to play a major role in the pathogenesis of ischemia and reperfusion injury in the liver [35]. Furthermore, the distribution of the XO among tissues varies, with very low activity detected in the human heart, where it is located in the endothelium only, but not in the

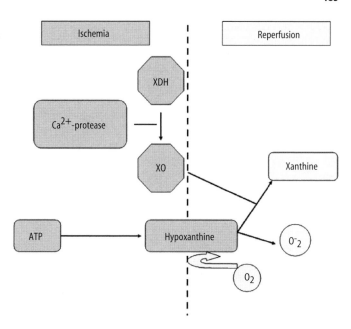

Figure 20.4. Formation of superoxide anion (O_2^-) by xanthine oxidase (XO). During ischemia, xanthine dehydrogenase (XDH) is converted to XO by a Ca^{2+}-dependent protease. At the same time, adenosine triphosphate (ATP) is degraded to hypoxanthine. During reperfusion, in the presence of large quantities of oxygen (O_2) and hypoxanthine, XO produces large amounts of O_2^-.

myocytes [36]. Interestingly, elevated plasma levels of XO have been reported in patients subjected to ischemia and reperfusion-induced limb tourniquet [37,38], liver transplantation [39], or small intestine [40]. These circulating levels may bind to endothelial cells of distant sites and contribute to initiate oxidative damage in organs remote from the original ischemic tissue [31]. Therefore, because XO is present mainly in endothelial cells and as a circulating form in the plasma, XO-derived free radicals may play a role in mediating neutrophil adhesion by activating signal transduction pathways to the endothelium rather than directly inducing tissue damage.

Oxidative Burst from the Infiltrated Neutrophils: The NAD(P)H Oxidase

Secondary to endothelial activation, the local accumulation and activation of neutrophils significantly enhances local production of reactive oxygen species. Neutrophils contain the complex enzyme NAD(P)H oxidase, which is a rich source of both superoxide and the potent oxidizing and chlorinating agent HOCl [4].

Nitric Oxide and Nitrosative Stress

Nitric oxide is a highly reactive gas and is synthesized from L-arginine by a family of enzymes known as NO synthase (NOS). Three isoforms of NOS has been identified: neuronal (nNOS or type 1), inducible (iNOS or type 2) and endothelial (eNOS or type 3) [41]. The eNOS and nNOS isoforms are constitutively expressed and calcium/calmodulin dependent and produce A low amount of NO. The iNOS isoform is a calcium/calmodulin-independent enzyme that is responsible for a high output of NO and is expressed in almost every cell type in response to inflammatory cytokines and growth factors during diverse pathologic conditions, including sepsis, hemorrhagic shock, trauma, and ischemia.

Under normal conditions, the constitutive forms of NOS release low concentrations of NO, which are critical to normal physiology. For example, the nNOS-derived NO acts as a neurotransmitter and a second messenger. The eNOS-derived NO is the physiologic mediator of vascular tone. Once formed by vascular endothelial cells, NO diffuses to adjacent smooth muscle cells and activates soluble guanylate cyclase, producing cyclic guanosine monophosphate and reducing intracellular calcium concentration, thus resulting in vasodilatation. The endothelium-derived NO also scavenges oxygen free radicals, inhibits platelet aggregation and leukocyte adherence, and inhibits smooth muscle proliferation, thus maintaining normal tissue perfusion and vascular permeability. In the cardiomyocytes, under physiologic conditions, both constitutive forms of NOS (type 1 and 3) have been described to release NO, which regulates cardiac function through direct effects on several aspects of cardiomyocyte contractility, from the fine regulation of excitation–contraction coupling (with positive inotropic and lusitropic effects) to modulation of (presynaptic and postsynaptic) autonomic signaling and mitochondrial respiration [41,42]

It is well established that ischemia and reperfusion results in alteration of the NO pathway, which can be summarized in two main events: (1) impairment of eNOS activity and (2) induction of iNOS (Figure 20.5). After prolonged ischemia, and immediately at the onset of reperfusion, the burst of oxidants and the release of proinflammatory cytokines cooperate to reduce NO production from the constitutive eNOS by scavenging effects and by reducing eNOS mRNA stability and expression, respectively [43,45]. Thus, reduction of NO release from the reperfusion-injured endothelium impairs vascular relaxation to endothelium-dependent vasodilators and predisposes the vascular endothelium to platelet aggregation and leukocyte adhesion. This early attenuation of

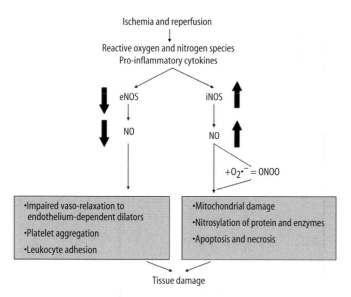

Figure 20.5. Impairment of nitric oxide (NO) synthesis during ischemia and reperfusion. Oxygen and nitrogen reactive species and several inflammatory mediators may reduce NO production from the constitutive endothelial nitric oxide synthase (eNOS), thus impairing vascular relaxation to endothelium-dependent vasodilators and predisposing the endothelium to platelet aggregation and leukocyte adhesion. In severe ischemia and reperfusion, high levels of NO may be produced by inducible nitric oxide synthase (iNOS). Cytotoxic effects may be mediated directly by NO and/or indirectly by peroxynitrite (ONOO), which is formed from the reaction of NO with superoxide. Nitric oxide and peroxynitrite may inhibit the mitochondrial respiratory chain, induce nitrosylation of proteins and enzymes, and cause cell apoptosis and/or necrosis.

endothelium-dependent vasodilatation has been considered a sensitive marker of endothelial dysfunction after ischemia and reperfusion in the heart and other vascular beds. Because of the very important effects of NO on vascular tone and thrombogenicity, drugs that can modulate NO levels have been used as therapeutic agents for the various angina syndromes for a long time and are also used in congestive heart failure and for patients with left ventricular dysfunction. Nitrovasodilators, such as nitroprusside, which acts by donating NO spontaneously, or glyceryl trinitrite and isosorbide dinitrate, which release NO after metabolic conversions, are able to activate guanylate cyclase and elevate cyclic guanosine monophosphate in the vasculature, thus providing favorable hemodynamic effects, including vasodilatation, reduction of myocardial work, and reduction of oxygen consumption 46].

However, in severe ischemia and reperfusion high levels of NO are produced by iNOS and may be responsible for potentially noxious effects. Cytotoxic effects may be mediated directly by NO and/or indirectly by reactive NO-derived byproducts. In fact, when NO is produced in massive outburst, it reacts with superoxide to form the toxic oxidant ONOO. Peroxynitrite causes oxidation of sulfhydryls, lipid peroxidation, and RNA and DNA breakage [8,9,14]; reacts with thiols; inhibits the mitochondrial respiratory chain by inactivating complexes I to III; and induces nitration of tyrosine residues in proteins to form nitrotyrosine, thus altering protein structure and function. In the highly oxidative milieu of the reperfused tissue, in addition to ONOO, several other chemical reactions, involving nitrite, hypochlorous acid, and peroxidases, can induce tyrosine nitration and contribute to tissue damage [9]. Furthermore, NO can react with oxygen to yield other reactive intermediates. The nitrosative reactive species contribute then to cell dysfunction and death. The deleterious effects are mainly related to mitochondrial damage, collapse of the energetic capacity, and induction of apoptosis by releasing proteins from the mitochondria and necrosis by lysis of plasma membrane [5–9]. However, the role of NO in ischemia and reperfusion injury is not completely known because several experimental studies with inhibitors of NO synthesis have reported controversial data [5]. It appears that multiple factors, such as NO concentration, redox status of the cell, NO-superoxide radical ratio, and length of ischemia will determine whether NO serves as a cytoprotective or cytotoxic agent. Certainly, in acute conditions of ischemia, small amounts of the endothelium-derived NO are important for the regulation of microvascular permeability and maintenance of local perfusion. On the contrary, in severe prolonged ischemia and reperfusion, overproduction of NO may mediate deleterious effects.

Other Sources

It has been suggested that the ischemia and reperfusion–induced calcium overload activates phospholipases, which degrade cell membrane phospholipids, releasing arachidonic acid [4]. Formation of prostaglandins and leukotrienes from arachidonic acid involves electron transfer that can initiate the formation of free radicals. Autooxidation of catecholamines may also contribute to oxygen free radicals, especially in ischemic myocardium, where catecholamines are released in abundance [4]. In ischemia-induced neurodegenerative disorders, the metabolism of dopamine produces reactive oxygen species (peroxide, superoxide, and hydroxyl radical) and a potent reactive quinone moiety [47]. However, the precise contribution of arachidonic acid metabolites and oxidation of catecholamines in reperfusion-induced oxidative stress is not completely known.

Alteration of Antioxidant Mechanisms

Decreased antioxidant activity may also contribute to the increase of reactive species. Under physiologic conditions, several cellular mechanisms counterbalance the production of reactive species, including enzymatic and nonenzymatic pathways [48]. The enzymatic pathways are catalase and glutathione peroxidase, which coordinate the catalysis of hydrogen peroxide to water, and superoxide dismutase, which facilitates the formation of H_2O_2 from superoxide. The nonenzymatic pathways include intracellular antioxidants such as vitamins C, E, and β-carotene, ubiquinone, glutathione, lipoic acid, urate, and cysteine. Thioredoxin and thioredoxin reductase form an additional redox regulatory system because they catalyze the regeneration of antioxidant molecules, such as ubiquinone (Q10), lipoic acid, and ascorbic acid. However, these defense mechanisms fail when the reperfusion-induced robust generation of reactive species exceeds the cellular antioxidant activity [28]. In addition, intracellular levels of glutathione decline with a concomitant accumulation of the oxidized and inactive form of glutathione (GSSG). Maladaptative decreases of other nonenzymatic antioxidants may also occur. For instance, plasma levels of ascorbate [49] and atria levels of vitamin E are reduced in patients after cardiopulmonary bypass [28,50]. Antioxidant capacity is also reduced in the plasma or in the venous effluent of reperfused myocardium in patients with short episodes of myocardial ischemia [51].

Endothelial Dysfunction and Neutrophil Infiltration

The event of reperfusion is frequently associated with early endothelial dysfunction. The dysfunction appears to be triggered by the endothelial generation of a large burst of oxidant molecules and amplified by accumulation of neutrophils into injured tissue. Secondary to oxidative stress and impairment of the NO pathways, vascular permeability increases and leads to edema formation and enhancement of interstitial pressure. When these detrimental changes occur in capillaries and arterioles, the local circulation of blood may be impaired, a phenomenon known as *no-reflow*. In the earliest stages of reperfusion after ischemia, neutrophils moving out of the circulation into inflamed tissue play a physiologic role in the destruction of foreign antigens and remodeling of injured tissue. Nevertheless, neutrophils may augment damage to vascular and parenchymal cellular elements by the release of proteolytic enzymes (elastase, collagenase, cathepepsin, hyaluronidase), free radicals, and proinflammatory mediators. Furthermore, neutrophils physically plug capillaries and small arterioles, thereby contributing to the no-reflow phenomenon and exacerbating the ischemic damage [52,53].

Expression of Adhesion Molecules on Endothelial Surface: Loss of Endothelial Barrier Function

The localization of neutrophils to reperfused tissue after ischemia involves a sequence of three complex steps coordinated by endothelial adhesion molecules, which are recognized by specific receptors on the leukocyte membrane (Figure 20.6). Three families of adhesion molecules have been identified: the selectins, the immunoglobulin gene superfamily and the integrins [54]. The initial interaction between leukocytes and endothelium is transient, resulting in the *rolling* of leukocytes along the vessel wall. Leukocyte rolling is promoted by the selectin family of adhesion glycoproteins, which are found on endothelial cells (P- and E-selectin), leukocytes (L-selectin), and platelets (P-selectin). P-selectin is constitutively expressed and located within Weibel-Palade bodies in the vascular endothelium and platelets. Therefore, it is rapidly translocated to the cell surface after exposure to hydrogen peroxide, ONOO, thrombin, histamine, or complement. E-selectin

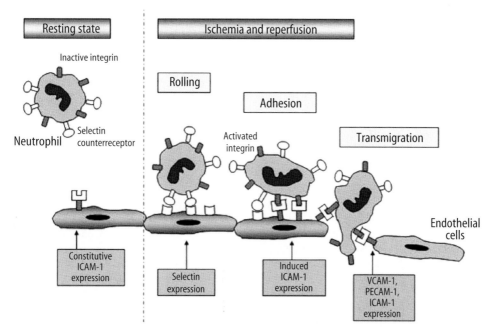

FIGURE 20.6. Kinetics of neutrophil interaction with endothelium and infiltration into parenchymal tissue. During resting state no interaction exists between neutrophils and endothelium: the endothelium expresses low levels of intercellular adhesion molecule-1 (ICAM-1), whereas neutrophils express inactive integrins and low levels of selectin counterreceptors. After ischemia and reperfusion, a sequence of three complex steps coordinates neutrophil infiltration. The initial step is the *rolling* of neutrophils along the vessel wall and is promoted by selectins. The rolling neutrophils then become activated by local factors generated by the endothelium, resulting in their *adhesion* to the vessel wall. Finally, this firm attachment allows the *transmigration* of the neutrophil from the endothelium into the tissue. Adhesion and transmigration are mediated by the interaction of β_2- and β_1-integrins on the surface of neutrophils with immunoglobulin gene superfamily members, such as ICAM-1, VCAM-1 and PECAM-1.

is synthesized after stimulation with proinflammatory cytokines (tumor necrosis factor-α and interleukin-1) and expressed on the endothelial cells after several hours after ischemia and reperfusion injury. The corresponding ligands for selectins on the surface of the leukocyte are sialylated Lewis[x] and A blood group antigens. In addition to endothelial cells, leukocytes also express a selectin (L-selectin), which participates in low affinity interactions with P- and E-selectin during the rolling phase [54,55].

The rolling leukocytes then become activated by local factors generated by the endothelium, resulting in their arrest and *firm adhesion* to the vessel wall. The list of activating factors includes cytokines, chemoattractants (e.g., leukotriene B4, C5a, platelet activating factor), and chemoattractive chemokines, which bind to and activate integrins on leukocyte. Finally, this firm attachment allows the *transmigration* or *diapedesis* of the leukocyte from the endothelium into the tissue [55].

Firm adhesion and transmigration are mediated by the interaction of β_2-integrin (also known as CD11/CD18) and β_1-integrin on the surface of leukocytes with immunoglobulin gene superfamily members expressed by endothelium [54]. The intercellular adhesion molecules (ICAMs), ICAM-1, ICAM-2 and ICAM-3, the vascular cellular adhesion molecule-1 (VCAM-1), and the platelet–endothelial cell adhesion molecule (PECAM) are members of the immunoglobulin superfamily. The CD11/CD18 family of integrins is the counterreceptor for ICAM-1 and ICAM-2, whereas VCAM-1 binds to the integrin *very late activation antigen-4* (VLA4 group/ β_1-integrin) found on leukocytes [56].

Intercellular adhesion molecule-1 is constitutively expressed (at low levels) on the surface of endothelial cells and is responsible for the firm adhesion of neutrophils. Its surface expression is enhanced during inflammation in vivo on endothelial cells after exposure to oxidants or cytokines, with maximal expression occurring within 4 hr and persisting at least 24 hr [56]. In addition to endothelial cells, ICAM-1 is also present on leukocyte, epithelial cells, cardiomyocytes, and fibroblasts, thus contributing to the tissue margination of leukocytes [57].

Vascular cellular adhesion molecule-1 is not constitutively expressed on unstimulated endothelial cells. Exposure to inflammatory mediators or cytokines results in rapid upregulation. The VCAM-1 message levels reach a sustained high level by 2 to 3 hr and gradually diminish over several days [56,58]. Because VCAM-1 binds circulating monocytes and lymphocytes expressing the VLA4 group, the relatively delayed and sustained VCAM-1 response to cytokine may correspond to the switch to preferential adhesion and infiltration of mononuclear leukocytes typical of chronic inflammatory processes.

In this complex machinery of leukocyte trafficking, platelets also accumulate in the vessels, resulting in further impairment of endothelial function and microcirculation. In fact, circulating platelets roll and adhere to the endothelium or subendothelial matrix using similar adhesion molecules and release substances that are able to cause further chemotaxis and migration of circulating leukocytes [59].

Because the abnormal sequestration of leukocytes is a central component in the development of reperfusion injury, therapeutic agents that block leukocyte–endothelial interactions, such as antibodies raised against adhesion molecules, have been used to inhibit the inflammatory response in a number of animal models of myocardial, splanchnic, cerebral, and liver reperfusion damage after ischemia [60]. In the clinical setting, however, very few studies have tested the efficacy of antibodies against adhesion molecules in

organ transplantation, hemorrhagic shock, and myocardial infarction with minor or unsatisfactory results [57,60–63].

Loss of Endothelial Barrier: The Injury Vicious Cycle

Therefore, production of oxygen and nitrogen reactive species, endothelial injury, activation of neutrophil-attractive factors, and neutrophil infiltration (leading to further production of reactive species and proteolytical enzymes) constitute a vicious cycle, which is ultimately responsible for endothelial and parenchymal injury. In the early phase of reperfusion (1–3 hr after reperfusion), neutrophils are present mainly in the intravascular space (attached to the endothelium) and play an important role in the endothelial injury associated with reperfusion. At later stages neutrophils migrate into the tissues and exacerbate parenchymal damage. In this positive feedback cycle, reactive species activate a variety of oxidant processes, such as activation of signal transduction pathways, induction of peroxidation, and DNA injury.

Complement Activation

The complement system is an important pathway of innate immune defense and inflammation [64]. It is composed of more than 30 plasma proteins, glycoproteins, and soluble or membrane bound receptors. The complement system can be activated by three pathways: classic, lectin binding, and alternative (Figure 20.7). The classic pathway is initiated by antigen/antibody complex and/ or inflammatory proteins such as C-reactive protein and serum amyloid protein. The alternative pathway is initiated by surface molecules containing carbohydrates and lipids. The lectin-binding pathway is initiated by the binding of mannose-binding lectin protein (MBL) resulting in activation of MLB-associated serineproteases (MASPs). Data from numerous experimental animal studies of ischemia and reperfusion injury in different organ systems as well as clinical studies support the concept that activation of complement is a crucial pathogenetic event of tissue injury [65,66]. All three pathways are activated in ischemia and reperfusion injury and seem to be involved in an organ-dependent manner [67]. Complement activation has been demonstrated in myocardial infarction, ischemia of the intestine, hind limb, kidney, liver, hemorrhagic shock, and sepsis. In the case of cardiopulmonary bypass procedure, contact of blood with artificial surfaces of the bypass equipment can also activate complement proteins. Under physiologic conditions, endothelial cells contain proteins (decay accelerating factor and membrane cofactor protein), which protect against complement injury. However, endothelial dysfunction during reperfusion may alter these protective mechanisms.

Complement activation results in a unidirectional cascade of enzymatic and biochemical reactions mediated by serine proteases, leading to the formation of biologically active factors. In this cascade, the two terminal byproducts of complement activation, C5a and the complex C5b-C59, also known as the terminal membrane attack complex (MAC), are believed to mediate tissue injury. C5a is one of the most proinflammatory peptides with pleiotropic functions (Table 20.2). C5a serves as a powerful *chemoattractant* for neutrophils, monocytes, and macrophages, where it binds on the C5aR receptor and causes activation of adhesion molecules, thus increasing their adhesiveness and aggregation. C5a stimulates oxidative burst in neutrophils, the release of lysosomal enzymes, and proinflammatory cytokines in macrophages and monocytes, and it activates the coagulation pathway [65]. C5a can also bind to

FIGURE 20.7. Activation pathways of the complement system. The classical pathway is initiated by antigen-antibody complexes and/or inflammatory proteins such as C-reactive protein and serum amyloid protein. The lectin pathway is initiated by serum mannose binding lectins (MLB), which are capable of binding mannose components of bacteria resulting in activation of MLB-associated serine-proteases (MASPs). The alternative pathway is initiated by surface molecules of microbial pathogens, artificial surfaces or protein debris of the injured tissue. These three pathways converge at the generation of the opsonizing protein C3b. C3b fragments in turn bind to their C3 convertases leading to the activation of the C5 component, which is cleaved to yield large amounts of C5a and C5b. C5a is a potent pro-inflammatory peptide, which serves as a chemoattractant for neutrophils, monocytes and macrophages, promoting their oxidative burst and release of lysosomal enzymes and pro-inflammatory mediators. C5b initiates the formation of the membrane attack complex (MAC) with the complement proteins C6, C7, C8, and C9. This complex ultimately disrupts the phospholipid bilayer of target cells, leading to cell lysis and death by the formation of transmembrane channels.

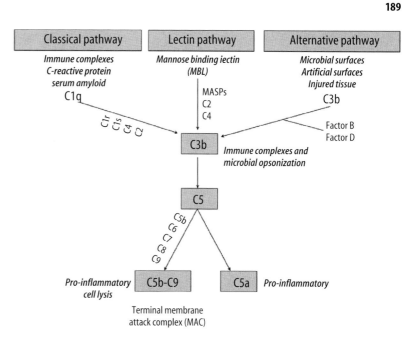

specific C5aR receptor in epithelial cells and activate the release of inflammatory mediators, such as cytokines [68]. C5a and MAC cause changes in the circulation and the vascular wall because they induce expression of adhesion molecules on endothelial cells and decrease the release of NO, causing vasoconstriction [69,70], thus amplifying the loss of vascular homeostasis and the endothelial dysfunction [67]. C5a and MAC activate platelets and favor the formation of procoagulant thrombin [65]. C3a and C5a, as well as C4a, also have *anaphylatoxin activity*. Anaphylatoxins cause increased vascular permeability, smooth muscle contraction, and mast cell degranulation.

Although numerous experimental studies have demonstrated beneficial effects of complement inhibition in ischemia and reperfusion–induced injury, there have been only a few clinical trials so far. Two recent human clinical studies tested a novel C5 complement monoclonal antibody, pexelizumab, combined with thrombolytic therapy [71] or angioplasty [72] after myocardial infarction. No significant effects of the C5 antibody against preexisting myocardial infarcts were found in both trials. However, a 70% reduction in 90-day mortality rate was observed when patients were treated with a bolus and continued infusion of pexelizumab [72]. These preliminary data may suggest that inhibition of the complement pathway may offer a therapeutic target in various reperfusion-induced clinical conditions.

Cellular and Molecular Defenses Against Cell Injury

During ischemia and reperfusion, cellular and molecular defense mechanisms are also deployed in order to counteract the inflammatory response and reflect the attempt of the cell to adapt within the hypoxic and dysmetabolic environment. These cytoprotective mechanisms have generated particular interest in the research field, because they may provide a reasonable base for developing novel therapeutic approaches for the reperfusion injury.

Hypoxia Inducible Factor-1

Deficiency of oxygen directly activates the nuclear transcription factor hypoxia inducible factor-1 (HIF-1), which regulates gene expression of several mediators that render the cell capable to survive and function within a hypoxic environment. Under normoxic conditions, this factor is unstable and inactive; however, during hypoxia HIF-1 is stabilized and binds to the promoter regions of many cytoprotective genes. The list of genes includes genes for glucose transporters and glycolytic enzymes, thereby enhancing the capacity for the anaerobic metabolism, and angiogenic growth factors for capillary formation and revascularization [73].

TABLE 20.2. Proinflammatory activities of C5a and membrane attack complex.

Leukocyte activation	Platelet activation	Endothelial dysfunction	Other effects
Chemoattraction	Thromboxane release	Adhesion molecules expression	Cyclooxygenase and lipooxygenase activation
CD11b expression			
Oxidative burst	P-selectin expression	Prothrombinase activation	Platelet-derived growth factor release
Proteases release	von Willebrand factor	Reduction of nitric oxide	
Histamine release	and IIb/IIIa release		Cell lysis
Cytokine production	Prothrombinase activation		
Prostaglandin release			
Thromboxane release			

The Heat Shock Response

The heat shock response is a highly conserved cellular response to injury. This cellular defense mechanism is characterized by the increased expression of heat shock proteins (HSPs) that provide cytoprotection from inflammatory insults, including oxidative stress, viral infection, and ischemia–reperfusion injury. In eukaryotic cells, the production of HSPs is regulated at the nuclear level by the transcription heat shock factor-1 (HSF-1). Under physiologic conditions, HSF-1 is a phosphorylated monomer located mainly in the cytoplasm. Activation of HSF-1 is induced by a variety of environmental stresses in the presence of elevated intracellular calcium and active protein kinases. Once activated, HSF-1 is translocated into the nucleus, forms trimers, and binds to DNA to drive transcription of HSPs [74]. The function of HSPs has been linked to their role as molecular chaperones. These macromolecules bind to denatured or misfolded proteins, promoting their correct refolding, preservation, or degradation [75]. Their cytoprotective mechanisms have been proven in several experimental studies. For instance, the HSP70 directly protects against myocardial damage, improves metabolic recovery, and reduces infarct size in hearts of transgenic mice subjected to ischemia and reperfusion [75,76]. Another important HSP is the HSP32, also known as heme-oxygenase 1 (HO-1). The cytoprotective HO-1 has been documented as a successful therapeutic strategy in a number of transplantation models. The beneficial effect of HO-1 is mediated through an antioxidant mechanism. Heme-oxygenase 1 removes a prooxidant (heme) while generating a putative antioxidant (bilirubin), carbon monoxide, and iron ions [77].

The Reperfusion Injury Salvage Kinase Pathway

Ischemia and reperfusion have also been shown to activate antiapoptotic kinase signaling cascades, such as the kinases phosphoinositide-3 kinase (PI3K)-Akt and ERK 1/2, which have been implicated in cellular survival and are referred to as the *reperfusion injury salvage kinase* (RISK) pathways [78]. These kinases regulate cell proliferation, differentiation, and survival. Although chronic activation of these pathways has been implicated in cardiac hypertrophy, activating these prosurvival kinases at the time of reperfusion or during ischemic preconditioning has been demonstrated to confer cardioprotection against reperfusion injury. The cardioprotective mechanism of Akt seems to be related to the targeting of apoptotic modulators. For example, Akt inhibits the proapoptotic proteins BAD and BAX, thus preventing the release of mitochondrial cytochrome c in response to an apoptotic stimulus and influences the activity of caspases [78].

The Ischemic Preconditioning Response

Of particular biologic and clinical relevance is the phenomenon known as *ischemic preconditioning response*. As noted originally in 1986 [79], multiple brief ischemic episodes (i.e., preconditioning) protect the heart from a subsequent sustained ischemic insult. Human clinical trials using ischemic preconditioning have been successfully carried out in the fields of cardiac, hepatic, and pulmonary surgery. Epidemiologic data exist to support the existence of preconditioning-induced neuroprotection in humans. Human skeletal muscle has been preconditioned experimentally, as have human proximal tubule renal cells. Additionally, preconditioning is not confined to one organ but can also limit infarct size in remote,

nonpreconditioned organs (*remote preconditioning*). At present, there is no evidence for ischemic preconditioning occurring in the human intestine, although animal studies attest to the possibility [80,81].

The protective effects of preconditioning occur in a well-described biphasic kinetic. Tissue protection appears within minutes and lasts only 2 to 3 hr (early phase or first window of protection) but reappears 24 hr after the preconditioning stimulus (late phase or second window of protection) [82]. Within the early phase, cytoprotective mechanisms depend mainly on post-translational modifications of preexisting cellular proteins. Late preconditioning is a genetic reprogramming of the organ that involves the simultaneous activation of multiple stress-responsive genes and de novo synthesis of several proteins, which ultimately results in the development of a protective phenotype. Sublethal ischemic insults release chemical signals (NO, adenosine, and reactive oxygen species) that trigger a series of signaling events (e.g., activation of protein kinases and NFκB) and culminates in increased synthesis of iNOS, COX-2, HO-1, superoxide dismutase, and probably other cytoprotective proteins.

Conclusion

In clinical therapy of acute infarction of an organ or tissue, reperfusion has proved to be the only way to limit infarct size by restoring the fractional uptake of oxygen to maintain the rate of cellular oxidation. However, restoration of flow is accompanied by the detrimental manifestations of reperfusion injury, which influences the degree of recovery. Reperfusion injury refers to an extremely complex situation that had not occurred during the preceding ischemic period. The existence of such damage has clinical relevance, as it would imply the possibility of improving recovery with specific interventions applied only at the time of reperfusion. Therefore, knowledge of the precise sequence of biochemical and molecular events of reperfusion could lead to rational treatments designed to prevent or delay cell death. However, at the present time, there is no simple answer to the question of what determines cell death and the failure to recover cell function after reperfusion. The analysis of the current experimental data suggests the existence of a self-amplifying vicious cycle, which is governed by reactive species and involves cellular effectors (endothelial and parenchymal cells, neutrophils, platelets), inflammatory mediators, and components of the coagulation and complement cascade. In this cycle, endogenous cytoprotective mechanisms also intervene to counteract inflammation. As described throughout this chapter, the current experimental research has raised the exciting prospect that pharmacologic intervention aimed to interrupt the various levels of this vicious cycle (such as the use of antioxidants, antibodies against adhesion molecules, inhibition of PARP-1, and NFκB, induction of HSPs or ischemic preconditioning) may ameliorate cell dysfunction and prevent death. However, the predictability of in vivo experimentation in animals and its extrapolation to humans is a function of the genetic kinship. Large clinical trials are needed to determine whether these novel therapeutic interventions may be beneficial to the patient.

References

1. Acierno LJ. Adolph Fick: mathematician, physicist, physiologist. Clin Cardiol 2000;23:390–391.

2. Jakob SM. Clinical review: splanchnic ischaemia. Crit Care 2002;6: 306–612.

3. Tegtmeyer H, King LM, Jones BE. Energy substrate metabolism, myocardial ischemia, and targets for pharmacotherapy. Am J Cardiol 1998;82:54K–60K.

4. Ferrari R, Guardigli G, Mele D, Percoco GF, Ceconi C, Curello S. Oxidative stress during myocardial ischaemia and heart failure. Curr Pharm Des 2004;10:1699–1711.

5. Ferdinandy P, Schulz R. Nitric oxide, superoxide, and peroxynitrite in myocardial ischaemia–reperfusion injury and preconditioning. Br J Pharmacol 2003;138:532–543.

6. Ischiropoulos H. Biological selectivity and functional aspects of protein tyrosine nitration. Biochem Biophys Res Commun 2003;305: 776–783.

7. Giordano FJ. Oxygen, oxidative stress, hypoxia, and heart failure. J Clin Invest 2005;115:500–508.

8. Alvarez B, Radi R. Peroxynitrite reactivity with amino acids and proteins. Amino Acids 2003;25:295–311.

9. Halliwell B. Free radicals, proteins and DNA: oxidative damage versus redox regulation. Biochem Soc Trans 1996;24:1023–1027.

10. Szabó C, Dawson VL. Role of poly(ADP-ribose) synthetase in inflammation and ischaemia–reperfusion. Trends Pharmacol Sci 1998;19:287–298.

11. Zingarelli B. Importance of poly (ADP-ribose) polymerase activation in myocardial reperfusion injury. In: Szabó C, ed. Cell Death: The Role of Poly (ADP-Ribose) Polymerase. Boca Raton, FL: CRC Press; 2000:41–60.

12. D'Amours D, Desnoyers S, D'Silva I, Poirier GG. Poly(ADP-ribosyl)ation reactions in the regulation of nuclear functions. Biochem J 1999;342: 249–268.

13. Chiarugi A. Poly(ADP-ribose) polymerase: killer or conspirator? The "suicide hypothesis" revisited. Trends Pharmacol Sci 2002;23:122–129.

14. Zingarelli B, O'Connor M, Wong H, Salzman AL, Szabó C. Peroxynitrite-mediated DNA strand breakage activates poly-adenosine diphosphate ribosyl synthetase and causes cellular energy depletion in macrophages stimulated with bacterial lipopolysaccharide. J Immunol 1996;156:350–358.

15. Zingarelli B, Salzman AL, Szabó C. Genetic disruption of poly (ADP-ribose) synthetase inhibits the expression of P-selectin and intercellular adhesion molecule-1 in myocardial ischemia/reperfusion injury. Circ Res 1998;83:85–94.

16. Zingarelli B, Hake PW, O'Connor M, Denenberg A, Kong S, Aronow BJ. Absence of poly(ADP-ribose)polymerase-1 alters nuclear factor-κB activation and gene expression of apoptosis regulators after reperfusion injury. Mol Med 2003;9:143–153.

17. Zingarelli B, Hake PW, O'Connor M, Denenberg A, Wong HR, Kong S, Aronow BJ. Differential regulation of activator protein-1 and heat shock factor-1 in myocardial ischemia and reperfusion injury: role of poly(ADP-ribose) polymerase-1. Am J Physiol Heart Circ Physiol 2004; 286:H1408–H1415.

18. Thannickal VJ, Fanburg BL. Reactive oxygen species in cell signaling. Am J Physiol Lung Cell Mol Physiol 2000;279:L1005–L1028.

19. Yoshizumi M, Tsuchiya K, Tamaki T. Signal transduction of reactive oxygen species and mitogen-activated protein kinases in cardiovascular disease. J Med Invest 2001;48:11–24.

20. Chang L, Karin M. Mammalian MAP kinase signalling cascades. Nature 2001;410:37–40.

21. Zingarelli B, Sheehan M, Wong HR. Nuclear factor-κB as a therapeutic target in critical care medicine. Crit Care Med 2003;31: S105–S111.

22. Shaulian E, Karin M. AP-1 as a regulator of cell life and death. Nat Cell Biol 2002;4:E131–E136.

23. Karin M, Takahashi T, Kapahi P, Delhase M, Chen Y, Makris C, Rothwarf D, Baud V, Natoli G, Guido F, Li N. Oxidative stress and gene expression: the AP-1 and NF-κB connections. Biofactors 2001;15:87–89.

24. Clemens JA, Stephenson DT, Dixon EP, Smalstig EB, Mincy RE, Rash KS, Little SP. Global cerebral ischemia activates nuclear factor-κB prior to evidence of DNA fragmentation. Brain Res Mol Brain Res 1997; 48:187–196.

25. Zwacka RM, Zhou W, Zhang Y, Darby CJ, Dudus L, Halldorson J, Oberley L, Engelhardt JF. Redox gene therapy for ischemia/reperfusion injury of the liver reduces AP1 and NF-κB activation. Nat Med 1998;4:698–704.

26. Chang CK, Albarillo MV, Schumer W. Therapeutic effect of dimethyl sulfoxide on ICAM-1 gene expression and activation of NF-κB and AP-1 in septic rats. J Surg Res 2001;95:181–187.

27. Valen G, Hansson GK, Dumitrescu A, Vaage J. Unstable angina activates myocardial heat shock protein 72, endothelial nitric oxide synthase, and transcription factors NF-κB and AP-1. Cardiovasc Res 2000;47:49–56.

28. Marczin N, El-Habashi N, Hoare GS, Bundy RE, Yacoub M. Antioxidants in myocardial ischemia-reperfusion injury: therapeutic potential and basic mechanisms. Arch Biochem Biophys 2003;420:222–236.

29. Hellsten-Westing Y. Immunohistochemical localization of xanthine oxidase in human cardiac and skeletal muscle. Histochemistry 1993; 100:215–222.

30. Harrison R. Structure and function of xanthine oxidoreductase: where are we now? Free Radic Biol Med 2002;33:774–797.

31. Meneshian A, Bulkley GB. The physiology of endothelial xanthine oxidase: from urate catabolism to reperfusion injury to inflammatory signal transduction. Microcirculation 2002;9:161–175.

32. Bulger EM, Maier RV. Antioxidants in critical illness. Arch Surg 2001;136:1201–1207.

33. Godber BLJ, Doel JJ, Sapkota GP, Blake DR, Stevens CR, Eisenthal R, Harrison R. Reduction of nitrite to nitric oxide catalyzed by xanthine oxidoreductase. J Biol Chem 2000;275:7757–7763.

34. Li H, Samouilov A, Liu X, Zweier JL. Characterization of the magnitude and kinetics of xanthine oxidase-catalyzed nitrite reduction. Evaluation of its role in nitric oxide generation in anoxic tissues. J Biol Chem 2001;276:24482–24489.

35. Brass CA. Xanthine oxidase and reperfusion injury: major player or minor irritant? Hepatology 1995;21:1757–1760.

36. de Jong JW, van der Meer P, Nieukoop AS, Huizer T, Stroeve RJ, Bos E. Xanthine oxidoreductase activity in perfused hearts of various species, including humans. Circ Res 1990;67:770–773.

37. Friedl HP, Smith DJ, Till GO, Thomson PD, Louis DS, Ward PA. Ischemia-reperfusion in humans. Appearance of xanthine oxidase activity. Am J Pathol 1990;136:491–495.

38. Mathru M, Dries DJ, Barnes L, Tonino P, Sukhani R, Rooney MW. Tourniquet-induced exsanguination in patients requiring lower limb surgery. An ischemia-reperfusion model of oxidant and antioxidant metabolism. Anesthesiology 1996;84:14–22.

39. Pesonen EJ, Linder N, Raivio KO, Sarnesto A, Lapatto R, Hockerstedt K, Makisalo H, Andersson S. Circulating xanthine oxidase and neutrophil activation during human liver transplantation. Gastroenterology 1998;114:1009–1015.

40. Terada LS, Dormish JJ, Shanley PF, Leff JA, Anderson BO, Repine JE. Circulating xanthine oxidase mediates lung neutrophil sequestration after intestinal ischemia-reperfusion. Am J Physiol 1992;263:L394–L401.

41. Bian K, Murad F. Nitric oxide (NO)—biogeneration, regulation, and relevance to human diseases. Front Biosci 2003;8:d264–d278.

42. Massion PB, Feron O, Dessy C, Balligand JL. Nitric oxide and cardiac function: ten years after, and continuing. Circ Res 2003;93:388–398.

43. Ma XL, Weyrich AS, Lefer DJ, Lefer AM. Diminished basal nitric oxide release after myocardial ischemia and reperfusion promotes neutrophil adherence to coronary endothelium. Circ Res 1993;72:403–412.

44. de Frutos T, Sanchez de Miguel L, Farre J, Gomez J, Romero J, Marcos-Alberca P, Nunez A, Rico L, Lopez-Farre A. Expression of an endothelial-type nitric oxide synthase isoform in human neutrophils: modification by tumor necrosis factor-alpha and during acute myocardial infarction. J Am Coll Cardiol 2001;37:800–807.

45. Schulz R, Kelm M, Heusch G. Nitric oxide in myocardial ischemia/reperfusion injury. Cardiovasc Res 2004;61:402–413.

46. Abrams J. Beneficial actions of nitrates in cardiovascular disease. Am J Cardiol 1996;77:31C–37C.

47. Stokes AH, Hastings TG, Vrana KE. Cytotoxic and genotoxic potential of dopamine. J Neurosci Res 1999;55:659–665.

48. Nordberg J, Arner ES. Reactive oxygen species, antioxidants, and the mammalian thioredoxin system. Free Radic Biol Med 2001;31:1287–1312.

49. Ballmer PE, Reinhart WH, Jordan P, Buhler E, Moser UK, Gey KF. Depletion of plasma vitamin C but not of vitamin E in response to cardiac operations. J Thorac Cardiovasc Surg 1994;108:311–320.

50. Barsacchi R, Pelosi G, Maffei S, Baroni M, Salvatore L, Ursini F, Verunelli F, Biagini A. Myocardial vitamin E is consumed during cardiopulmonary bypass: indirect evidence of free radical generation in human ischemic heart. Int J Cardiol 1992;37:339–343.

51. Buffon A, Santini SA, Ramazzotti V, Rigattieri S, Liuzzo G, Biasucci LM, Crea F, Giardina B, Maseri A. Large, sustained cardiac lipid peroxidation and reduced antioxidant capacity in the coronary circulation after brief episodes of myocardial ischemia. J Am Coll Cardiol 2000;35:633–639.

52. Seal JB, Gewertz BL. Vascular dysfunction in ischemia–reperfusion injury. Ann Vasc Surg 2005;19:572–584.

53. Rezkalla SH, Kloner RA. No-reflow phenomenon. Circulation 2002;105:656–662.

54. Carlos TM, Harlan JM. Leukocyte–endothelial adhesion molecules. Blood 1994;84:2068–2101.

55. Lawrence MB, Springer TA. Leukocytes roll on a selectin at physiologic flow rates: distinction from and prerequisite for adhesion through integrins. Cell 1991;65:859–873.

56. Malik AB, Lo SK. Vascular endothelial adhesion molecules and tissue inflammation. Pharmacol Rev 1996;48:213–229.

57. Yonekawa K, Harlan JM. Targeting leukocyte integrins in human diseases. J Leukocyte Biol 2005;77:129–140.

58. Collins T, Read MA, Neish AS, Whitley MZ, Thanos D, Maniatis T. Transcriptional regulation of endothelial cell adhesion molecules: NF-κB and cytokine-inducible enhancers. FASEB J 1995;9:899–909.

59. Gawaz M. Role of platelets in coronary thrombosis and reperfusion of ischemic myocardium. Cardiovasc Res 2004;61:498–511.

60. Anaya-Prado R, Toledo-Pereyra LH, Lentsch AB, Ward PA. Ischemia/reperfusion injury. J Surg Res 2002;105:248–258.

61. Rhee P, Morris J, Durham R, Hauser C, Cipolle M, Wilson R, Luchette F, McSwain N, Miller R. Recombinant humanized monoclonal antibody against CD18 (rhuMAb CD18) in traumatic hemorrhagic shock: results of a phase II clinical trial. Traumatic Shock Group. J Trauma 2000;49:611–620.

62. Baran KW, Nguyen M, McKendall GR, Lambrew CT, Dykstra G, Palmeri ST, Gibbons RJ, Borzak S, Sobel BE, Gourlay SG, Rundle AC, Gibson CM, Barron HV; Limitation of Myocardial Infarction Following Thrombolysis in Acute Myocardial Infarction (LIMIT AMI) Study Group. Double-blind, randomized trial of an anti-CD18 antibody in conjunction with recombinant tissue plasminogen activator for acute myocardial infarction: limitation of myocardial infarction following thrombolysis in acute myocardial infarction (LIMIT AMI) study. Circulation 2001;104:2778–2783.

63. Faxon DP, Gibbons RJ, Chronos NA, Gurbel PA, Sheehan F; HALT-MI Investigators. The effect of blockade of the CD11/CD18 integrin receptor on infarct size in patients with acute myocardial infarction treated with direct angioplasty: the results of the HALT-MI study. J Am Coll Cardiol 2002;40:1199–1204.

64. Mastellos D, Morikis D, Isaacs SN, Holland MC, Strey CW, Lambris JD. Complement: structure, functions, evolution, and viral molecular mimicry. Immunol Res 2003;27:367–386.

65. Guo RF, Ward PA. Role of C5a in inflammatory responses. Annu Rev Immunol 2005;23:821–852.

66. Arumugam TV, Shiels IA, Woodruff TM, Granger DN, Taylor SM. The role of the complement system in ischemia–reperfusion injury. Shock 2004;21:401–409.

67. Hart ML, Walsh MC, Stahl GL. Initiation of complement activation following oxidative stress. In vitro and in vivo observations. Mol Immunol 2004;41:165–171.

68. Riedemann NC, Guo RF, Sarma VJ, Laudes IJ, Huber-Lang M, Warner RL, Albrecht EA, Speyer CL, Ward PA. Expression and function of the C5a receptor in rat alveolar epithelial cells. J Immunol 2002;168:1919–1925.

69. Park KW, Tofukuji M, Metais C, Comunale ME, Dai HB, Simons M, Stahl GL, Agah A, Sellke FW. Attenuation of endothelium-dependent dilation of pig pulmonary arterioles after cardiopulmonary bypass is prevented by monoclonal antibody to complement C5a. Anesth Analg 1999;89:42–48.

70. Cable DG, Hisamochi K, Schaff HV. A model of xenograft hyperacute rejection attenuates endothelial nitric oxide production: a mechanism for graft vasospasm? J Heart Lung Transplant 1999;18:177–184.

71. Mahaffey KW, Granger CB, Nicolau JC, Ruzyllo W, Weaver WD, Theroux P, Hochman JS, Filloon TG, Mojcik CF, Todaro TG, Armstrong PW; COMPLY Investigators. Effect of pexelizumab, an anti-C5 complement antibody, as adjunctive therapy to fibrinolysis in acute myocardial infarction: the COMPlement inhibition in myocardial infarction treated with thromboLYtics (COMPLY) trial. Circulation 2003;108:1176–1183.

72. Granger CB, Mahaffey KW, Weaver WD, Theroux P, Hochman JS, Filloon TG, Rollins S, Todaro TG, Nicolau JC, Ruzyllo W, Armstrong PW; COMMA Investigators. Pexelizumab, an anti-C5 complement antibody, as adjunctive therapy to primary percutaneous coronary intervention in acute myocardial infarction: the COMPlement inhibition in Myocardial infarction treated with Angioplasty (COMMA) trial. Circulation 2003;108:1184–1190.

73. Williams RS, Benjamin IJ. Protective responses in the ischemic myocardium. J Clin Invest 2000;106:813–818.

74. Stephanou A, Latchman DS. Transcriptional regulation of the heat shock protein genes by STAT family transcription factors. Gene Expr 1999;7:311–319.

75. Knowlton AA, Sun L. Heat-shock factor-1, steroid hormones, and regulation of heat-shock protein expression in the heart. Am J Physiol Heart Circ Physiol 2001;280:H455–H464.

76. Okubo S, Wildner O, Shah MR, Chelliah JC, Hess ML, Kukreja RC. Gene transfer of heat-shock protein 70 reduces infarct size in vivo after ischemia/reperfusion in the rabbit heart. Circulation 2001;103:877–881

77. Abraham NG, Kappas A. Heme oxygenase and the cardiovascular-renal system. Free Radic Biol Med 2005;39:1–25.

78. Hausenloy DJ, Yellon DM. New directions for protecting the heart against ischaemia–reperfusion injury: targeting the Reperfusion Injury Salvage Kinase (RISK)-pathway. Cardiovasc Res 2004;61:448–460.

79. Murry CE, Jennings RB, Reimer KA. Preconditioning with ischemia: a delay of lethal cell injury in ischemic myocardium. Circulation 1986;74:1124–1136.

80. Mallick IH, Yang W, Winslet MC, Seifalian AM. Ischemia-reperfusion injury of the intestine and protective strategies against injury. Dig Dis Sci 2004;49:1359–1377.

81. Pasupathy S, Homer-Vanniasinkam S. Surgical implications of ischemic preconditioning. Arch Surg 2005;140:405–410.

82. Stein AB, Tang XL, Guo Y, Xuan YT, Dawn B, Bolli R. Delayed adaptation of the heart to stress: late preconditioning. Stroke 2004;35:2676–2679.

Index

Printed in the United States